Image-Guided Musculoskeletal Intervention

Image-Guided Musculoskeletal Intervention

- **Jeffrey J. Peterson, MD**
  Assistant Professor of Radiology
  Mayo Medical School
  Mayo Clinic
  Jacksonville, Florida

- **Douglas S. Fenton, MD**
  Assistant Professor of Radiology
  Mayo Medical School
  Mayo Clinic
  Jacksonville, Florida

- **Leo F. Czervionke, MD**
  Associate Professor of Radiology
  Mayo Medical School
  Mayo Clinic
  Jacksonville, Florida

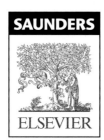

SAUNDERS

ELSEVIER

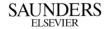

SAUNDERS
ELSEVIER

1600 John F. Kennedy Blvd.
Ste 1800
Philadelphia, PA 19103-2899

Image-Guided Musculoskeletal Intervention   ISBN: 978-1-4160-2905-2

Notice

Knowledge and best practice in this field are constantly changing. As new research and experience broaden our knowledge, changes in practice, treatment and drug therapy may become necessary or appropriate. Readers are advised to check the most current information provided (i) on procedures featured or (ii) by the manufacturer of each product to be administered, to verify the recommended dose or formula, the method and duration of administration, and contraindications. It is the responsibility of the practitioner, relying on their own experience and knowledge of the patient, to make diagnoses, to determine dosages and the best treatment for each individual patient, and to take all appropriate safety precautions. To the fullest extent of the law, neither the Publisher nor the Authors assume any liability for any injury and/or damage to persons or property arising out or related to any use of the material contained in this book.

The Publisher

Library of Congress Cataloging-in-Publication Data

Peterson, Jeffrey J.
  Image-guided musculoskeletal intervention / Jeffrey J. Peterson, Douglas S. Fenton, Leo F. Czervionke. —
1st ed.
    p. ; cm.
  Includes bibliographical references.
  ISBN 978-1-4160-2905-2
    1. Musculoskeletal system—Diseases—Diagnosis. 2. Musculoskeletal system—Imaging.
    3. Musculoskeletal system—Surgery. I. Fenton, Douglas S. (Douglas Scott). II. Czervionke, Leo F.
    III. Mayo Foundation for Medical Education and Research. IV. Title.
    [DNLM: 1. Joint Diseases—surgery. 2. Joints—surgery. 3. Surgery, computer-assisted.
    WE 312 P485i 2008]
  RC925.7.I4354 2008
  616.7'075—dc22

                                                                                    2006100781

Acquisitions Editor: Todd Hummel
Editorial Assistant: Colleen McGonigal
Publishing Services Manager: Tina Rebane
Project Manager: Norm Stellander
Design Direction: Gene Harris

Printed in China

Last digit is the print number: 9 8 7 6 5 4 3 2 1

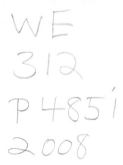

Thank you to my colleagues and mentors,
Mark Kransdorf, Laura Bancroft, and Tom Berquist,
for all of their encouragement and contributions.

Thanks to Doug Fenton and Leo Czervionke
for their tireless efforts in editing this book.

Thanks to my parents, Mary Kay and Jim,
for their inspiration and support.

Most importantly, thank you to my wife, Julie,
for her fortitude, endless love, and devotion.

Contributors

Kirkland W. Davis, MD
Associate Professor of Radiology
University of Wisconsin School of Medicine and Public
  Health
Director of Fluoroscopic Musculoskeletal Interventions
Department of Radiology, Musculoskeletal Division
University of Wisconsin Hospitals and Clinics
Madison, Wisconsin
Foreword

James K. DeOrio, MD
Director, Foot and Ankle Fellowship
Professor of Orthopedic Surgery
Department of Orthopedic Surgery
Mayo Clinic
Jacksonville, Florida
Chapter 7: *A Foot and Ankle Surgeon's Perspective*

Gavan P. Duffy, MD
Assistant Professor of Orthopedic Surgery
Department of Orthopedic Surgery
Mayo Clinic
Jacksonville, Florida
Chapter 5: *A Hip Surgeon's Perspective*

Peter M. Murray, MD
Consultant and Chair, Division of Education
Associate Professor of Orthopedic Surgery
Department of Orthopedic Surgery
Mayo Clinic
Jacksonville, Florida
Chapter 3: *An Elbow Surgeon's Perspective*
Chapter 4: *A Hand Surgeon's Perspective*

Mary I. O'Connor, MD
Chair and Associate Professor of Orthopedic Surgery
Department of Orthopedic Surgery
Mayo Clinic
Jacksonville, Florida
Chapter 8: *An Orthopedic Oncology Surgeon's
  Perspective*

Cedric J. Ortiguera, MD
Assistant Professor of Orthopedic Surgery
Department of Orthopedic Surgery
Mayo Clinic
Jacksonville, Florida
Chapter 2: *A Shoulder Surgeon's Perspective*
Chapter 6: *A Knee Surgeon's Perspective*

Image Acknowledgements

Laura W. Bancroft, MD
Associate Professor of Radiology
Department of Radiology
Mayo Clinic
Jacksonville, Florida

Douglas P. Beall, MD
Associate Professor of Orthopedic Surgery
Department of Orthopedic Surgery
University of Oklahoma
Chief of Radiology Services
Department of Radiology
Clinical Radiology of Oklahoma
Oklahoma City, Oklahoma

Thomas H. Berquist, MD, FACR
Professor of Radiology
Department of Radiology
Mayo Clinic
Jacksonville, Florida

Mark J. Kransdorf, MD, FACR
Professor of Radiology
Department of Radiology
Mayo Clinic
Jacksonville, Florida

Thomas Magee, MD
Radiologist in Chief
Department of Radiology
Neuroskeletal Imaging
Melbourne, Florida

Foreword

There is an ever-expanding need for image-guided musculoskeletal interventions. Some of these procedures are designed solely to facilitate further imaging studies, such as magnetic resonance arthrograms and computed tomography arthrograms. Other procedures, such as anesthetic joint injections, joint aspirations, and biopsies, are stand-alone diagnostic tests. Still others are therapeutic, including administration of local anesthetics and corticosteroids to joints, bursae, and tendon sheaths; viscosupplementation; and image-guided ablations. As some procedures, such as conventional arthrography, lose popularity due to evolving technology and techniques, other procedures take their place. With the continued expansion of the field of image-guided interventions in the musculoskeletal system, there is an urgent need for adequate training of general and musculoskeletal radiologists and other practitioners to perform these procedures.

Dr. Peterson has compiled an invaluable resource for training and maintenance of expertise in these interventions. In Chapters 2 through 7, Dr. Peterson addresses specific joints or regions of musculoskeletal anatomy. For each joint, he exhausts the specific structures to be injected and the various approaches to each injection, with exquisite diagrams and accompanying spot images demonstrating the approaches and appearance after injection. Chapter 8 includes similar step-by-step instructions, with ample illustrations, for performing image-guided biopsy in the extremities and radiofrequency ablation of osteoid osteomas.

If the text ended there, it would be a welcome resource for those who are learning, teaching, and performing these procedures. However, each chapter provides much more than just procedural techniques. Each chapter also includes introductory historical background information that explains the origins of each of these procedures. Next, the regional anatomy is explained in detail, with copious and elegant diagrams and clearly labeled accompanying radiographs and magnetic resonance and computed tomography studies. The discussion of compartment anatomy in Chapter 8 is particularly helpful in the performance of biopsies. Not only are the approaches to the various joints and body parts examined, but Dr. Peterson extensively discusses indications and contraindications, equipment, injection mixtures and volumes, possible complications, and post-procedure care. Additionally, sample dictations and appropriate CPT codes are provided for each procedure to assist in some of the more mundane technical details. As a final bonus, each chapter ends with case examples that place these procedures into practical settings.

Image-Guided Musculoskeletal Intervention is a thorough but concise treatment of the topic. It is the first broad treatment of the topic in the modern era of musculoskeletal radiology and is sure to be a cherished reference for many years to come. With its emphasis on both everyday injections, such as those of the knee, hip, and shoulder joints, as well as less routine injections, such as acromioclavicular and carpometacarpal joint injections and tenograms, this guide will be valuable as a training aid for residents and fellows who have little experience with these techniques, as well as a reference to assist the experienced practitioner in performing the less common procedures. I look forward to purchasing several copies of *Image-Guided Musculoskeletal Intervention* for our reading rooms, to accompany the copies of *Image-Guided Spine Intervention* we already own.

Kirkland W. Davis, MD

Preface

Image-guided musculoskeletal interventions play a vital role in the diagnosis and treatment of musculoskeletal pathology. First introduced in 1905 with examinations of the knee, image-guided joint interventions have evolved greatly over the last century. From the early days of image-guided therapeutic injections and conventional arthrography to modern MR arthrography, diagnostic and therapeutic injections of the joint have passed through several phases of evolution. In the 1960s and 1970s fluoroscopic joint injections developed into a commonly performed procedure allowing visualization of intraarticular structures previously unable to be visualized nonoperatively. In the late 1980s with the introduction of MR arthrography, indications for image-guided injections significantly changed. Conventional arthrography for the most part has been replaced in favor of MR or CT arthrography. Post-injection MR or CT provide multiplanar images that allow visualization of intraarticular structures in any plane. Today MR and CT arthrography are the gold standard techniques for evaluating internal derangement in many joints and are rivaled in accuracy only by diagnostic arthroscopy.

While there have been significant changes in diagnostic interventions through the years, the utility of therapeutic injections has remained constant. Therapeutic joint and bursal injections continue to play an important role in the treatment of orthopedic disease and to confirm the origin of symptomatology. Joint aspirations continue to be widely used for diagnosing infectious and other intraarticular processes. In addition to joint interventions, image-guided percutaneous biopsy has become a mainstay of oncologic evaluation of both osseous and soft tissue lesions. Evolution of image technology and improvement in needle design have allowed image-guided biopsy to become a valuable tool for diagnosing lesions involving the musculoskeletal system. We are now in the early stages of another revolution in treatment of musculoskeletal disease with the introduction of image-guided radiofrequency ablation and cryotherapy, which have great promise for the future.

Image-guided intervention is a dynamic field with an ever-changing landscape. The aim of this book is to provide an update of the current utility and techniques for image-guided interventions. Obviously, there are many approaches for performing the various procedures outlined in this book. This text is not intended to define the only way to perform these procedures, but merely to outline the techniques utilized at our institution that have proven successful for us. There are many injection mixtures that can be used for image-guided joint injections and different approaches for needle placement. There are other needle designs and radiofrequency ablation and cryotherapy techniques besides those described in the chapter devoted to image-guided biopsies and radiofrequency ablation. I encourage you to experiment with the various techniques and approaches for these procedures. One should remain open to trying new techniques and methods that other colleagues in this dynamic field are using; this allows you to continually refine your skills and find the techniques that work best for you, in order to provide optimal patient care.

This book has been organized into chapters covering a given joint or region and the interventions relevant to that area. The final chapter describes image-guided biopsy and radiofrequency ablation. A concerted effort has been made to organize each chapter in a consistent and orderly fashion and to describe every aspect of the interventional procedure in detail. The organization is similar to the preceding book by Fenton and Czervionke entitled *Image-Guided Spine Intervention*. Each chapter begins with a discussion of the background of the procedure and how it evolved through the years. Relevant anatomy is then discussed in detail, as this information is essential to both the performance of the procedure as well as image interpretation. Patient selection and contraindications are then described in detail, including the various indications for the injections applicable to the given region. The procedural section follows and outlines the equipment and supplies necessary for each procedure. Next is a list of the various injection mixtures and volumes that we use for various injections. Again, the injection mixtures we recommend are not meant to be rigid but instead a recommendation based on our practice. Methodology follows with a step-by-step illustrated review of the techniques we utilize to perform the various interventions. Potential complications and routine post-procedure care are then presented and followed by sample dictations for selected procedures. A few interesting cases are shared with the reader including the clinical, imaging, and operative findings. The most current procedural terminology (CPT) codes are listed, followed by recent and historical references. Finally, a brief perspective, authored by a fellowship-trained orthopedic surgeon in each of the various specialties, describes the importance of these procedures from the perspective of the clinician. This section emphasizes various situations and scenarios in which image-guided interventions are beneficial to their patients.

Jeffrey J. Peterson, MD

Contents

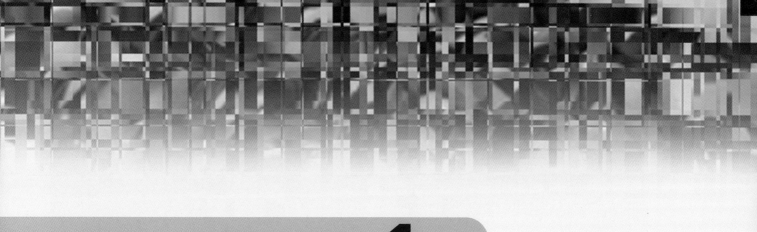

Chapter 1

Procedural Similarities

■ Douglas S. Fenton, MD
■ Jeffrey J. Peterson, MD

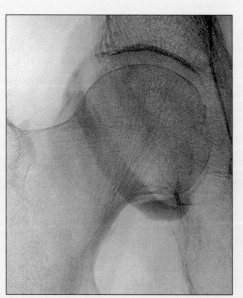

Although the interventional procedures described in this book are arranged by anatomic location, there are enough similarities within the various procedures to warrant a separate chapter describing the things that are in common. Although it is tempting to make each chapter a stand-alone entity, the large areas of overlap behooves us to consolidate the similarities into a single preliminary chapter rather than have the reader read the same thing over and over.

   This chapter focuses on consent, contraindications, medications used during the procedure, standard equipment necessary for the procedure, preparing the patient, methodology, potential complications, follow-up/discharge instructions, and Current Procedural Terminology (CPT) codes. If there is something within these sections that is unique to a particular injection, it will be discussed in that body part's chapter.

CONSENT

The procedure, risks, potential complications, and alternative tests should be explained to the patient and informed consent should be obtained. The patient should be questioned regarding any preexisting drug allergies.

CONTRAINDICATIONS[1]

* Coagulopathy (International Normalized Ratio [INR] >1.5 or platelets < 50,000/mm^3)
* Pregnancy (because of the teratogenic effects of radiation)
* Systemic infection or skin infection over the puncture site
* Severe allergy to any component of the injectate
* The patient has received the maximum amount of steroid including systemic steroids allowed for a given time period, unless the injection is to be performed without steroid

MEDICATIONS

Iodinated contrast media should be used to confirm intra-articular needle position for diagnostic and therapeutic injections and for the purposes of intra-articular imaging with diagnostic arthrography. Either ionic or nonionic iodinated contrast media can be used safely.[2] Nonionic contrast agents have the advantage of a decreased incidence of allergic reactions and have been reported to be associated with a lower incidence of transient synovitis in reaction to the intra-articular contrast media.[3–5] Unfortunately, nonionic agents are significantly more expensive than ionic contrast media. The incidence of allergic reactions with intra-articular administration of contrast media is rare, much lower than the incidence of allergic reaction to intravenous iodinated contrast media.[3,6] Iodinated contrast medium is often administered to patients with a known allergy to iodinated contrast material without precipitating an allergic reaction, although this should be avoided if possible.[6] For patients without a history of allergy, ionic agents can be used with minimal risk of precipitating an allergic reaction. For patients with multiple drug allergies or questionable allergies to iodinated contrast agents, nonionic contrast media are the agents of choice. For patients with known contrast allergies, the patient may be premedicated and nonionic contrast agents used. The following is a typical premedication regimen.

At 12 hours and 2 hours prior to radiographic contrast administration:

1. 20 to 50 mg prednisone by mouth
2. 150 mg ranitidine by mouth
3. 50 mg diphenhydramine by mouth

Immediately prior to injection of radiographic contrast material:

1. 25 to 50 mg diphenhydramine (optional)

For patients with severe allergies to iodinated contrast media, gadolinium-based agents can be utilized. Although less dense than iodinated contrast media, gadolinium can be seen under fluoroscopy and can be used to guide injections (Fig. 1-1). Unfortunately, gadolinium is significantly more expensive than iodinated contrast media.

Anesthetic agents are also very useful for both diagnostic and therapeutic injections. Anesthetic agents are key diagnostic agents in injections of the musculoskeletal joints. Patients often benefit from the temporary relief of pain afforded by the inclusion of anesthetic agents in the injection solution.[7,8] The two agents most commonly utilized are

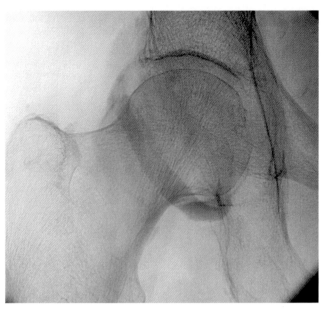

Figure 1-1 ■ Hip injection performed with gadopentetate dimeglumine (MR contrast, Magnevist, Berlex Laboratories, Wayne, NJ) in a patient with allergy to iodinated contrast media. Gadolinium is less dense than iodinated contrast media but adequate for visualization for image-guided injections.

lidocaine and bupivacaine.[7] Lidocaine provides immediate but temporary anesthesia lasting 1 to 2 hours; bupivacaine has a slower onset of action but provides longer lasting pain relief, lasting up to 24 hours. The lengths of action can vary depending on joint integrity and adjacent vascularity. A mixture of lidocaine and bupivacaine may be used to take advantage of the immediate affects of lidocaine and the long-lasting effects of bupivacaine.

A gadolinium-based contrast agent is added to the solution for MR arthrography.[9] Gadolinium is a strong paramagnetic contrast agent, and only small amounts are necessary for the desired effect.[8,10] From 0.1 to 0.2 mL of gadolinium is added to the solution. A 1-mL tuberculin syringe is used to draw up the gadolinium contrast agent, which is then added to the solution. The Food and Drug Administration (FDA) considers intra-articular administration of gadolinium an off-label use and therefore institutional review board approval may be required for its use.

We have found that articular cartilage is less well demonstrated when increasing concentrations of iodinated contrast material are included in the injection solution for MR arthrography. For this reason, we routinely dilute the iodinated contrast medium with sterile saline by half, which makes the solution typically just dense enough to ensure adequate intra-articular needle positioning with fluoroscopy.

Epinephrine can be effective for CT and MR arthrography in cases in which imaging will not be performed immediately following the injection. When post-procedural delay is anticipated, 0.3 mL of 1:1000 epinephrine can be added to the injection solution without loss of image quality.[9] Epinephrine acts to increase the quality of the arthrogram by reducing the egress of contrast material from the joint. Epinephrine causes vasoconstriction of the synovial vessels, which in turn decreases the amount of contrast material absorbed by the synovium and thereby decreases the amount of reactive intra-articular fluid formed in response to the injection, which can dilute the contrast agent.

Anesthetics

- Lidocaine hydrochloride 1% MPF (Xylocaine-MPF 1%, AstraZeneca LP, Wilmington, DE)
- Bupivacaine hydrochloride 0.25% or 0.5% MPF (Sensorcaine MPF injection 0.25%, AstraZeneca LP, Wilmington, DE)
- Local anesthetics should be from single-use vials and be free of paraben (MPF) and phenol in order to prevent flocculation of the steroid.[11]

Steroids

- Methylprednisolone sodium succinate 40 mg/mL (Solu-Medrol)
- Triamcinolone acetonide injectable 40 mg/mL (Kenalog-40, Apothecon, Princeton, NJ)
- Betamethasone sodium phosphate and betamethasone acetate 6 mg/mL (Celestone Soluspan, Schering Corporation, Kenilworth, NJ)

Contrasts

- Ionic iodinated myelographic contrast 60% strength (Reno-60 diatrizoate meglumine injection, Bracco Diagnostics, Incorporated, Princeton, NJ)
- Nonionic iodinated myelographic contrast 300 mg/mL (Omnipaque [Iohexol] injection, Nycomed Incorporated, Princeton, NJ)
- Gadopentetate dimeglumine (MR contrast, Magnevist, Berlex Laboratories, Wayne, NJ)
- Gadodiamide (MR contrast, Omniscan, Amersham Health Incorporated, Princeton, NJ).

STANDARD EQUIPMENT[1]

- Spinal needle, 22-gauge, 3.5-inch (Quincke type point, Becton Dickinson & Co., Franklin Lakes, NJ)
- Luer-Lock syringe containing injection mixture (size dependent on individual joint; see individual chapters)
- Control 12-mL syringe with 25-gauge, 1.5-inch needle containing 8 mL 1% lidocaine for local anesthesia and 2 mL 8.4% sodium bicarbonate injectable (1 mEq/mL) to alleviate burning pain associated with anesthetic
- Sterile 4 × 4 gauze pads
- Povidone-iodine (Betadine) and alcohol for preparation
- Sterile towels or aperture drape
- Needles, 18-gauge, 1.5-inch, to draw up lidocaine and medication
- Surgical hat, mask, sterile gloves
- Adhesive bandages
- Lead apron
- Multidirectional C-arm fluoroscopy with film archiving capability

IMAGING REVIEW

Prior to injection, routine radiographic images of the joint to be injected are obtained and reviewed.[12] Prior radiographic examinations can identify any preexisting pathologic conditions or anatomic variations, which may affect the technique of the procedure and aid in diagnosis.

PREPARING THE PATIENT

The patient should be placed on the fluoroscopic table in a position that will allow the physician to best perform the procedure. Ideal positioning per body part is discussed in the individual chapters. Some patients are not able to obtain ideal positioning and therefore a compromise is necessary. The patient should be placed in a position that can be comfortably maintained throughout the procedure.

A large area around the puncture site is then cleansed with the Betadine-alcohol solution.[12] One should ensure that the Betadine has dried prior to the alcohol wipe. The bactericidal properties of Betadine are greatest when it has dried, which usually takes between 2 and 3 minutes. When the skin has been cleansed, the puncture site is dressed with sterile towels or an aperture sheet. The fluoroscope is then brought into position over the puncture site for a general overview.

METHODOLOGY

Injection

The fluoroscopic image should be collimated to minimize radiation exposure to the surrounding tissues and physician. The solution to be injected into the articulation should then be drawn up in a syringe. The choice of agents to be included in the solution depends on the examination to be performed. Examples of solutions are listed under the medications section of each chapter. Flexible tubing should then be placed on the syringe and the solution should be advanced through the tubing to the tip. Any air bubbles should be expelled from the syringe and tubing. A metallic object such as a clamp can be used to identify the precise location of the injection. The clamp or needle can be moved until, using fluoroscopy, it overlies the ideal needle puncture site. This area is then marked.

Local anesthesia of the skin and underlying subcutaneous tissue is then obtained. This is typically performed with 1% lidocaine with 8.4% sodium bicarbonate buffer (4:1 lidocaine–sodium bicarbonate). A 0.5- or 1.5-inch 25-gauge needle is used to anesthetize the skin. This anesthetic needle can also be left at the puncture site, disconnected from the syringe, and used to gauge the position of the planned puncture site relative to the target site. The needle should be vertically oriented, seen end on with fluoroscopy, with the needle positioned directly over the target site. If the planned puncture site is concordant with the target site, the 25-gauge needle can be removed and exchanged for the needle to be utilized for the injection. The needles utilized for various injections are delineated in the respective chapters. The needle is then inserted through the skin. It is important to make your initial skin puncture (excluding the numbing needle) your only puncture because the risk of infection

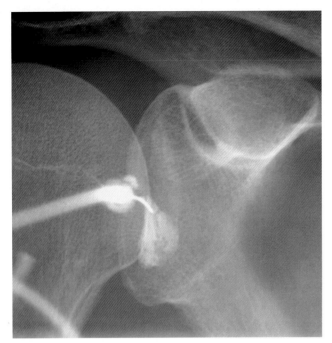

Figure 1-2 ■ Extra-articular needle position. Contrast material collecting at the needle tip, necessitating repositioning of the needle.

increases the more often you puncture the skin. Fluoroscopy is then used to check the needle position. Alterations in needle position can then be made to place the needle at the target site. This additional movement should be minimal and performed with care, as damage to the articular cartilage or other surrounding structures can result from overaggressive placement and manipulation of the needle. When the needle has been properly positioned, the stylet of the spinal needle is withdrawn. The syringe and tubing containing the solution to be injected into the joint are then connected to the indwelling needle. A small test injection should be performed to ensure appropriate intra-articular placement of the needle. If resistance to injection is met, the needle may be embedded in articular cartilage and the needle should be withdrawn slightly. If contrast material collects at the needle tip, the needle is extra-articular and needs to be repositioned (Fig. 1-2). If contrast flows freely away from the needle tip, the injection can then be administered. The entire injection should be performed under continuous fluoroscopic monitoring.

The volume of injection depends upon the indication for the injection. For conventional arthrography, the joint should be maximally distended to allow contrast material to extend into small rents or tears, which may not fill if the joint is not adequately distended. With conventional arthrography, the joint should be injected until resistance is met because of fullness of the joint or the patient experiences discomfort related to fullness of the joint. This volume varies depending on the joint, tendon sheath, or bursa injected. Typically, less distention is necessary with CT or MR arthrography than conventional arthrography. Overdistention of the articulation leads to leakage from the joint puncture site and possible capsular rupture prior to imaging, which markedly hinders image quality with both MR and CT.

The needle is withdrawn following the injection. Fluoroscopic evaluation of the joint should then be performed.

Dynamic fluoroscopic evaluation may be indicated for certain joints, such as the shoulder, in which both internal and external rotation positioning is necessary. Spot films of the joint, bursa, or tendon sheath should be obtained in each of these positions. For CT and MR arthrography, manipulation of the joint should be kept to a minimum to avoid extravasations from the joint prior to imaging. For conventional arthrography, vigorous exercise of the joint may be useful followed by additional fluoroscopic evaluation, as many small tears may become evident only after increased intra-articular pressure related to exercise and positional changes forces contrast material into small defects.

Aspiration

For most joints, aspiration is very similar to joint injection; however, when the needle is in place, a 60-mL syringe and tubing are connected to the needle and the aspiration of the joint is performed. If no fluid is withdrawn, repositioning of the needle within the joint can be helpful. If still no fluid can be aspirated, the joint is washed with nonbacteriostatic saline and reaspirated. Nonbacteriostatic saline is drawn up into a separate syringe and tubing and is administered into the joint through the indwelling needle. The syringe tubing is then exchanged for the 60-mL syringe and tubing and the nonbacteriostatic saline is reaspirated.

The aspirated fluid or nonbacteriostatic saline wash is then sent for aerobic and anaerobic culture. If enough fluid is present, Gram stain and additional analysis of the fluid can be performed depending upon the specific clinical situation.

POTENTIAL COMPLICATIONS[1]

- Bleeding
- Infection (cellulitis, septic arthritis, or osteomyelitis)
- Drug-related allergic reactions
- Transient synovitis
- Transitory extremity weakness
- Transitory extremity paresthesia
- Vascular injury
- Embolic events from particulate steroid entering vessels
- Vasovagal reactions
- Pneumothorax (procedures near the lung)

FOLLOW-UP/DISCHARGE INSTRUCTIONS[1]

Immediate

1. The patient should be observed for 15 minutes following injection.
2. Blood pressure, pulse, heart rate, and respiratory rate are monitored as necessary.

Discharge

1. An adhesive bandage may be placed on the puncture site. The bandage should remain dry for at least 24 hours, at which point it can be removed.

2. The patient is instructed to continue taking his or her prescription medication, although pain medication may be tapered as indicated.
3. A discharge sheet should be given to the patient outlining the following:
   a. Which procedure was performed
   b. Procedure-related symptoms that typically resolve in 7 to 10 days
      • Pain at the needle puncture site(s)
      • Mild increase in joint stiffness with a feeling of fullness in the joint
      • Deep pain in the joint
   c. Treatment for mild post-procedure symptoms
      • Rest the joint for 1 to 2 days
      • Avoid movements that worsen the pain
      • Use cold compresses to the area that hurts
   d. Signs and symptoms of infection
      • Fever
      • Chills
      • Swelling or drainage from the puncture site(s)
      • New joint pain that is different from the usual pain
   e. Signs and symptoms of possible more serious problems
      • Decreased range of motion of the joint
      • Increasing pain
      • Motor dysfunction of the extremity
   f. Physician name and contact number if the patient has any concerns or if any problem were to arise as a result of the procedure
   g. Advice to schedule a follow-up appointment with the referring physician in 7 to 10 days

CURRENT PROCEDURAL TERMINOLOGY (CPT) CODES[13]

CPT codes change often and sometimes are valid only for certain states or regions. It is best to consult with coding experts to make sure that coding for one's procedures is legitimate and complete. Below is a sample of codes that are being used for musculoskeletal injection procedures at this writing.

Surgery

General

10021 Fine-needle aspiration; without imaging guidance
10022 with imaging guidance
(For radiologic supervision and interpretation, see 76942, 77002, 77012, 77021)
(For percutaneous needle biopsy other than fine-needle aspiration, see 20206 for muscle)

Musculoskeletal System

General

Excision

20200 Biopsy, muscle; superficial
20205 deep

20206 Biopsy, muscle, percutaneous needle
(If imaging guidance is performed, see 76942, 77012, 77021)
(For fine-needle aspiration, use 10021 or 10022)
20220 Biopsy, bone, trocar, or needle; superficial (e.g., ilium, sternum, spinous process, ribs)
20225 deep (e.g., vertebral body, femur)
(For bone marrow biopsy, use 38221)
(For radiologic supervision and interpretation, see 77002, 77012, 77021)

Introduction or Removal

(For injection procedure for arthrography, see anatomic area)
20526 Injection, therapeutic (e.g., local anesthetic, corticosteroid), carpal tunnel
20550 Injection(s); single tendon sheath, or ligament, aponeurosis (e.g., plantar "fascia")
20600 Arthrocentesis, aspiration and/or injection; small joint or bursa (e.g., fingers, toes)
20605 intermediate joint or bursa (e.g., temporomandibular, acromioclavicular, wrist, elbow or ankle, olecranon bursa)
20610 major joint or bursa (e.g., shoulder, hip, knee joint, subacromial bursa)
(if imaging guidance is performed, see 76942, 77002, 77012, 77021)
20612 Aspiration and/or injection of ganglion cyst(s) any location
(To report multiple ganglion cyst aspirations/injections, use 20612 and append modifier 59)
20615 Aspiration and injection for treatment of bone cyst

Other Procedures

20982 Ablation, bone tumor(s) (e.g., osteoid osteoma, metastasis), radiofrequency, percutaneous, including computed tomographic guidance

Shoulder

Clavicle, scapula, humerus head and neck, sternoclavicular joint, acromioclavicular joint, and shoulder joint.

Excision

23065 Biopsy, soft tissue of shoulder area; superficial
23066 deep

Introduction or Removal

23350 Injection procedure for shoulder arthrography or enhanced CT/MRI shoulder arthrography
(For radiographic arthrography, radiologic

supervision and interpretation, use 73040. Fluoroscopy [77002] is inclusive of radiographic arthrography)

(When fluoroscopy-guided injection is performed for enhanced CT arthrography, use 23350, 77002, and 73201 or 73202)

(When fluoroscopy-guided injection is performed for enhanced MR arthrography, use 23350, 77002, and 73222 or 73223)

(For enhanced CT or enhanced MRI arthrography, use 77002 and either 73201, 73202, 73222, or 73223)

Humerus (Upper Arm) and Elbow

Elbow area includes head and neck of radius and olecranon process.

Excision

24065 Biopsy, soft tissue of upper arm or elbow area; superficial

24066 deep (subfascial or intramuscular)

(For needle biopsy of soft tissue, use 20206)

Introduction or Removal

24220 Injection procedure for elbow arthrography

(For radiologic supervision and interpretation, use 73085. Do not report 77002 in addition to 73085)

(For injection for tennis elbow, use 20550)

Forearm and Wrist

Radius, ulna, carpal bones and joints.

Excision

25065 Biopsy, soft tissue of forearm and/or wrist; superficial

25066 deep (subfascial or intramuscular)

(For needle biopsy of soft tissue, use 20206)

Introduction or Removal

25246 Injection procedure for wrist arthrography

(For radiologic supervision and interpretation, use 73115. Do not report 77002 in addition to 73115)

Pelvis and Hip Joint

Including head and neck of femur.

Excision

27040 Biopsy, soft tissue of pelvis and hip area; superficial

27041 deep, subfascial or intramuscular

(For needle biopsy of soft tissue, use 20206)

Introduction or Removal

27093 Injection procedure for hip arthrography; without anesthesia

(For radiologic supervision and interpretation, use 73525. Do not report 77002 in addition to 73525)

27095 with anesthesia

(For radiologic supervision and interpretation, use 73525. Do not report 77002 in addition to 73525)

Femur (Thigh Region) and Knee Joint

Including tibial plateaus.

Excision

27323 Biopsy, soft tissue of thigh or knee area; superficial

27324 deep (subfascial or intramuscular)

(For needle biopsy of soft tissue, use 20206)

Introduction or Removal

27370 Injection procedure for knee arthrography

(For radiologic supervision and interpretation, use 73580. Do not report 77002 in addition to 73580)

Leg (Tibia and Fibula) and Ankle Joint

Excision

27613 Biopsy, soft tissue of leg or ankle area; superficial

27614 deep (subfascial or intramuscular)

(For needle biopsy of soft tissue, use 20206)

Introduction or Removal

27648 Injection procedure for ankle arthrography

(For radiologic supervision and interpretation, use 73615. Do not report 77002 in addition to 73615)

Hemic and Lymphatic Systems

Bone Marrow or Stem Cell Services/Procedures

38220 Bone marrow; aspiration only

38221 biopsy, needle or trocar

Radiology

Upper Extremities

73040 Radiologic examination, shoulder, arthrography, radiologic supervision and interpretation

(Do not report 77002 in conjunction with 73040)

73085 Radiologic examination, elbow; arthrography, radiologic supervision and interpretation

(Do not report 77002 in conjunction with 73085)

73115 Radiologic examination, wrist; arthrography, radiologic supervision and interpretation

(Do not report 77002 in conjunction with 73115)

73200 Computed tomography, upper extremity; without contrast material

73201 with contrast material(s)

73202 without contrast material, followed by contrast material(s) and further sequences

(To report 3D rendering, see 76376, 76377)

73221 Magnetic resonance (e.g., proton) imaging, any joint of upper extremity; without contrast material(s)

73222 with contrast material(s)

73223 without contrast material, followed by contrast material(s) and further sequences

Lower Extremities

73525 Radiologic examination, hip; arthrography, radiologic supervision and interpretation

(Do not report 73525 in conjunction with 77002)

73580 Radiologic examination, knee; arthrography, radiologic supervision and interpretation

(Do not report 73580 in conjunction with 77002)

73615 Radiologic examination, ankle, arthrography, radiologic supervision and interpretation

(Do not report 73615 in conjunction with 77002)

73700 Computed tomography, lower extremity; without contrast material

73701 with contrast material(s)

73702 without contrast material, followed by contrast material(s) and further sequences

73721 Magnetic resonance (e.g., proton) imaging, any joint of lower extremity; without contrast material

73722 with contrast material(s)

73723 without contrast material(s), followed by contrast material(s) and further sequences

Other Procedures

76376 3D rendering with interpretation and reporting of computed tomography, magnetic resonance imaging, ultrasound, or other tomographic modality; not requiring image postprocessing on an independent workstation

(Use 76376 in conjunction with code(s) for base imaging, procedure(s))

76377 requiring image postprocessing on an independent workstation

(Use 76376 in conjunction with code(s) for base imaging, procedure(s))

Ultrasonic Guidance Procedures

76942 Ultrasonic guidance for needle placement (e.g., biopsy, aspiration, injection, localization device), imaging supervision and interpretation

(Do not report 76942 in conjunction with 43232, 43237, 43242, 45341, 45342, or 76975)

Fluoroscopic Guidance

77002 Fluoroscopic guidance for needle placement (e.g., biopsy, aspiration, injection, localization device)

(See appropriate surgical code for procedure and anatomic location)

(77002 includes all radiographic arthrography with the exception of supervision and interpretation for CT and MR arthrography)

(Do not report 77002 in addition to 70332, 73040, 73085, 73115, 73525, 73580, 73615)

Computed Tomography Guidance

77012 Computed tomography guidance for needle placement (e.g., biopsy, aspiration, injection, localization device), radiologic supervision and interpretation

Magnetic Resonance Guidance

77021 Magnetic resonance guidance for needle placement (e.g., for biopsy, needle aspiration, injection, or placement of localization device) radiologic supervision and interpretation.

References

1. Fenton DS, Czervionke LF. Image-Guided Spine Intervention. Philadelphia: WB Saunders, 2003.
2. Kaplan P, Tu H, Lydiatt D, et al. Temporomandibular joint arthrography of normal subjects: Prevalence of pain with ionic versus nonionic contrast agents. Radiology 1985; 156:825–826.
3. Cochran ST, Bomyea K, Sayre JW. Trends in adverse events after IV administration of contrast media. AJR Am J Roentgenol 2001; 176:1385–1388.
4. Hall FM, Rosenthal DI, Goldberg RP, Wyshak G. Morbidity from shoulder arthrography: Etiology, incidence, and prevention. AJR Am J Roentgenol 1981; 136:59–62.
5. Hall FM, Goldberg RP, Wyshak G, Kilcoyne RF. Shoulder arthrography: Comparison of morbidity after use of various contrast media. Radiology 1985; 154:339–341.
6. Newberg AH, Munn CS, Robbins AH. Complications of arthrography. Radiology 1985; 155:605–606.
7. Berquist TH. Diagnostic and therapeutic injections as an aid to musculoskeletal diagnosis. Semin Intervent Radiol 1993; 10:326–344.
8. Hodge JC. Musculoskeletal Imaging Diagnostic and Therapeutic Procedures. Montreal: Karger Landes Systems, 1997, pp 1–23.
9. Resnick D. Diagnosis of Bone and Joint Disorders, 4th ed. Philadelphia: WB Saunders, 2002, pp 193–318.
10. Rafii M, Minkoff J. Advanced arthrography of the shoulder with CT and MR imaging. Radiol Clin North Am 1998; 36:609–633.
11. Physicians' Desk Reference, 60th ed. Montvale, NJ: Medical Economics Company, 2006.
12. Freiberger RH, Kaye JJ. Arthrography. Norwalk, CT: Appleton Century Crofts, 1979, pp xii, 1–3.
13. CPT 2007, CPT Intellectual Property Services. Chicago: American Medical Association, 2007.

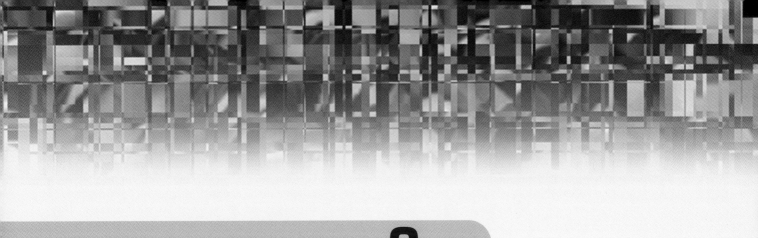

Chapter **2**

Shoulder Injections

■ Jeffrey J. Peterson, MD

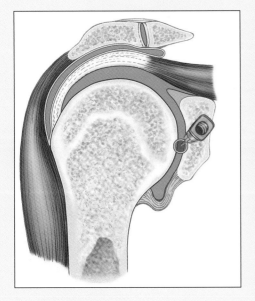

BACKGROUND

The first reports of shoulder arthrography date back to 1933, when air was used as an intra-articular contrast medium to evaluate for distortions in the shoulder capsule after shoulder dislocations.[1,2] Utilization of iodinated contrast media soon followed to evaluate for defects in the rotator cuff.[2,3] Improved techniques, better equipment, and the use of newer contrast media have resulted in better image quality, allowing shoulder arthrography to evolve for more than 75 years.

Today, several imaging techniques are available to evaluate the shoulder joint and adjacent structures. The introduction of magnetic resonance (MR) imaging has revolutionized the evaluation of the shoulder joint. Although the indications for shoulder arthrography have been redefined, there is still an important role for arthrography for both diagnostic and therapeutic purposes.[2] Conventional arthrography continues to be a useful tool for the evaluation of rotator cuff pathology.[4,5] Computed tomography (CT) and MR arthrography can reveal subtle pathology involving the glenoid labrum and articular cartilage of the shoulder joint.[6,7]

Therapeutic injections continue to have an important role in the treatment of shoulder symptoms and of adhesive capsulitis.[8] Therapeutic injections are useful not only for the glenohumeral joint but also for other articulations of the shoulder girdle including the acromioclavicular joints and sternoclavicular articulations. These injections are also described in this chapter.

ANATOMIC CONSIDERATIONS

Understanding the normal anatomy of the shoulder and its variations is critical for the successful performance of shoulder interventions and subsequent interpretation of the resultant images. The anatomy of the shoulder is complex.[9,10] The shoulder joint is capable of a wide range of motion. In fact, the shoulder joint has a wider range of motion than any other joint in the body and is capable of a remarkable combination of movements.[11] This mobility, however, occurs at the expense of joint stability.[11,12]

The glenohumeral joint is a multiaxial ball-and-socket joint.[11] The osseous components include the proximal humerus and the scapula. The hemispheric humeral head represents the ball and the pear-shaped glenoid portion of the scapula represents the socket of this joint.[11,12] The greater tuberosity of the humerus arises from the lateral aspect of the humeral head, and the lesser tuberosity arises anteriorly. The muscles of the rotator cuff insert upon these bone prominences. The supraspinatus, infraspinatus, and teres minor muscles insert upon the greater tuberosity and the subscapularis inserts upon the lesser tuberosity (Fig. 2-1).[13]

The coracoacromial arch consists of the acromion and the coracoid process of the scapula as well as the intervening coracoacromial ligament, which surround and protect the rotator cuff musculature and provide stabilization of the shoulder joint superiorly (Fig. 2-2).[11] Unfortunately, this stabilizing arch can restrict range of motion and limit the space for the rotator cuff musculature and tendons during abduction of the arm. This has been termed rotator cuff impingement.[14] There is variation in the acromial shape with three described types.[15] The type 1 acromion has a flat undersurface. The type 2 acromion has a curved undersurface, and the type 3 acromion has an inferior bend or hook at its anterior end.[15] The type 3 acromion has a higher incidence of rotator cuff impingement (Fig. 2-3).[15]

The soft tissue components of the shoulder joint include the articular cartilage, the glenoid labrum, the joint capsule, and the synovial membrane.[12] The joint capsule surrounds the articulation and is reinforced by the rotator cuff muscles and several ligaments.[11] The capsule is thin and lax, facilitating the wide range of motion of the shoulder joint.[12] Laterally, the capsule attaches to the anatomic neck of the humerus and medially to the margin of the glenoid just peripheral to

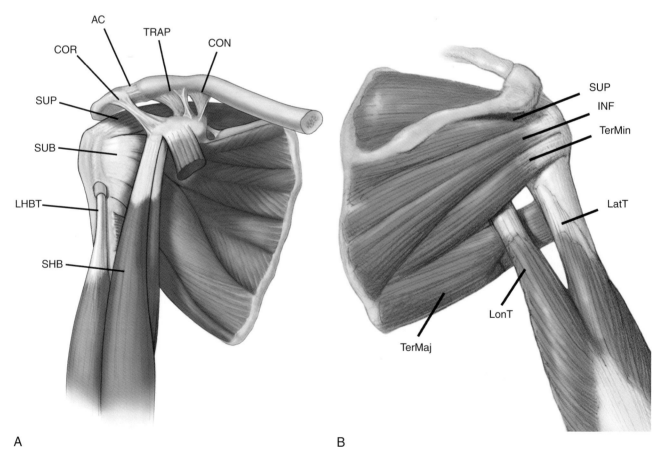

A   B

Figure 2-1 ■ Anterior (*A*) and posterior (*B*) views of the shoulder depicting the osseous and muscular anatomy of the shoulder. Anterior (*A*): SUB = subscapularis muscle and tendon; SUP = supraspinatus muscle and tendon; AC = acromioclavicular articulation; COR = coracoacromial ligament; TRAP = trapezoid component of coracoclavicular ligament; CON = conoid component of coracoclavicular ligament; LHBT = long head biceps tendon; SHB = short head biceps. Posterior (*B*): SUP = supraspinatus muscle and tendon; INF = infraspinatus muscle and tendon; TerMin = teres minor muscle and tendon; TerMaj = teres major muscle and tendon; LonT = long head triceps; LatT = lateral head triceps.

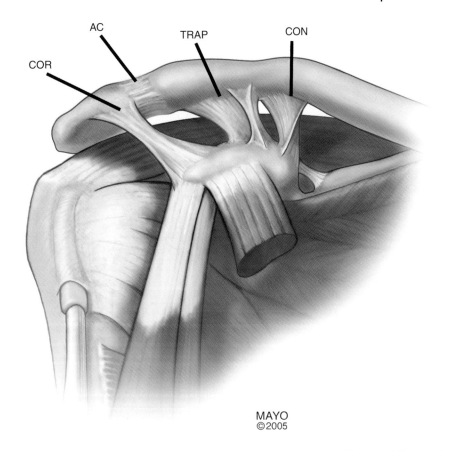

MAYO
©2005

Figure 2-2 ■ Anatomy of the coracoacromial arch. COR = coracoacromial ligament; AC = acromio-clavicular articulation; TRAP = trapezoid component of coracoclavicular ligament; CON = conoid component of coracoclavicular ligament.

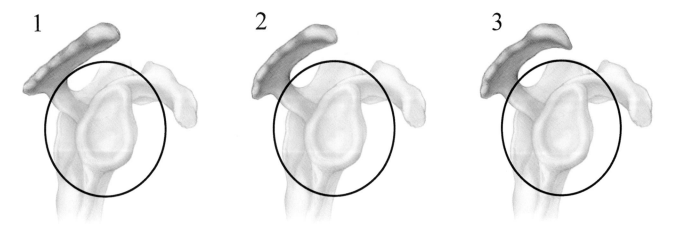

Figure 2-3 ■ Variations in acromial arch shape. Type 1 = flat undersurface. Type 2 = curved undersurface. Type 3 = inferior bend or hook at its anterior end.[15]

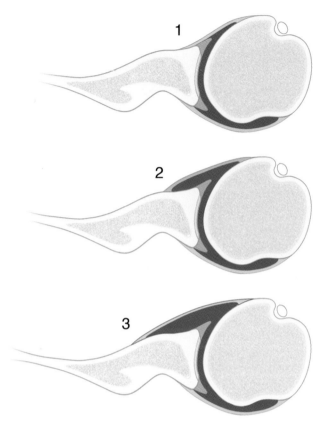

Figure 2-4 ■ Variations in anterior capsular attachments. With type 1 insertions, the anterior capsule attaches to the margin of the glenoid at the base of the glenoid labrum. With type 2 and type 3, insertions the capsular insertion extends progressively more medially.[16]

the glenoid labrum.[11] There is variation of the anterior capsular insertion upon the glenoid.[11] Three types of anterior capsular insertions have been described (Fig. 2-4).[16] In a type 1 insertion, the anterior capsule attaches to the margin of the glenoid at the base of the glenoid labrum (Fig. 2-5).

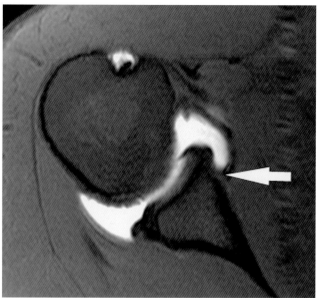

Figure 2-6 ■ Type 2 capsule *(arrow).*

This is the most common and most stable configuration. With type 2 and type 3 insertions, the capsular insertion extends progressively more medially (Figs. 2-6 and 2-7). Medial insertions of the capsule are associated with increased instability of the glenohumeral joint.[16] The synovial membrane lines the inner margins of the joint capsule.[12]

The glenohumeral ligaments (Fig. 2-8) are important accessory stabilizers of the glenohumeral joint. They serve to reinforce the anterior aspect of the glenohumeral joint capsule and to prevent excessive external rotation of the shoulder joint. These are divided into the superior, middle, and inferior glenohumeral ligaments, although these ligaments are inconstant structures of variable size (Figs. 2-9, 2-10, and 2-11).[17] The inferior glenohumeral ligament is the

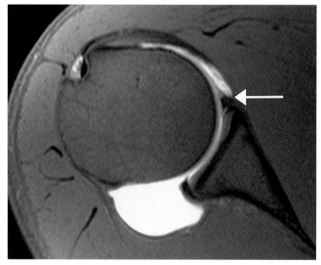

Figure 2-5 ■ Type 1 capsule *(arrow).*

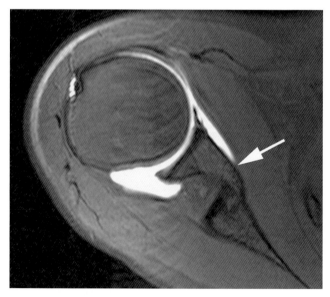

Figure 2-7 ■ Type 3 capsule *(arrow).*

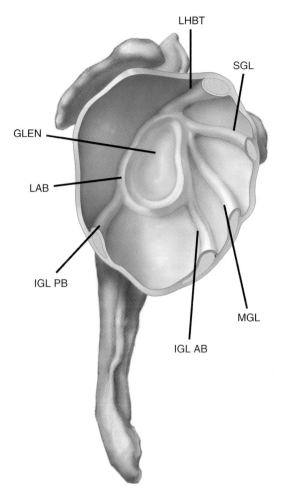

Figure 2-8 ■ Lateral view of the labral capsular ligamentous complex of the shoulder with depiction of the glenohumeral ligaments and the long head of the biceps tendon. GLEN = glenoid process of scapula; LAB = glenoid labrum; SGL = superior glenohumeral ligament; MGL = middle glenohumeral ligament; IGL AB = inferior glenohumeral ligament anterior band; IGL PB = inferior glenohumeral ligament posterior band; LHBT = long head biceps tendon.

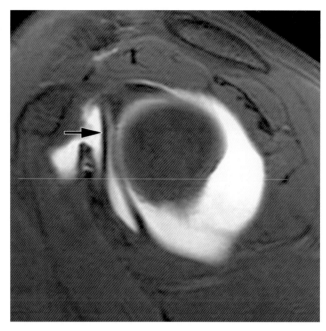

Figure 2-10 ■ Sagittal image depicting the middle glenohumeral ligament *(arrow)*.

most constant and also the thickest ligament. The middle glenohumeral ligament has the most variation. Rather than distinct structures, the glenohumeral ligaments represent thickening of the glenohumeral joint capsule as identified from the inside of the joint.[17]

Hyaline articular cartilage lines the articular surfaces of the humeral head and glenoid (Fig. 2-12), and the glenoid labrum, composed of fibrocartilage, is firmly applied to the periphery of the glenoid and serves to deepen the glenoid cavity (Fig. 2-13).[11] The articular cartilage is thickest at its center and diminishes in thickness toward the periphery,

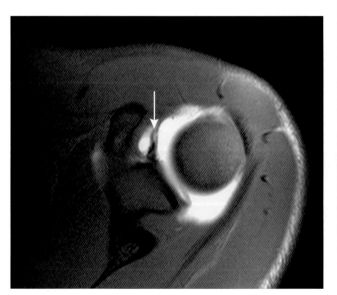

Figure 2-9 ■ Axial image demonstrating the superior glenohumeral ligament *(arrow)*.

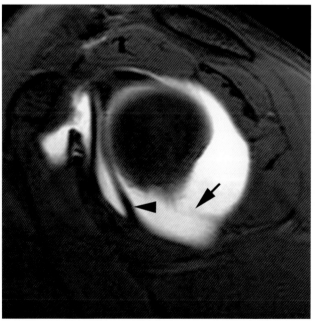

Figure 2-11 ■ Sagittal image demonstrating both the anterior band *(arrowhead)* and the posterior band *(arrow)* of the inferior glenohumeral ligament.

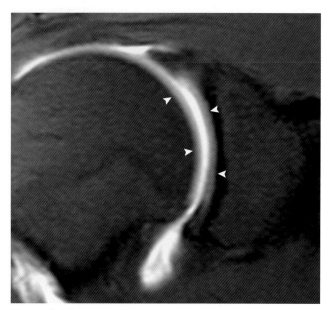

Figure 2-12 ■ Coronal image of the glenohumeral articulation that depicts the articular hyaline cartilage of the humeral head and glenoid *(arrowheads)*.

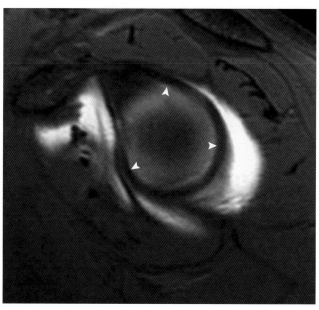

Figure 2-13 ■ Sagittal image revealing the glenoid labrum *(arrowheads)* firmly attached to the margin of the glenoid. The labrum serves to deepen the articular surface of the glenoid fossa.

whereas the labrum is thickest at the margins of the joint and is more thin centrally.[13] The primary function of the glenoid labrum is to deepen the shallow bony glenoid fossa, which results in increased stability of the joint.[12] The labrum displays significant variation in size and morphology, and occasionally portions of the labrum may be absent (Figs. 2-14 and 2-15).[9,10]

The long head of the biceps tendon originates from the supraglenoid tubercle of the superior glenoid and extends intra-articularly to penetrate the rotator cuff at the rotator cuff interval between the subscapularis and supraspinatus muscles (Fig. 2-16).[18] The long head of the biceps then extends inferiorly through the bicipital groove of the anterior humerus. The long head of the biceps and its surrounding

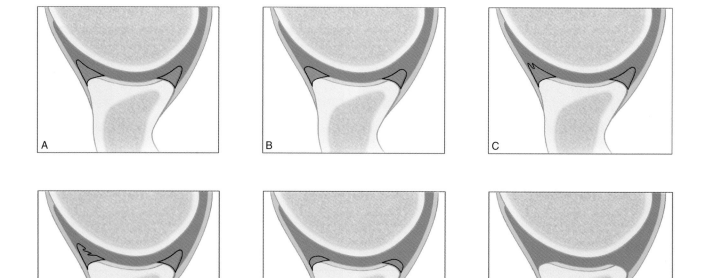

Figure 2-14 ■ Morphologic variations in glenoid labral anatomy. *A*, Triangular labrum. *B*, Rounded labrum. *C*, Notched labrum. *D*, Cleaved labrum. *E*, Flat labrum. *F*, Absent labrum.

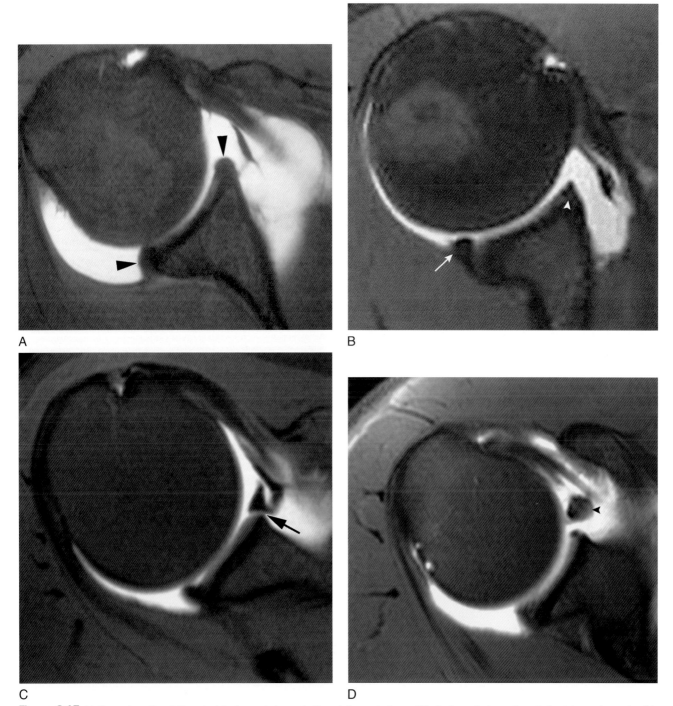

A

B

C

D

Figure 2-15 ■ Examples of variations in labral morphology. *A,* Rounded morphology of both the anterior and posterior labrum *(arrowheads).* *B,* Rounded morphology of the posterior labrum *(arrow)* with near-complete absence of the anterior labrum *(arrowhead). C,* Sublabral foramen *(arrow)* with portions of the anterosuperior labrum that are not adherent to the underlying anterosuperior glenoid. *D,* Buford complex with near absence of the anterior glenoid labrum associated with a thickened middle glenohumeral ligament *(arrowhead).*

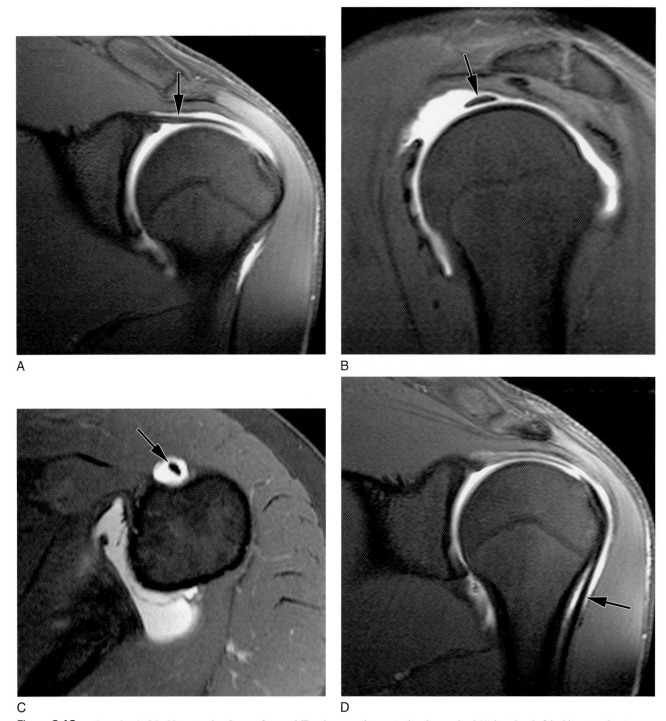

A

B

C

D

Figure 2-16 ■ Long head of the biceps tendon. Images from an MR arthrogram demonstrating the proximal (*A*) long head of the biceps tendon *(arrow-head)* originating from the supraglenoid tubercle, passing adjacent to the superior labrum and anterolaterally through the glenohumeral joint (*B*) *(arrow-head)*. Distally (*C*) the long head of the biceps tendon exits the joint through the rotator cuff interval and extends inferiorly through the bicipital groove of the humerus *(arrow)* (*D*) into the upper arm *(arrow)*.

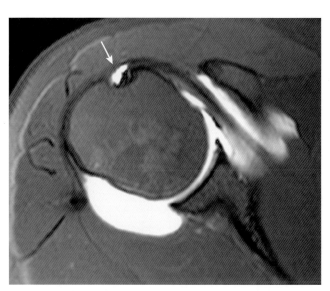

Figure 2-17 ■ Transverse humeral ligament *(arrow)* traversing the bicipital groove that contains the long head of the biceps tendon.

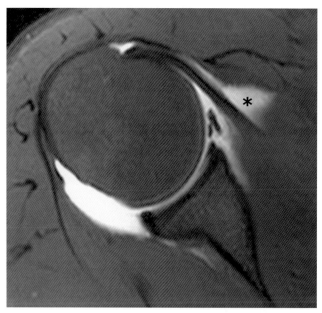

Figure 2-19 ■ The subscapular recess of the glenohumeral articulation *(asterick).*

tendon sheath are maintained in the bicipital groove by the transverse humeral ligament (Fig. 2-17). The long head of the biceps then continues inferiorly into the upper arm along with the short head of the biceps, which arises from the coracoid process of the scapula.[18]

Three predominant recesses can be seen about the shoulder joint, the axillary recess (Fig. 2-18), the subscapular recess (Fig. 2-19), and the sheath for the long head of the biceps tendon (Fig. 2-20).[12] Although variable in size and morphology, these recesses can typically be easily identified with arthrography. The axillary recess is formed by a focus of redundant capsular tissue found between the anterior and posterior bands of the glenohumeral ligaments (Fig. 2-21).[11] The subscapular recess is a small focus of redundant capsular tissue, which wraps around the superior margin of the subscapularis muscle just beneath the coracoid process of

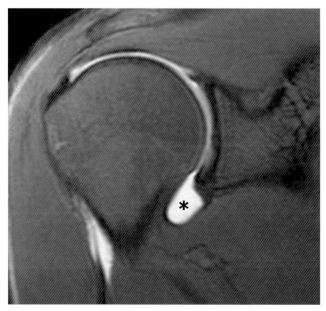

Figure 2-18 ■ The axillary recess of the glenohumeral articulation *(asterick).*

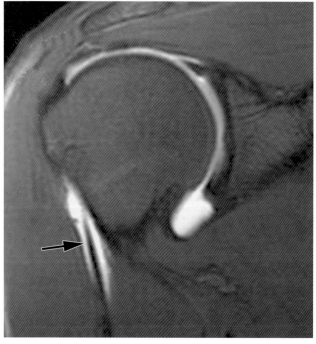

Figure 2-20 ■ The long head of the biceps tendon sheath surrounding the proximal long head of the biceps tendon *(arrow).*

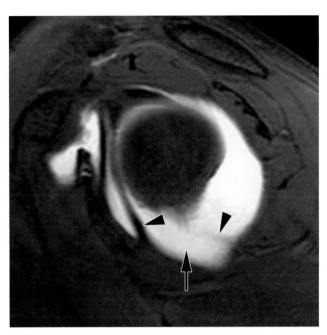

Figure 2-21 ■ The axillary recess *(white arrow)* consists of redundant capsular tissue between the anterior and posterior bands of the inferior glenohumeral ligament *(black arrowheads)*.

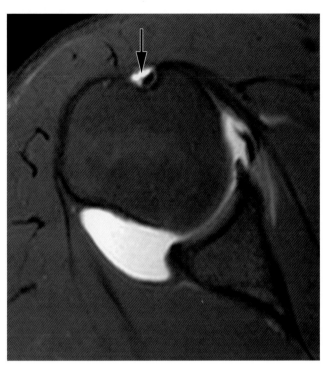

Figure 2-23 ■ The long head of the biceps tendon sheath surrounds the proximal long head of the biceps tendon as it passes inferiorly through the bicipital groove of the humerus *(arrow)*.

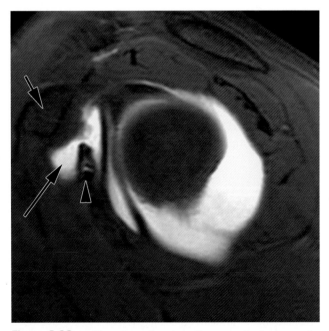

Figure 2-22 ■ The subscapular recess *(long arrow)* extends over the superior margin of the subscapularis muscle and tendon *(arrowhead)* beneath the coracoid process *(short arrow)*.

the scapula medial to the glenoid (Fig. 2-22).[11] The biceps tendon sheath extends along the long head of the biceps tendon as it passes through the bicipital groove of the antero-lateral proximal humerus (Fig. 2-23).[18]

The four muscles that make up the rotator cuff are the subscapularis muscle, the supraspinatus muscle, the infraspinatus muscle, and the teres minor muscle (see Fig. 2-1). The subscapularis muscle arises from the anterior aspect of the scapula with a broad fan-shaped origin, coursing laterally over the anterior aspect of the glenohumeral articulation to insert upon the lesser tuberosity of the humerus (Fig. 2-24).[13] The supraspinatus is located superior to the glenohumeral articulation originating from the superior aspect of the scapula above the level of the spine of the scapula (Fig. 2-25).[12] The infraspinatus muscle originates from the posterior scapula below the spine of the scapula (Fig. 2-26).[12] The teres minor also arises from the posterior scapula just below the origin of the infraspinatus (Fig. 2-27).[31] The supraspinatus, the infraspinatus, and the teres minor muscles all attach to the greater tuberosity of the humeral head.[13]

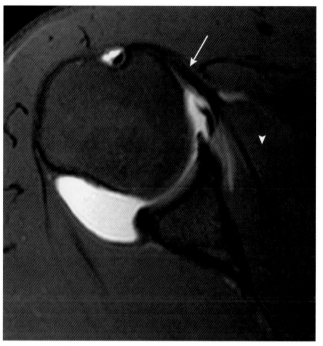

A

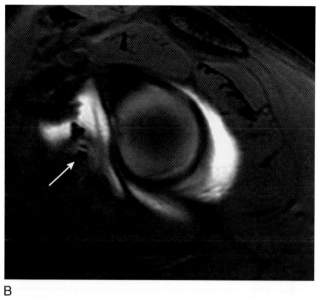

B

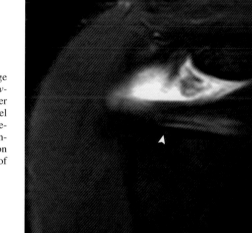

C

Figure 2-24 ■ The subscapularis muscle and tendon. *A,* Axial image demonstrates the subscapularis muscle belly anterior to the scapula *(arrowhead)* with the subscapularis tendon distally inserting upon the lesser tuberosity of the proximal humerus *(arrow). B,* Sagittal image at the level of the glenoid depicting the subscapularis muscle and tendon *(arrow)* anterior to the glenohumeral joint. *C,* Coronal image depicting the broad fan-shaped muscle belly of the subscapularis *(arrow)* with the distal tendon extending anterior to the shoulder, inserting upon the lesser tuberosity of the humerus *(arrowhead).*

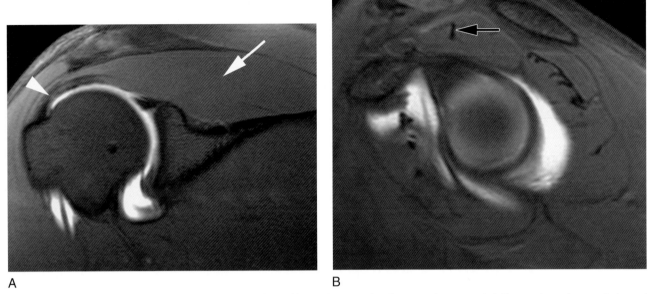

A
B

Figure 2-25 ■ The supraspinatus muscle and tendon. *A*, Coronal image demonstrating the supraspinatus muscle belly superior to the scapula *(arrow)* with the supraspinatus tendon extending superior to the glenohumeral joint to insert upon the greater tuberosity of the humerus *(arrowhead)*. *B*, Sagittal image at the level of the glenoid depicts the supraspinatus muscle and tendon superior to the glenohumeral articulation *(arrow)*.

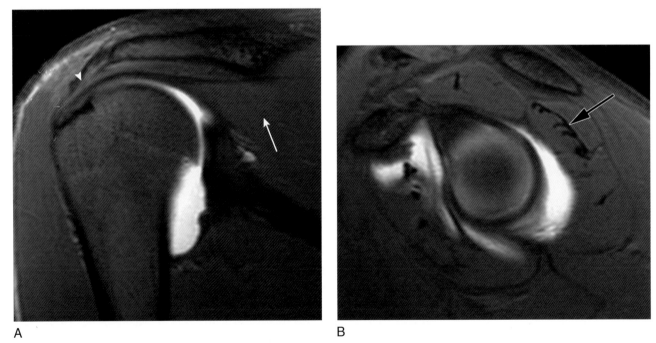

A
B

Figure 2-26 ■ The infraspinatus muscle and tendon. *A*, Coronal image demonstrating the infraspinatus muscle belly *(arrow)* posterior to the superior aspect of the scapula with the infraspinatus tendon *(arrowhead)* extending posteriorly and superiorly over the glenohumeral joint to insert upon the greater tuberosity of the humerus. *B*, Sagittal image at the level of the glenoid depicts the infraspinatus muscle and tendon *(arrow)* posterior and superior to the glenohumeral articulation.

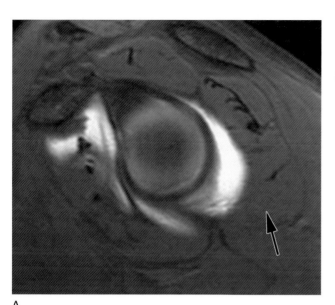

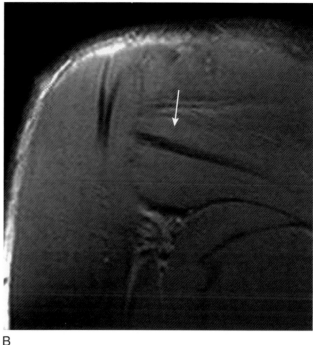

A   B

Figure 2-27 ■ The teres minor muscle and tendon. *A*, Sagittal image at the level of the glenoid depicting the teres minor muscle and tendon *(arrow)* posterior to the glenohumeral articulation. *B*, Coronal image showing the teres minor muscle and tendon *(arrow)* passing posterior to the shoulder.

PATIENT SELECTION

The introduction of MR imaging has led to alterations in the indications for shoulder arthrography. Prior to MR, arthrography was the only readily available diagnostic imaging study that could be used to reliably detect internal derangement of the shoulder. MR has now replaced conventional arthrography for the detection of rotator cuff pathology. However, arthrography still has a role in diagnosing rotator cuff tears and other derangements of the shoulder.[2,19]

Conventional Arthrography

Conventional arthrography is commonly performed to evaluate for rotator cuff tears in patients who have contraindications to MR imaging or patients who cannot tolerate the MR examination (Fig. 2-28). Arthrography can also be used to evaluate and treat adhesive capsulitis, as many patients report relief of symptoms following shoulder joint injections related to distention of the contracted capsule and rupture of the intra-articular adhesions (Fig. 2-29).[8] Occasionally, shoulder joint injections are performed solely for therapeutic purposes for the relief of symptoms related to the glenohumeral articulation.

Both single- and double-contrast conventional shoulder arthrography allow reliable detection of rotator cuff pathology including full-thickness rotator cuff tears and articular surface partial-thickness tears (Fig. 2-30).[13] Bursal surface

partial-thickness tears are not demonstrated with conventional shoulder arthrography. The glenoid labrum can be visualized and labral pathology may be seen with conventional arthrographic images.[20] Using double-contrast arthrography, one is often better able to identify and diagnose glenoid labral pathology.[13]

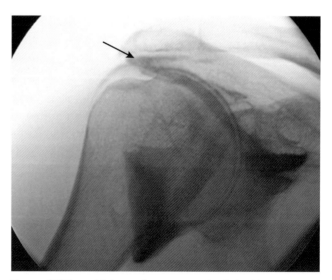

Figure 2-28 ■ AP image from a conventional shoulder arthrogram depicts a small focal full-thickness rotator cuff tear *(arrow)* involving the distal supraspinatus tendon allowing contrast material to spill into the sub-acromial subdeltoid bursa.

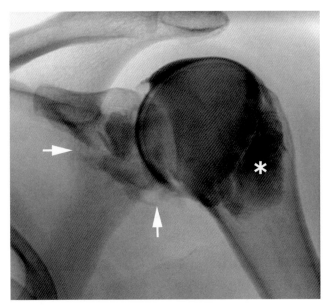

Figure 2-29 ■ AP image from a conventional arthrogram of the shoulder in a patient with adhesive capsulitis. The glenohumeral joint is small in volume, with absence of the axillary and subscapular recesses *(arrows)*, and extravasation from the lateral aspect of the joint *(asterick)*.

MR Arthrography

MR arthrography has proved to be the "gold standard" for diagnosing intra-articular pathology involving the glenohumeral articulation.[21] Distention of the glenohumeral joint by instillation of gadolinium contrast agent significantly improves detection of internal derangement of the shoulder joint. MR arthrography is superior to conventional MR imaging and conventional double-contrast arthrography for the detection of glenolabral pathology (Fig. 2-31).[21] Intra-articular administration of contrast medium prior to MR imaging also allows more precise evaluation of the articular cartilage of the humeral head and the glenoid (Fig. 2-32).[22] MR arthrography is also useful for evaluation of rotator cuff tears (Fig. 2-33).[19] Evaluation of other intra-articular processes such as synovial abnormalities and detection of loose bodies can also be performed with MR arthrography of the shoulder (Fig. 2-34).[23]

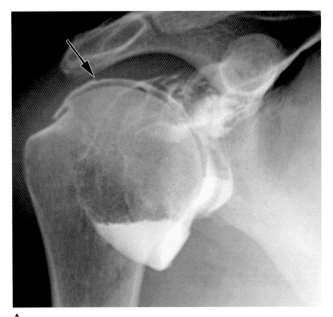

A

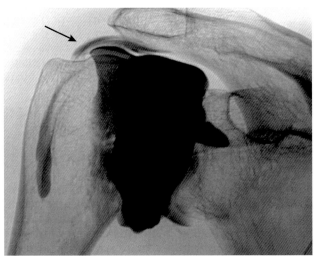

B

Figure 2-30 ■ Examples of partial-thickness rotator cuff tears. *A,* Double-contrast conventional shoulder arthrogram depicting contrast extending into a small defect *(arrow)* in the undersurface of the supraspinatus compatible with a small partial-thickness articular surface rotator cuff tear. *B,* Image from a conventional shoulder arthrogram demonstrating contrast extending into a defect in the undersurface of the distal supraspinatus tendon with significant intrasubstance extension of the tear *(arrow).* There was no communication demonstrated with the overlying subacromial subdeltoid bursa. Arthroscopy confirmed a complex articular surface partial-thickness supraspinatus tear.

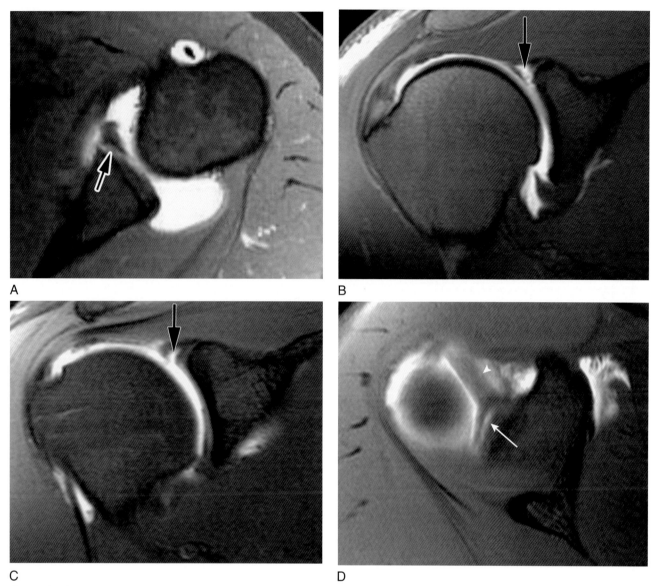

Figure 2-31 ■ Examples of glenoid labral tears. *A*, Axial image depicting abnormal extension of contrast into the substance of the anteroinferior labrum *(arrow)* compatible with a cartilaginous Bankart lesion in a patient with anterior glenohumeral instability. *B*, Coronal image showing a complex tear of the superior labrum *(arrow)* with marked abnormal contrast extension into the substance of the labrum. *C*, Coronal image depicting a tear of the superior labrum *(arrow)* associated with a small partial-thickness tear *(arrowhead)* of the distal supraspinatus tendon. *D*, Axial image in the same patient demonstrating the superior labral tear *(arrow)* extending posterior to the long head of the biceps tendon origin *(arrowhead)*.

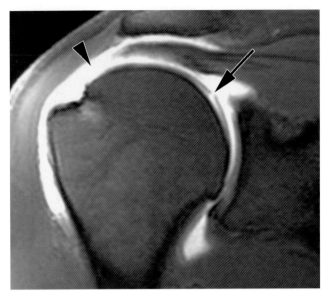

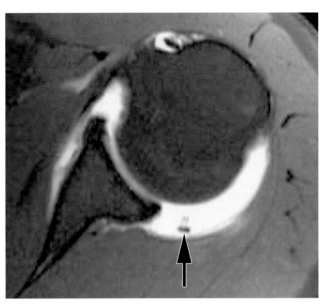

Figure 2-32 ■ Coronal image depicting a focal chondral defect involving the articular cartilage of the humeral head *(arrow)* in a patient with a full-thickness supraspinatus tear *(arrowhead).*

Figure 2-34 ■ Iatrogenic loose body. Axial image revealing a small loose tack in the posterior aspect of the shoulder joint *(arrow)* in a patient with prior repair of a superior labral tear.

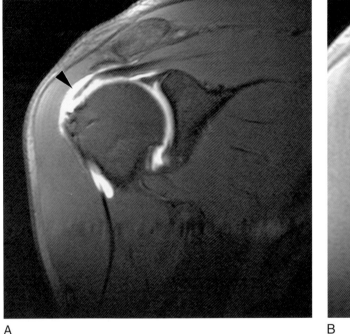

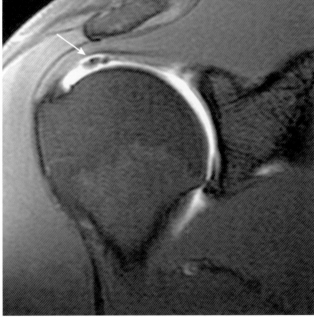

A

B

Figure 2-33 ■ Rotator cuff pathology seen with MR arthrography. *A,* Coronal image showing a full-thickness rotator cuff tear involving the distal supraspinatus tendon with contrast extending into the subacromial subdeltoid bursa *(arrowhead). B,* Coronal image showing a partial-thickness rotator cuff tear involving the undersurface of the distal supraspinatus tendon *(arrow).*

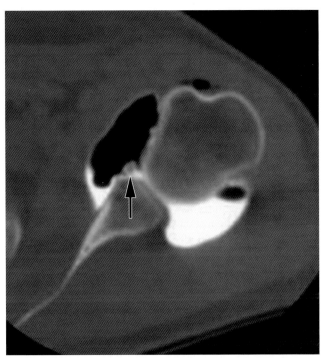

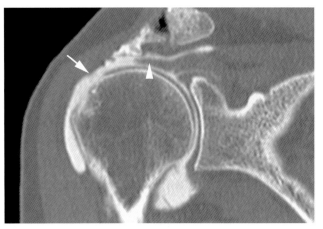

Figure 2-36 ■ Coronal reformatted image from a CT arthrogram of the shoulder in a patient with a full-thickness rotator cuff tear involving the distal supraspinatus tendon with contrast seen filling the subacromial subdeltoid bursa *(arrow)*. There is retraction of the torn supraspinatus tendon to the level of the acromion *(arrowhead)*.

Figure 2-35 ■ Axial image from a double-contrast CT arthrogram of the shoulder depicting a Bankart lesion *(arrow)* with contrast and air extending beneath the anteroinferior labrum in a patient with anterior glenohumeral instability.

tion.[19] Diagnostic indications for acromioclavicular joint injections are limited.

Sternoclavicular Joint Injection

Therapeutic injections of the sternoclavicular articulation are performed for relief of pain (Fig. 2-37). Diagnostic indications for sternoclavicular joint injections are limited. Aspiration of the sternoclavicular joint can be useful to evaluate for septic arthritis.

CT Arthrography

CT arthrography can be substituted for MR arthrography when MR imaging is contraindicated or in patients who cannot tolerate the examination. Either single- or double-contrast technique can be used. CT arthrography, like MR arthrography, can be a valuable tool in evaluating the glenoid labrum (Fig. 2-35). CT arthrography can also be used to evaluate for full-thickness or articular surface partial-thickness rotator cuff tears (Fig. 2-36).[2] Articular cartilage abnormalities are exquisitely demonstrated with CT arthrography. Intra-articular pathology such as synovial pathology and loose bodies can also be detected with CT arthrography.[2]

Subacromial Bursal Injection

Subacromial bursal injections can be performed for both diagnostic and therapeutic purposes. Often, subacromial injections of anesthetic agents and steroids are performed for therapeutic purposes in patients with subacromial bursitis.[2] Opacification of the subacromial bursa can be utilized for diagnostic purposes to evaluate the bursal surface of the rotator cuff and to evaluate for rotator cuff impingement.[2]

Acromioclavicular Joint Injection

Acromioclavicular joint injections are performed for therapeutic purposes in patients with pain related to this articula-

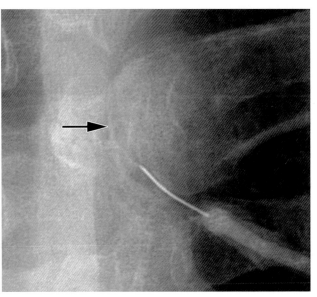

Figure 2-37 ■ Image from a left sternoclavicular joint injection with a 25-gauge needle in place and a small amount of the injectate *(arrow)* within the joint cavity. The sternoclavicular joint is very small in volume.

CONTRAINDICATIONS

- Coagulopathy (caution in patients with International Normalized Ratio [INR] >1.5 or platelets < 50,000/mm³)
- Pregnancy (because of teratogenic effects of radiation)
- Systemic infection or skin infection over the puncture site
- Severe allergy to any component of the injectate
- The patient has received the maximum amount of steroid including systemic steroids allowed for a given time period unless the injection is to be performed without steroid

PROCEDURE

Equipment/Supplies

Procedural

- Spinal needle, 22-gauge, 3.5-inch (Quincke-type point, Becton Dickinson, Franklin Lakes, NJ)
- Luer-Lock (10- or 20-mL) syringe containing injection mixture
- Sterile tubing to connect injection solution to spinal needle
- Control 12-mL syringe with 25-gauge, 1.5-inch needle containing 8 mL 1% lidocaine for local anesthesia and 2 mL 8.4% sodium bicarbonate injectable (1 mEq/mL) to alleviate burning pain associated with anesthetic
- Sterile 4 × 4 gauze pads

- Povidone-iodine (Betadine) and alcohol for preparation
- Sterile towels or fenestrated drape for draping
- Needle, 18-gauge, 1.5-inch, to draw up lidocaine and medication
- Sterile gloves
- Adhesive bandage

Injection Volume

The typical glenohumeral joint volume is approximately 12 to 18 mL.[2] A 20-mL syringe is sufficient for glenohumeral injections. The volume of the glenohumeral injection depends upon the indication for the injection. For conventional arthrography, the joint is maximally distended to allow contrast material to extend into small rents or tears, which may not fill if the joint is not adequately distended. With conventional arthrography, the joint is injected until resistance is met when the joint is full or the patient experiences discomfort related to fullness of the joint. This typically occurs at approximately 15 mL in a normal-size patient. Less joint distention is necessary for CT or MR arthrography compared with conventional arthrography. Overdistention of the joint leads to leakage from the joint puncture site (Fig. 2-38) or possible capsular rupture prior to imaging, which markedly hinders image quality with both MR and CT. A volume of 12 mL is adequate to distend the shoulder articulation in most patients. Subacromial bursa injections require a smaller joint volume, typically about 3 to 4 mL.[2] The acromioclavicular

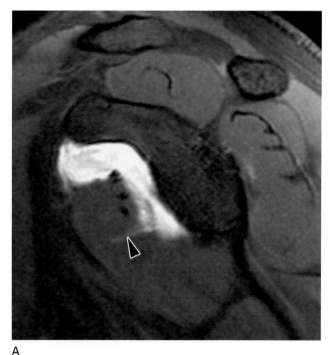 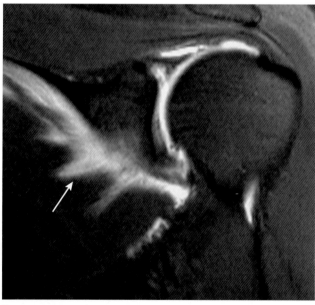

A   B

Figure 2-38 ■ Extravasation seen with MR arthrography. *A*, A small amount of gadolinium is not uncommonly seen extending along the needle tract *(arrowhead)*. *B*, Coronal image showing significant extravasation *(arrow)* anterior to the shoulder joint following MR arthrography related to overdistention of the joint.

joint is a very small joint with a volume of 1 mL.[19] The sterno-clavicular articulation is similar in size with a volume of only 1 mL.[24]

Injection Mixtures

Conventional Arthrography: Single Contrast

DIAGNOSTIC OR THERAPEUTIC

(14 to 18 mL total injected joint volume)
- 20-mL syringe
- 10 mL iodinated contrast (Reno-60, Omnipaque 300)
- 8 to 10 mL anesthetic agent (bupivacaine hydrochloride 0.5%, lidocaine hydrochloride 1% MPF)
- Optional: 0 to 2 mL steroid (methylprednisolone sodium succinate [Solu-Medrol 40 mg/mL, Depo-Medrol 40 mg/mL], triamcinolone [Kenalog-40], betamethasone sodium phosphate and betamethasone acetate [Celestone Soluspan 6 mg/mL])

Conventional Arthrography: Double Contrast

(14 to 18 mL total injected joint volume)
- 20-mL syringe
- 4 mL iodinated contrast (Reno-60, Omnipaque 300)
- Optional: 0 to 2 mL anesthetic agent (bupivacaine 0.5%, lidocaine 1%)
- 10 to 12 mL room air

CT Arthrography: Single Contrast

(12 mL total injected joint volume)
- 20-mL syringe
- 10 mL iodinated contrast (Reno-60, Omnipaque 300)
- 8 to 10 mL anesthetic agent (bupivacaine 0.5%, lidocaine 1%)
- Optional: 0 to 2 mL steroid (Solu-Medrol, Kenalog, Celestone)

CT Arthrography: Double Contrast

(14 to 18 mL total injected joint volume)
- 20-mL syringe
- 4 mL iodinated contrast (Reno-60, Omnipaque 300)
- Optional: 0 to 2 mL anesthetic agent (bupivacaine 0.5%, lidocaine 1%)
- 10 to 12 mL room air

MR Arthrography

(12 mL total injected joint volume)
- 20-mL syringe
- 5 mL iodinated contrast (Reno-60, Omnipaque 300)
- 10 mL anesthetic agent (bupivacaine 0.5%, lidocaine 1%)
- 5 mL 0.9% normal saline
- 0.1 to 0.2 mL gadodiamide or gadopentetate dimeglumine MR contrast (Omniscan, Magnevist)

Subacromial Bursa

(3 to 4 mL total injected joint volume)
- 10-mL syringe
- 5 mL iodinated contrast (Reno-60, Omnipaque 300)
- 4 to 5 mL anesthetic agent (bupivacaine 0.5%, lidocaine 1%)
- Optional: 0 to 1 mL steroid (Solu-Medrol, Kenalog, Celestone)

Acromioclavicular Articulation

(1 mL total injected joint volume)
- 10-mL syringe
- 5 mL iodinated contrast (Reno-60, Omnipaque 300)
- 4 to 5 mL anesthetic agent (bupivacaine 0.5%, lidocaine 1%)
- Optional: 0 to 1 mL steroid (Solu-Medrol, Kenalog, Celestone)

Sternoclavicular Articulation

(1 mL total injected joint volume)
- 10-mL syringe
- 5 mL iodinated contrast (Reno-60, Omnipaque 300)
- 4 to 5 mL anesthetic agent (bupivacaine 0.5%, lidocaine 1%)
- Optional: 0 to 1 mL steroid (Solu-Medrol, Kenalog, Celestone)

Methodology

Glenohumeral Joint Injection

ANTERIOR APPROACH

Prior to shoulder interventions, routine radiographic images of the shoulder are obtained and reviewed. The images should include anteroposterior (AP) views in both internal and external rotation. The patient is then placed on the fluoroscopy table in the supine position. Additional preliminary fluoroscopic evaluation of the joint in both internal and external arm rotation should also be performed before proceeding with the arthrogram to evaluate the dynamics of the shoulder joint (Fig. 2-39). The arm is then externally rotated with supination of the forearm and wrist. This serves to open the glenohumeral articulation anteriorly. Joint fluid shifts to the anterior aspect of the joint, further distending the capsule anteriorly, facilitating entry of the needle into the joint. A weight, such as a beanbag, can then be placed in the patient's palm, which passively stabilizes the patient's arm and allows the patient to relax the musculature of the shoulder and arm.

The target site for a glenohumeral joint injection using the anterior approach is the junction of the middle and inferior thirds of the anterior aspect of the glenohumeral joint (Figs. 2-40 and 2-41). The injection is made slightly closer to the humeral head than the glenoid.

The 25-gauge local anesthetic needle is then positioned directly over the target site (Fig. 2-42). If the planned punc-

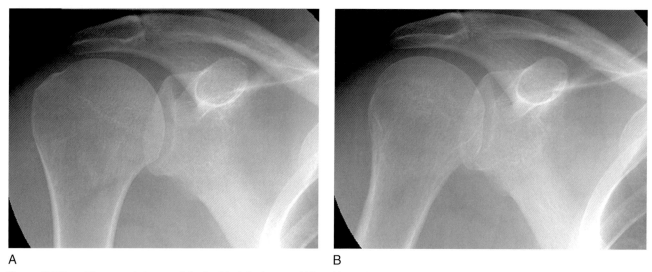

A   B

Figure 2-39 ■ Fluoroscopic images of the shoulder in both external (*A*) and internal (*B*) rotation. Fluoroscopic evaluation of the shoulder is performed prior to shoulder arthrography to evaluate the dynamics of the shoulder joint.

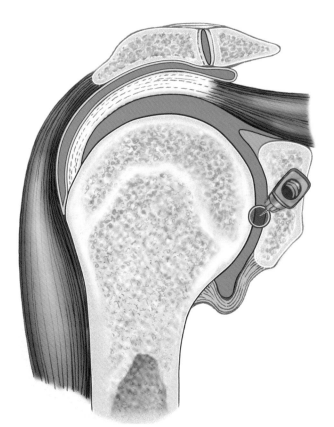

Figure 2-40 ■ Target site for glenohumeral joint injection at the junction of the middle and inferior third of the anterior aspect of the glenohumeral joint.

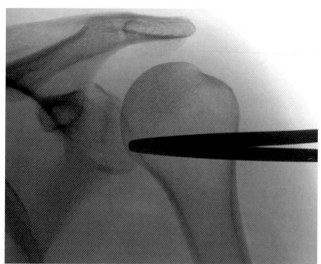

Figure 2-41 ■ The target site for a shoulder joint injection is the junction of the middle and inferior third of the anterior aspect of the glenohumeral joint.

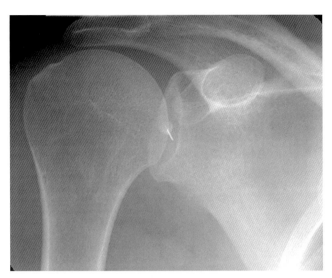

Figure 2-42 ▪ The 25-gauge needle used for local anesthesia can be used to gauge the position of the planned puncture site relative to the target site.

ture site is concordant with the target site, the 25-gauge needle can be removed and exchanged for a 22-gauge, 3.5-inch spinal needle. The spinal needle can then be advanced through the soft tissues overlying the glenohumeral articulation until contact is made with bone. It is not uncommon for the patient to experience discomfort when the needle enters the joint or makes contact with the periosteum of the bone. Fluoroscopy is then utilized to check the needle position (Fig. 2-43). Alterations in needle position can then be made to place the needle at the target site. The target site, located between the humeral head laterally and the glenoid medial-

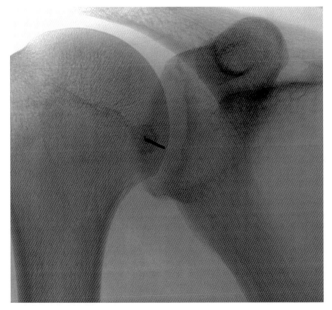

Figure 2-43 ▪ Positioning of the spinal needle is evaluated with fluoroscopy to guide entrance into the shoulder joint.

ly, can be felt by the resistance of these osseous structures to movement of the needle. Often the needle "engages the articulation" and allows further advancement. This additional movement should be minimal and performed with care as damage to the articular cartilage or labrum can result from overaggressive placement and manipulation of the needle while positioned in the glenohumeral joint. Often, with the joint opened anteriorly and the capsule distended anteriorly related to the external rotation of the arm, placement of the needle at the junction of the anterior glenoid and humeral head is sufficient and further advancement between the glenoid and humeral head is not necessary.

Once the needle has been properly positioned, the stylet of the spinal needle is withdrawn. The syringe and tubing containing the solution to be injected into the shoulder joint are then connected to the indwelling needle. A small test contrast injection is performed to ensure appropriate intra-articular placement of the needle. If resistance to injection is met, the needle may be embedded in articular cartilage and the needle is withdrawn slightly. If contrast material collects at the needle tip, the needle is extra-articular and needs to be repositioned. If contrast material flows freely away from the needle tip, the injection can be administered. The entire injection is performed under continuous fluoroscopic monitoring, especially if a rotator cuff tear is suspected, as contrast medium can rapidly fill the subacromial subdeltoid bursa. Obtaining early images may be helpful in this situation.

The volume of injection depends upon the indication for the injection. For conventional arthrography, the joint is maximally distended to allow contrast to extend into small rents or tears, which may not fill if the joint is not adequately distended. With conventional arthrography, the joint is injected until resistance is met because of fullness of the joint or the patient experiences discomfort related to fullness of the joint. This typically occurs at approximately 15 mL in a normal-size patient. Less distention is necessary with CT or MR arthrography compared with conventional arthrography. Overdistention of the articulation leads to leakage from the joint puncture site and possible capsular rupture prior to imaging, which markedly hinders image quality with both MR and CT. A volume of 12 mL is adequate to distend the shoulder articulation in most patients. Care is taken not to overdistend the joint.

The needle is withdrawn following the injection. Fluoroscopic evaluation of the joint should then be performed in both internal and external rotation. Spot films are obtained in each of these positions (Fig. 2-44). For CT and MR arthrography, manipulation of the joint is kept to a minimum to avoid extravasation from the joint prior to imaging. For conventional arthrography, vigorous exercise of the shoulder is performed followed by additional fluoroscopic evaluation, as many small tears become evident after increased intra-articular pressure related to exercise and positional changes force contrast material into small undersurface defects.

POSTERIOR APPROACH

A posterior approach to the glenohumeral injection is used to avoid occasional problems with extravasation from the anterior puncture site or inadvertent extra-articular injection

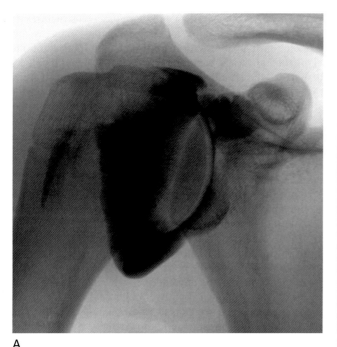

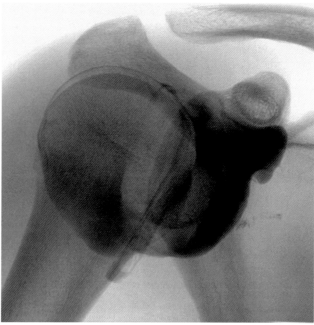

A
B

Figure 2-44 ■ Normal images following a shoulder joint injection in both external (*A*) and internal (*B*) rotation.

of contrast material anteriorly, which can present interpretive difficulties with CT or MR arthrography.[25] The procedure is similar to the anterior approach. The patient is placed on the fluoroscopic table in the prone position. The patient's arm is placed at the patient's side in the neutral position or internal rotation. A triangular foam pad is then placed under the

patient's torso to raise the shoulder that is to be injected (Fig. 2-45). This places the glenohumeral articulation in profile, allowing a direct puncture to be performed from the posterior approach (Fig. 2-46). Precise positioning using an obliquity that allows perfect tangential viewing of the glenohumeral articulation is critical for the posterior approach to the glenohumeral articulation.[25]

The remainder of the procedure is similar to the anterior approach. The target site is identified and marked (Fig. 2-47). The posterior aspect of the shoulder is prepared and draped

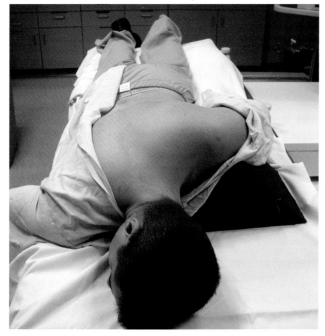

Figure 2-45 ■ Oblique positioning for posterior approach for a shoulder joint injection.

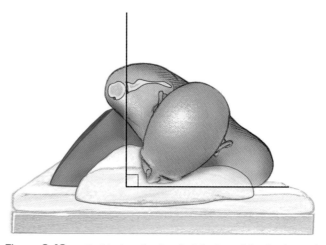

Figure 2-46 ■ Positioning of patient for injections of the glenohumeral joint using a posterior approach. A triangular foam pad is placed under the patient's torso to raise the shoulder to be injected. This brings the glenohumeral articulation in profile.

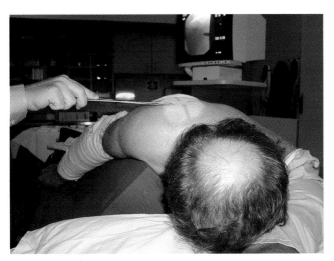

Figure 2-47 ▪ Posterior approach for a shoulder joint injection. The target site is identified with a metallic object.

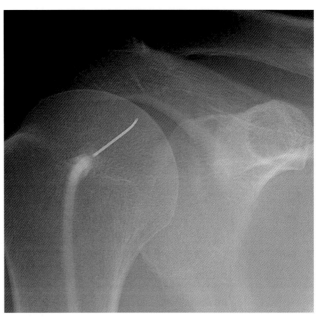

Figure 2-49 ▪ Glenohumeral joint injection utilizing the rotator cuff interval approach. The target site for the injection is the upper medial quadrant of the humeral head close to the articular joint line.

in sterile fashion. Local anesthesia is administered subcutaneously. A 22-gauge spinal needle is then advanced vertically into the shoulder joint (Fig. 2-48) and the injection is made.

ROTATOR CUFF INTERVAL APPROACH

Another anterior approach into the shoulder joint is through the rotator cuff interval. The rotator cuff interval is the anatomic separation of the rotator cuff between the anterior aspect of the supraspinatus and the superior aspect of the subscapularis related to the coracoid process of the scapula.[26] The radiographic target is the upper medial quadrant of the humeral head close to the articular joint line (Fig. 2-49).[26] The injection is performed with the shoulder joint in external rotation to avoid puncture of the long head of the biceps tendon. Using this approach, one avoids the labroligamentous structures of the anterior aspect of the joint and the subscapularis muscle and tendon (Fig. 2-50). A potential pitfall with this technique is that the subacromial-subdeltoid bursa

overlies the rotator cuff interval and therefore extravasation related to the injection or improper needle position may result in contrast material entering this overlying bursa.[27] Contrast within the subacromial-subdeltoid bursa may hinder the evaluation of full-thickness versus partial-thickness rotator cuff tears, and contrast within this bursa may be confused with a full-thickness tear.[27]

Glenohumeral Joint Aspiration

Glenohumeral joint aspiration is similar to glenohumeral joint injection. The same needle technique as that described previously for glenohumeral joint injection is used. When the

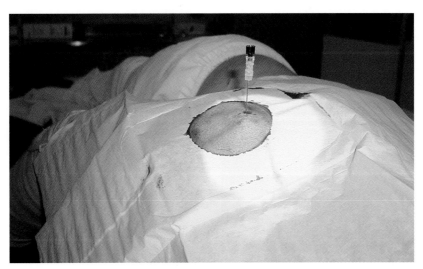

Figure 2-48 ▪ A 22-gauge spinal needle is advanced into the shoulder joint by a posterior approach under fluoroscopic guidance.

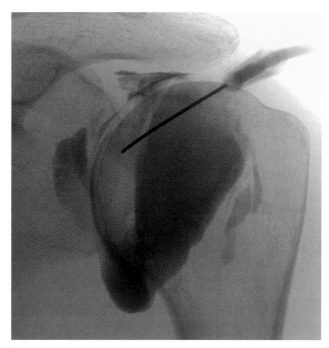

Figure 2-50 ▪ Glenohumeral joint injection performed using the rotator cuff interval technique.

needle is in place, a 60-mL syringe and connecting tube is attached to the needle hub, and the joint is aspirated (Fig. 2-51). If no fluid is obtained, an attempt is made to reposition the needle within the joint. If still no fluid is aspirated, the joint is washed with nonbacteriostatic saline and then re-aspirated. To accomplish this, nonbacteriostatic saline is drawn up into a separate 20-mL syringe and tubing and 10 mL is injected into the joint through the indwelling needle. The syringe tubing is then exchanged for a 60-mL syringe and tubing and the nonbacteriostatic saline is aspirated.

The aspirated fluid or nonbacteriostatic saline wash is sent for aerobic and anaerobic culture. If sufficient fluid is

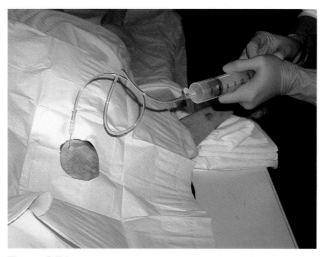

Figure 2-51 ▪ Glenohumeral joint aspiration. A 60-mL syringe and extension tubing are connected to the indwelling spinal needle and fluid is aspirated.

obtained, Gram stain and additional analysis of the fluid can be performed, depending upon the specific clinical situation.

Subacromial Joint Injection

Prior to injection, routine radiographic images of the shoulder are obtained and reviewed. Additional preliminary fluoroscopic evaluation of the joint in both internal and external arm rotation and with shoulder abduction should also be performed before proceeding with the injection. An anterior or posterior approach can be utilized for a subacromial bursa injection. The patient is placed in the supine position for the anterior approach or the prone position for the posterior approach. The target site using either approach is the undersurface of the acromion (Fig. 2-52).

A 22-gauge, 3.5-inch spinal needle is advanced through the soft tissues just below the acromion until contact is made with the undersurface of the acromion.[2] Fluoroscopy is used to check the needle position. Necessary alterations in needle position can then be made. Typically, after contact is made with the undersurface of the acromion, the needle is withdrawn 1 to 2 mm. The syringe and tubing containing the solution to be injected are connected to the indwelling 22-gauge needle. A small test injection is performed to ensure appropriate intrabursal placement of the needle. The bursal volume is variable but typically moderate sized and an injection of about 3 to 4 mL is usually sufficient. Little resistance to injection is encountered. Imaging is used to confirm proper

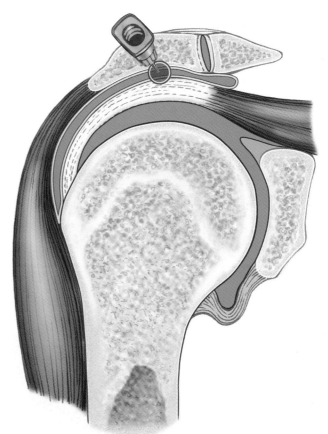

Figure 2-52 ▪ Target site for subacromial-subdeltoid bursal injection.

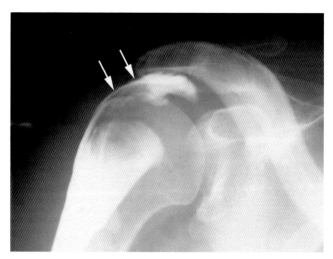

Figure 2-53 ▪ Fluoroscopic image following a therapeutic right subacromial subdeltoid bursal injection. There is evidence of mild synovitis with mild irregularity of the synovial margins (*arrows*).

position (Fig. 2-53). If contrast material collects at the needle tip, the needle is extra-articular and need to be repositioned. If contrast flows away from the needle tip delineating the bursal surface of the rotator cuff, the remainder of the injection mixture is given. The entire injection is performed under continuous fluoroscopic monitoring. The subdeltoid bursa typically also fills with subacromial injections, and the

morphology of the combination of the subacromial and subdeltoid bursa can be quite variable. The needle is withdrawn following the injection. Fluoroscopic evaluation of the joint should then be performed with a spot film obtained to document the injection.

Acromioclavicular Joint Injection

The patient is placed on the fluoroscopy table in the supine position. Additional preliminary fluoroscopic evaluation of the joint is performed noting any abnormal motion at the articulation, which would indicate acromioclavicular separation.

The target site for acromioclavicular injections is the midportion of the joint space, which is seen end on utilizing a direct anterior approach (Fig. 2-54).[19] The 1.5-inch, 25-gauge needle is advanced through the soft tissues overlying the acromioclavicular articulation until contact is made with bone. The patient commonly experiences discomfort when the needle enters the joint or makes contact with the periosteum of the bone. Fluoroscopy is utilized to verify the needle position (Fig. 2-55). Alterations in needle position can then be made. The articulation between the distal clavicle and the acromion can be very narrow. The needle is advanced between the clavicle and the acromion into the articulation. When the needle has been properly positioned, the syringe and tubing containing the solution to be injected are connected to the indwelling 25-gauge needle. A small test injection is performed to ensure appropriate intra-articular placement of the needle. The joint is very small, and resistance to injection is normal. Imaging must be used to confirm proper position. If contrast material collects at the needle tip, the needle is extra-articular and needs to be repositioned. If contrast flows away from the needle tip in a linear fashion along the joint line, the remainder of the injection mixture is given (Fig. 2-56). The acromioclavicular joint has a small volume typically requiring only a 1-mL injection.[24] The entire injection is performed under continuous fluoroscopic monitoring. Occasionally, large synovial cysts emanate from the acromioclavicular joint and can fill

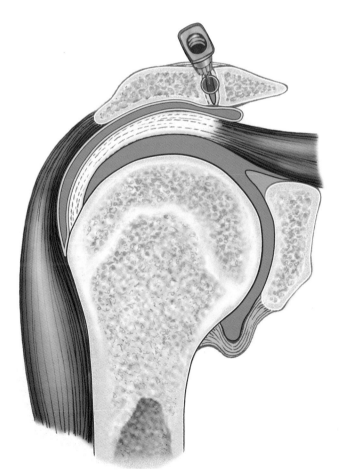

Figure 2-54 ▪ Target site for acromioclavicular joint injection.

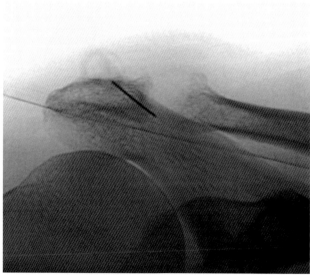

Figure 2-55 ▪ Fluoroscopic guidance is utilized to place the needle into the acromioclavicular joint.

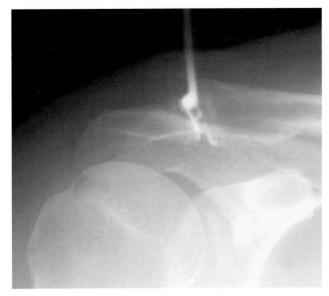

Figure 2-56 ■ Fluoroscopic images following a therapeutic acromio-clavicular joint injection.

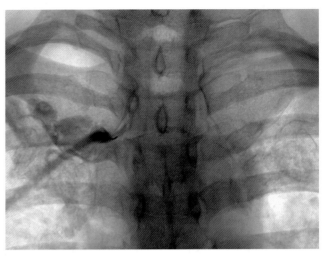

Figure 2-58 ■ The sternoclavicular joint injection performed under fluoroscopic guidance.

with contrast. The needle is withdrawn following the injection. Fluoroscopic evaluation of the joint should then be performed with a spot radiograph obtained to document the injection.

Sternoclavicular Joint Injection

The patient is placed on the fluoroscopy table in the supine position. Additional preliminary fluoroscopic evaluation of the joint is performed, and the fluoroscopic image is collimated to minimize radiation exposure to the surrounding tissues. A direct anterior approach is used for a sternoclavicular joint injection.

The target site for sternoclavicular injections is the middle to inferior portion of the articulation, which is seen en face using a direct anterior approach (Fig. 2-57).

If the planned puncture site is concordant with the target site, the 1.5-inch, 25-gauge needle can be advanced through the soft tissues overlying the sternoclavicular articulation until contact is made with bone. Fluoroscopy is then utilized to check the needle position and necessary alterations in needle position can be made. The articulation between the sternum and the proximal clavicle is typically very narrow. The needle is advanced between the sternum and the clavicle into the articulation, and when the needle has been properly positioned, the syringe and tubing containing the solution to be injected are connected to the indwelling 25-gauge needle. A small test injection is performed to ensure appropriate intra-articular placement of the needle. The joint is very small, and resistance to injection is normal. Imaging must be used to confirm proper position. If contrast collects at the needle tip, the needle is extra-articular and is repositioned. If contrast flows away from the needle tip in a linear fashion along the joint line, the remainder of the injection is made (Fig. 2-58). The sternoclavicular joint typically has a small

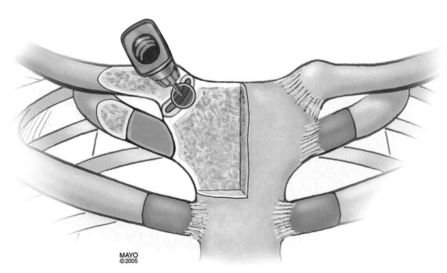

MAYO
©2005

Figure 2-57 ■ Target site for sternoclavicular joint injection.

volume, requiring only a 1-mL injection. The entire injection is performed under continuous fluoroscopic monitoring. The needle is withdrawn following the injection. Fluoroscopic evaluation of the joint should then be performed with a spot radiograph obtained to document the injection.

Sternoclavicular Aspiration

The needle is inserted using the same technique as for sternoclavicular injection. Aspiration is performed in the same manner described for glenohumeral joint aspiration with the exception that if fluid cannot be obtained, the sternoclavicular joint can be washed with 2 to 3 mL of nonbacteriostatic saline and aspirated.

POTENTIAL COMPLICATIONS

- Bleeding
- Infection (cellulitis, septic arthritis, or osteomyelitis)
- Drug-related allergic reactions
- Transient synovitis
- Transitory upper extremity weakness
- Transitory upper extremity paresthesia
- Vascular injury (subclavian/axillary artery or vein)
- Pneumothorax

POST-PROCEDURE CARE/FOLLOW-UP[28]

Immediate

1. The patient is observed for 15 minutes following injection.
2. Blood pressure, pulse, heart rate, and respiratory rate are monitored as necessary.

Discharge

1. An adhesive bandage may be placed on the puncture site. The bandage should remain dry for at least 24 hours, at which point it can be removed.
2. The patient is instructed to continue taking his or her prescription medication, although pain medication may be tapered as indicated.
3. A discharge sheet is given to the patient outlining the following:
   a. Which procedure was performed
   b. Procedure-related symptoms that typically resolve in 7 to 10 days
      - Pain at the needle puncture site(s)
      - Mild increase in shoulder stiffness with a feeling of fullness in the joint
      - Deep shoulder pain
   c. Treatment for mild post-procedure symptoms
      - Rest the shoulder for 1 to 2 days
      - Avoid movements that worsen the pain
      - Use cold compresses to the area that hurts
   d. Signs and symptoms of infection
      - Fever
      - Chills
      - Swelling or drainage from the puncture site(s)
      - New shoulder pain that is different from the usual pain
   e. Signs and symptoms of possible more serious problems
      - Decreased range of motion of the shoulder
      - Increasing pain
      - Motor dysfunction of the upper extremity
   f. Physician name and contact number if the patient has any concerns or if any problem were to arise as a result of the procedure
   g. Advice to schedule a follow-up appointment with the referring physician in 7 to 10 days.

SAMPLE DICTATIONS

Glenohumeral Injection

The procedure and potential complications were explained to the patient, and voluntary informed, signed consent was obtained. The patient was placed on the table in the supine position. Preliminary fluoroscopic evaluation of the shoulder was performed with both internal and external rotation as well as abduction. The skin overlying the glenohumeral articulation was prepared and draped in a sterile fashion. Local anesthesia was obtained with a 4:1 solution of 1% lidocaine and bicarbonate buffer. Under fluoroscopic guidance, a 22-gauge, 3.5-inch spinal needle was advanced into the glenohumeral articulation and a 12-mL solution containing iodinated contrast material (iohexol, 300 mg I/mL), 0.5% bupivacaine, and 0.1 mL of gadolinium (gadopentetate dimeglumine) was administered into the shoulder articulation. The needle was withdrawn. Post-injection fluoroscopic evaluation was performed, and appropriate spot films were obtained. The patient was sent to MR for additional imaging of the shoulder status after arthrography.

Acromioclavicular Joint Injection

The procedure and potential complications were explained to the patient, and voluntary informed, signed consent was obtained. The patient was placed on the table in the supine position. Preliminary fluoroscopic evaluation of the acromioclavicular articulation was performed. The skin overlying the acromioclavicular articulation was prepared and draped in a sterile fashion. Local anesthesia was obtained with 1% lidocaine with bicarbonate buffer. Under fluoroscopic guidance, a 22-gauge, 3.5-inch spinal needle was advanced into the acromioclavicular articulation and a 1-mL solution containing iodinated contrast material (iohexol, 300 mg I/mL), 0.5% bupivacaine, and corticosteroid (Solu-Medrol 40 mg/mL) was administered into the acromioclavicular joint. The needle was withdrawn. Post-injection fluoroscopic evaluation was performed and a spot film was obtained.

CASE REPORTS

CASE 1

Clinical Presentation

A 22-year-old left hand–dominant rugby player presented with left shoulder pain for 4 months. He does not recall a specific injury but states that he often has aches and pains following a rugby match. The patient has taken anti-inflammatory medications without relief and also has undergone physical therapy with no improvement. The patient reports normal range of motion but describes pain with abduction of the shoulder and internal rotation. He also complains of mild weakness of the shoulder.

On physical examination, the patient demonstrated shoulder pain with abduction with mild weakness but no paresthesias. The patient demonstrated bilateral range of motion to 160 degrees of abduction. Strength was normal and symmetric but there was a weakly positive left O'Brien test. The patient had a negative apprehension test with no apprehension about instability with passive abduction, extension, and external rotation of the shoulder. The patient was neurovascularly intact.

Imaging and Therapy

An MR arthrogram of the left shoulder was performed (Fig. 2-59). Axial T1-weighted images with fat saturation of the shoulder following intra-articular gadolinium administration revealed a torn posterior labrum with a small posterior paralabral cyst. The cyst was small but was extended medially toward the spinoglenoid notch. The cyst was near but not impinging upon the infraspinatus nerve. The patient reported significant short-term relief of shoulder joint pain following the injection that contained 0.5% bupivacaine.

The patient subsequently underwent arthroscopic surgical repair of the torn labrum. At arthroscopy, the posterior labrum was found to be focally torn at the 3 o'clock position with a small flap of the labrum able to be displaced into the joint. There was no medial displacement of the labrum. Intraoperative needle aspiration of the cyst was performed, revealing a small

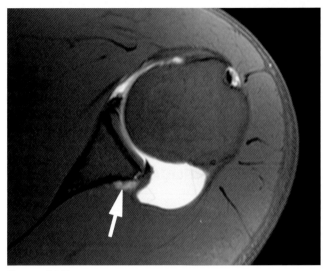

Figure 2-59 ■ Axial image from an MR arthrogram of the left shoulder depicting a posterior labral tear with an associated small posterior paralabral cyst *(arrow)* extending medially toward the spinoglenoid notch.

amount of fluid from tissues medial to the labral tear. The labral tear was then repaired with a single Mitek Panalok anchor with excellent anatomic apposition of the posterior labrum.

Results

The patient was treated with sling immobilization in external rotation for 4 weeks after the procedure, followed by a formal range of motion and strengthening program with excellent results. Shoulder pain and the sensation of weakness were eliminated. The patient returned to rugby the following season.

CASE 2

Clinical Presentation

A 41-year-old man presented with chronic left shoulder pain. The patient has an extensive surgical history including three previous shoulder surgeries. The patient has undergone two previous rotator cuff repair procedures and previous subtotal acromionectomy and an anterior inferior capsular shift procedure. The patient continues to have shoulder pain, especially with elevation and abduction of the shoulder. Physical examination demonstrated good shoulder strength with intact rotator cuff function. The patient did have a positive apprehension sign, suggesting glenohumeral instability.

Imaging and Therapy

An MR arthrogram was performed of the left shoulder; however, extensive artifact was seen related to the previous rotator cuff repairs (Fig. 2-60). This markedly

hindered the diagnostic capability and image quality. The repaired rotator cuff was intact, but the capsular labral ligamentous complex was not well evaluated. To salvage the examination, the patient was taken immediately from the MR scanner to the CT scanner and a CT arthrogram was performed. Iodinated contrast medium, in addition to gadolineim, was utilized for the injection and also made CT arthrography possible. The CT arthrogram showed some artifact related to the rotator cuff repair but to a lesser extent than the MR arthrogram. The labrum could be well visualized, and the superior glenoid labrum was found to be torn (Fig. 2-61). This was well seen with the CT arthrogram but not well appreciated with the MR arthrogram related to the artifact. The inclusion of iodinated contrast medium with the injection allowed salvage of the examination and a diagnostic study to be obtained.

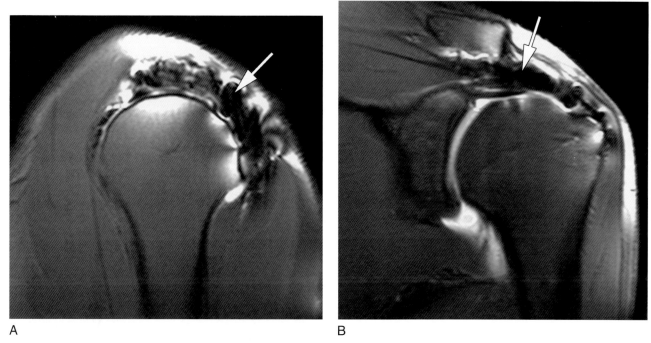

A   B

Figure 2-60 ■ Sagittal (*A*) and coronal (*B*) images from an MR arthrogram in a patient with prior rotator cuff repair depicting extensive susceptibility artifact *(arrows)* related to the prior surgery, which markedly hinders image quality.

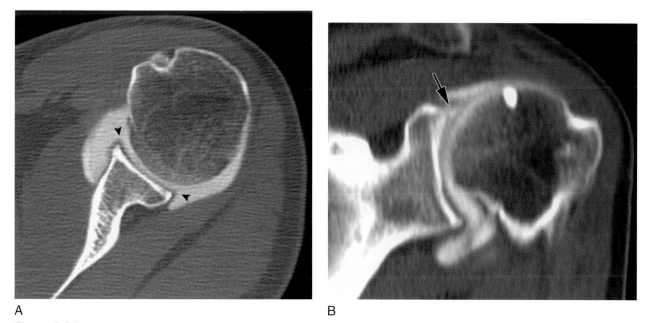

A   B

Figure 2-61 ■ CT arthrography obtained immediately following the MR examination depicts the anterior and posterior glenoid labrum *(arrows)* quite well (*A*). The coronal reformatted image (*B*) depicts a large tear *(arrow)* involving the superior glenoid labrum, which was not as well seen on the MR secondary to susceptibility artifact.

Results

The patient underwent arthroscopic repair of the superior glenoid labrum. Arthroscopy confirmed a type 2 superior labral tear from the 10 o'clock to the 2 o'clock position. A superior labral repair was performed with two Mitek Panalok suture anchors, which achieved a very stable repair. The shoulder was splinted with no range of motion for 4 weeks, followed by a formal range of motion and strengthening regimen. The patient reported significant improvement in shoulder symptoms following the procedure.

CASE 3

Clinical Presentation

A 38-year-old patient presented with severe shoulder pain with markedly limited range of motion. The patient reported no specific injury to the shoulder but stated that the shoulder had troubled her for several years. Physical examination confirmed limitation of shoulder joint motion diffusely with preserved rotator cuff function. There was no other specific evidence on physical examination for shoulder joint pathology. Previous MR of the shoulder demonstrated an intact rotator cuff with no evidence of glenoid labral tear. The diagnosis of frozen shoulder was made on the basis of clinical and physical examination findings.

Imaging and Therapy

Treatment was performed with image-guided intra-articular corticosteroid injection (Fig. 2-62). The joint was accessed utilizing the standard technique. The standard injection solution was utilized apart from the addition of 2 mL of corticosteroid. The joint volume was very small, holding only 8 mL prior to rupture. The injection had a very tight feel with significant resistance to injection. The axillary and subscapularis recesses were absent, and rupture of the posterolateral aspect of the joint capsule occurred at 8 mL of injected volume.

Results

The patient tolerated the procedure well. The patient reported some stiffness and discomfort related to the procedure for 1 to 2 hours following the procedure but subsequently noticed significant improvement in symptoms. The patient reported significant short-term relief of pain related to the intra-articular 0.5% bupivacaine administration. She also reported moderate long-term improvement in shoulder pain, presumably

related to a combination of anti-inflammatory effects of the steroid and the mechanical distention of the joint with rupture of intra-articular adhesions. The referring surgeon noticed a significant improvement in range of motion following the injection.

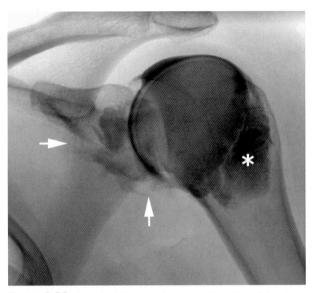

Figure 2-62 ▪ Image following therapeutic injection of the gleno-humeral joint in a middle-aged woman with adhesive capsulitis. The joint is very small in volume, with absence of the axillary and sub-scapularis bursae *(arrows)* and extravasation from the posterolateral aspect of the joint *(asterick)*. The patient reported significant improvement in symptoms following the injection related to capsular distention and rupture of intra-articular adhesions.

CURRENT PROCEDURAL TERMINOLOGY (CPT) CODES[29]

CPT codes change often and sometimes are valid only for certain states or regions. It is best to consult with coding experts to make sure that coding for one's procedures is legitimate and complete. Below is a sample of codes that are being used for shoulder injection procedures at this writing.

20610 Arthrocentesis, aspiration, and/or injection; major joint or bursa (e.g., shoulder, hip, knee joint, subacromial bursa)

(If imaging guidance is performed, see 76003, 76360, 76393, 76942)

23350 Injection procedure for shoulder arthrography or enhanced CT/MRI shoulder arthrography

(For radiographic arthrography, radiologic supervision, and interpretation, use 73030. Fluoroscopy ([76003] is inclusive of radiographic arthrography)

(When fluoroscopically guided injection is performed for enhanced CT arthrography, use 23350, 76003, and 73201 or 73202)

(When fluoroscopically guided injection is performed for enhanced MR arthrography, use 23350, 76003, and 73222 or 73223)

(For enhanced CT or enhanced MRI arthrography, use 76003 and either 73201, 73202, 73222, or 73223)

73020 Radiologic examination, shoulder; one view

73030 complete, minimum of two views

73040 Radiologic examination, shoulder; arthrography, radiologic supervision and interpretation

(Do not report 76003 in addition to 73040)

73050 Radiologic examination; acromioclavicular joints, bilateral, with or without weighted distraction

73060 humerus, minimum of three views

73200 Computed tomography, upper extremity; without contrast material

73201 with contrast material(s)

73202 without contrast material, followed by contrast material(s) and further sections

(To report three-dimensional [3D] rendering, see 76376, 76377)

73221 Magnetic resonance (e.g., proton) imaging, any joint of upper extremity; without contrast material(s)

73222 with contrast material(s)

73223 without contrast material(s), followed by contrast material(s) and further sequences

76003 Fluoroscopic guidance for needle placement (e.g., biopsy, aspiration, injection, localization device)

76360 Computed tomography guidance for needle placement (e.g., biopsy, aspiration, injection, or placement of localization device), radiologic supervision and interpretation

76376 3D rendering with interpretation and reporting of computed tomography, magnetic resonance imaging, ultrasound, or other tomographic modality; not requiring image postprocessing on an independent workstation

76377 requiring image postprocessing on an independent workstation

76393 Magnetic resonance guidance for needle placement (e.g., for biopsy, needle aspiration, injection, localization device), radiologic supervision and interpretation

76942 Ultrasonic guidance for needle placement (e.g., biopsy, aspiration, injection, localization device), imaging supervision and interpretation

References

1. Oberholzer J. Die Arthropneumonradiographie bei Habitueller Shulterluxation. Rontgenpraxis 1933; 5:589–590.
2. Rafii M, Minkoff J. Advanced arthrography of the shoulder with CT and MR imaging. Radiol Clin North Am 1998; 36:609–633.
3. Lindblom K. Arthrography and roentgenography in ruptures of tendons of the shoulder joint. Acta Radiol 1939; 20:548–562.
4. Freiberger RH, Kaye JJ. Arthrography. Norwalk, CT: Appleton Century Crofts, 1979, pp 1–3, 137–188.
5. Garcia JF. Arthrographic visualization of rotator cuff tears. Radiology 1984; 150:595–596.
6. Beltran J, Rosenberg ZS, Chandnani VP, et al. Glenohumeral instability: Evaluation with MR arthrography. Radiographics 1997; 17:657–673.
7. Rafii M, Firooznia H, Golimbu C. CT arthrography of shoulder instabilities in athletes. Am J Sports Med 1988; 16:352–361.
8. Buchbinder R, Green S. Effect of arthrographic shoulder joint distension with saline and corticosteroid for adhesive capsulitis. Br J Sports Med 2004; 38:384–385.
9. Neumann CH, Petersen SA, Jahnke AH. MR imaging of the labral-capsular complex: Normal variations. AJR Am J Roentgenol 1991; 157:1015–1021.
10. Park YH, Lee JY, Moon SH, et al. MR Arthrography of the labral capsular ligamentous complex in the shoulder: Imaging variations and pitfalls. AJR Am J Roentgenol 2000; 175:667–672.
11. Zlatkin MB. MRI of the Shoulder. New York: Raven Press, 1991, pp 21–39.
12. Berquist TH. MRI of the Musculoskeletal System, 5th ed. Philadelphia: Lippincott Williams & Wilkins, 2006, pp 557–656.
13. Resnick D. Diagnosis of Bone and Joint Disorders, 4th ed. Philadelphia: WB Saunders, 2002, pp 193-318, 3068-3146.
14. Cone RO, Resnick D, Danzig L. Shoulder impingement syndrome: Radiographic evaluation. Radiology 1984; 150:29–33.
15. Peh WC, Farmer TH, Totty WG. Acromial arch shape: Assessment with MR imaging. Radiology 1995; 195:501–505.
16. Zlatkin MB, Bjorkengren AG, Gylys-Morin V, et al. Cross-sectional imaging of the capsular mechanism of the glenohumeral joint. AJR Am J Roentgenol 1988; 150:151–158.
17. Kwak SM, Brown RR, Resnick D, et al. Anatomy, anatomic variations, and pathology of the 11- to 3-o'clock position of the glenoid labrum. AJR Am J Roentgenol 1998; 171:235–238.
18. Erickson SJ, Fitzgerald SW, Quinn SF, et al. Long bicipital tendon of the shoulder: Normal Anatomy And Pathologic Findings on MR imaging. AJR Am J Roentgenol 1992; 158:1091–1096.
19. Hodge JC. Musculoskeletal Imaging Diagnostic and Therapeutic Procedures. Montreal: Karger Landes Systems, 1997, pp 1–23.
20. Lee JHE, van Raalte V, Malian V. Diagnosis of SLAP lesions with Grashey-view arthrography. Skeletal Radiol 2003; 32:388–395.
21. Roger B, Skaf A, Hooper AW, et al. Imaging findings in the dominant shoulder of throwing athletes: Comparison of radiography, arthrography, CT arthrography, and MR arthrography with arthroscopic correlation. AJR Am J Roentgenol 1999; 172:1371–1380.
22. Guntern DV, Pfirrmann CWA, Schmid MR, et al. Articular cartilage lesions of the glenohumeral joint: Diagnostic effectiveness of MR

arthrography and prevalence in patients with subacromial impingement syndrome. Radiology 2003; 226:165–170.

23. Major NM, Banks MC. MR imaging of complications of loose surgical tacks in the shoulder. AJR Am J Roentgenol 2003; 180:377–380.

24. Berquist TH. Diagnostic and therapeutic injections as an aid to musculoskeletal diagnosis. Semin Interv Radiol 1993; 10:326–344.

25. Farmer KD, Hughes PM. MR arthrography of the shoulder: Fluoroscopically guided technique using a posterior approach. AJR Am J Roentgenol 2002; 178:433–434.

26. Depelteau H, Bureau NJ, Cardinal E, et al. Arthrography of the shoulder: A simple fluoroscopically guided approach for targeting the rotator cuff interval. AJR Am J Roentgenol 2004; 182:329–332.

27. Ehara S. Injection of rotator interval for shoulder arthrography. AJR Am J Roentgenol 2004; 183:1172–1173.

28. Fenton DS, Czervionke LF. Image Guided Spine Intervention. Philadelphia: WB Saunders, 2003.

29. CPT 2007, CPT Intellectual Property Services. Chicago: American Medical Association, 2007.

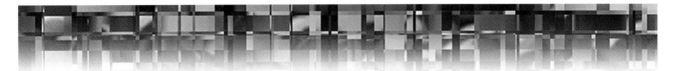

A Shoulder Surgeon's Perspective

Shoulder Injections

Cedric J. Ortiguera, MD

Shoulder injections play an extremely important role in the diagnostic and therapeutic management of shoulder disorders. Shoulder pain is a very common complaint seen by primary care physicians as well as the orthopedic specialist. Impingement syndrome, one of the most common disorders of the shoulder, is routinely treated with subacromial injection for both diagnostic and therapeutic purposes. Other helpful therapeutic injections that may prove useful include intra-articular acromioclavicular joint injections and glenohumeral injections. Injections in these areas of lidocaine or bupivacaine combined with a corticosteroid often give pain relief and when combined with a thorough nonoperative program are successful for many patients. In the setting where corticosteroids are contraindicated or refused by the patient, a subacromial lidocaine or bupivacaine injection is still helpful to confirm the diagnosis of impingement based on temporary pain relief.

With the advent of arthroscopy, much more is known about shoulder anatomy and pathology. Labral pathology in particular has seen a wealth of literature and descriptions of varying pathology in both traumatic and nontraumatic cases. Previously, diagnosis of these lesions required a careful history, physical examination, and diagnostic arthroscopy. Current utilization of MR arthrography for the shoulder yields sensitivity and specificity of well over 90%. In addition to labral pathology, MR arthrography has given us a better understanding of partial articular-sided rotator cuff tears as well as glenohumeral ligament pathology.

In the setting where MRI is contraindicated, evaluation of the rotator cuff with ultrasound has been reasonable, but this gives few data regarding the glenohumeral joint and labrum. Standard arthrography or CT arthrography can be helpful in these situations as well. Our current practice is to obtain MRI with arthrography when there is a concern for labral pathology. The advent of MR arthrography has improved our understanding of shoulder anatomy and pathology and reduced the need for unnecessary diagnostic arthroscopy.

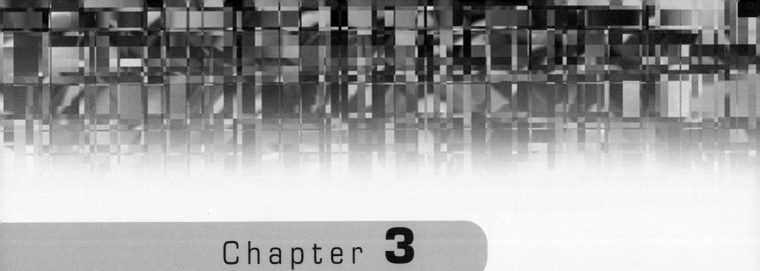

Chapter 3

Elbow Injections

- Jeffrey J. Peterson, MD

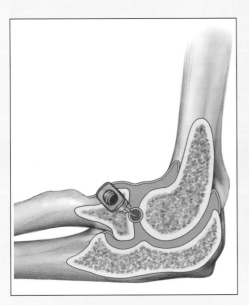

BACKGROUND

Elbow arthrography is not a commonly performed procedure but is occasionally obtained to evaluate the integrity of the joint capsule, or the articular cartilage of the elbow joint, or to assess for other intra-articular or synovium-based processes.[1,2] When performed properly, elbow injections are safe, painless, and relatively simple.

Elbow arthrography was originally described in 1952 by Lindblom[3] and further delineated by Arvidsson and Johansson in 1955.[4] Until the 1980s, conventional elbow arthrography remained the best procedure for evaluation of intra-articular pathology involving the elbow joint.[5] In the late 1980s magnetic resonance (MR) imaging of the elbow was introduced, and by the1990s, MR imaging became widely available. This dramatically reduced the indications for elbow arthrography. MR of the elbow proved superior to conventional arthrography in the evaluation of elbow joint disorders.[6] MR of the elbow is noninvasive, allows multiplanar imaging, and more precisely depicts the intra-articular structures of the elbow joint.

Today, conventional elbow arthrography is an uncommon procedure and most diagnostic injections of the elbow joint are performed for the purposes of computed tomography (CT) or MR arthrography.[7] CT and MR arthrography was introduced as a way to improve upon conventional CT and MR examinations of the elbow. CT or MR arthrography of the elbow remains a useful modality for evaluation of intra-articular pathology, synovium-based processes, or the capsular or ligamentous integrity of the elbow.[8,9] CT arthrography also precisely depicts a wide variety of intra-articular pathology about the elbow and is useful in patients who cannot undergo conventional MR examinations or in cases in which MR was equivocal.

ANATOMIC CONSIDERATIONS

The elbow joint is formed at the confluence of three osseous structures, the humerus, the radius, and the ulna (Fig. 3-1).[9,10] The distal aspect of the humerus consists of the capitellum and the trochlea, which articulate with the proximal radius and the proximal ulna, respectively. The radial head also articulates with the radial notch of the ulna, forming the proximal radioulnar articulation. The elbow articulation is composed of three distinct joints: the radiocapitellar, the ulnar-trochlear, and the proximal radioulnar joint. The trochlear notch of the ulna surrounds nearly 180 degrees of the trochlea, making the elbow joint one of the most stable articulations in the body (Fig. 3-2).[10]

The elbow joint capsule is thin anteriorly and posteriorly, having additional support anteriorly by the brachialis muscle and posteriorly by the triceps muscle.[2,10] Medially and laterally, the joint capsule is inseparable from the medial and lateral collateral ligaments of the elbow.[10] Several recesses are present in the elbow joint. The largest is the olecranon recess, also known as the posterior recess.[9,10] This is seen posterior to the elbow and is subdivided into the superior, medial, and lateral olecranon recesses (Fig. 3-3).[10] The olec-

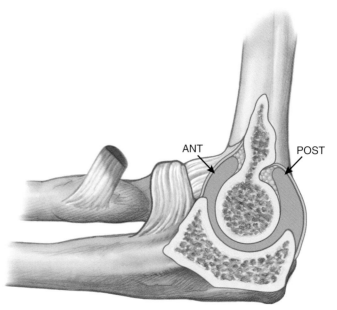

Figure 3-2 ■ Anterior and posterior recesses of the elbow joint. ANT = anterior recess; POST = posterior recess.

ranon recess is capacious, allowing marked flexion of the elbow joint.[9] The olecranon recess distends with extension.[9] The smaller anterior humeral recess (Fig. 3-4) is seen anterior to the elbow joint and is subdivided into the coronoid and radial fossae.[10] The annular recess is the most distal recess of the joint and surrounds the radial neck (Fig. 3-5).[10] The recesses for the ulnar collateral ligament and radial collateral ligament are seen deep to the

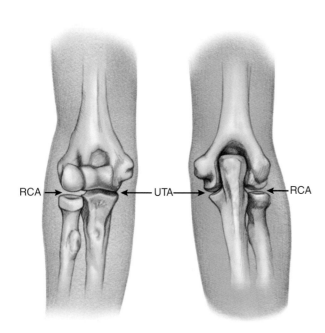

Figure 3-1 ■ Elbow joint—frontal view. RCA = radiocapitellar articulation; UTA = ulnar-trochlear articulation.

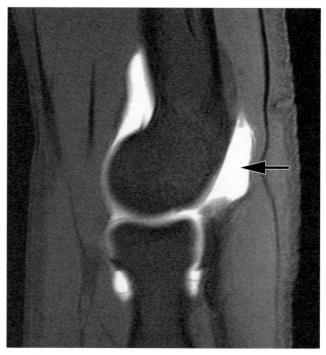

Figure 3-3 ■ The olecranon recess, also known as the posterior recess of the elbow joint *(arrow).* This is seen posterior to the distal humerus and is capacious, allowing marked flexion of the elbow joint.

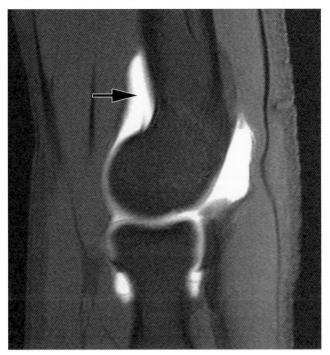

Figure 3-4 ■ Anterior humeral recess is seen anterior to the distal humerus *(arrow)*.

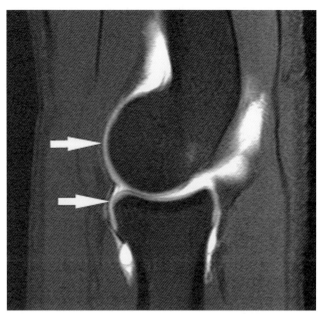

Figure 3-6 ■ Articular hyaline cartilage overlies the articular surfaces of the distal humerus and the proximal radius and ulna *(arrows)*.

ulnar collateral ligament and radial collateral ligament, respectively.[10]

Articular hyaline cartilage overlies the articular surfaces of the distal humerus and the proximal radius and ulna (Fig. 3-6).[9,10] The cartilage is fairly uniform in thickness and covers all of the articular surfaces apart from two small focal defects, which should not be misinterpreted as pathologic defects.[9] A normal cleft can be seen at the junction of the capitellum and the lateral epicondyle, which is referred to as the pseudodefect of the capitellum (Fig. 3-7).[11] Another

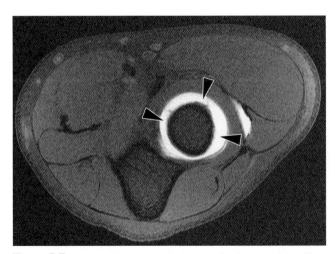

Figure 3-5 ■ The annular recess is the most distal recess of the elbow joint and surrounds the radial neck *(arrowheads)*.

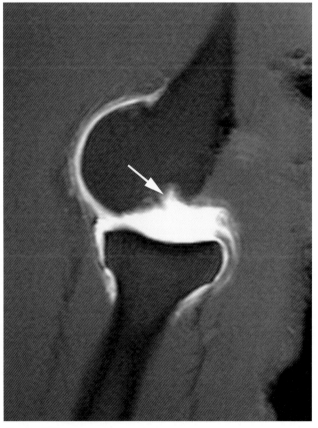

Figure 3-7 ■ Pseudodefect of the capitellum. Sagittal image from an MR arthrogram of the elbow depicting a small irregular cleft *(arrow)* seen at the junction of the posterior margin of the capitellum and the posterior aspect of the lateral epicondyle. This is a normal variation and should not be confused for pathology.

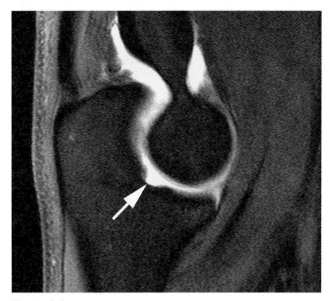

Figure 3-8 ■ Trochlear notch of the ulna. Sagittal image from an MR arthrogram of the elbow depicts a small transverse groove *(arrow)* seen at the junction of the coronoid and olecranon process, which is a normal developmental variation in anatomy.

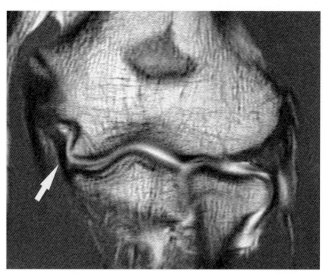

Figure 3-10 ■ Ulnar collateral ligament. The ulnar collateral ligament is composed of three distinct bands, the anterior band, the posterior band, and the transverse ligament. The anterior band is the dominant component and provides the most valgus stability *(arrow)*.

small transverse groove can be seen at the junction of the coronoid and olecranon processes and is referred to as the trochlear notch (Fig. 3-8).[9,12]

Additional stability of the elbow is provided by three prominent ligamentous complexes, the radial collateral ligament, the ulnar collateral ligament, and the annular ligament.[9] The ulnar collateral ligament is stronger than the radial collateral ligament and provides resistance to valgus stress.[8,10] The ulnar collateral ligament is composed of three

distinct bands: the anterior band, the posterior band, and the transverse ligament (Fig. 3-9).[9,13] The anterior band is the dominant component and provides the most valgus stability (Fig. 3-10).[14] The radial collateral ligament provides resistance to varus stress and is composed of four individual ligaments (Fig. 3-11), the radial collateral ligament proper, the accessory lateral collateral ligament, the lateral ulnar collateral ligament, and portions of the annular ligament (Fig. 3-12).[10] Disruption of the radial collateral ligament

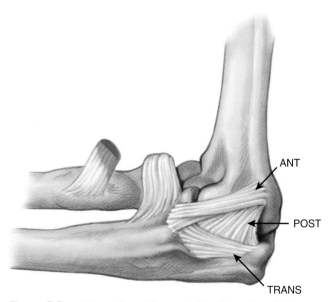

Figure 3-9 ■ Ulnar collateral ligaments. The ulnar collateral ligament is composed of three distinct bands, the anterior band (ANT), the posterior band (POST), and the transverse ligament (TRANS). The anterior band is the dominant component and provides the most valgus stability.

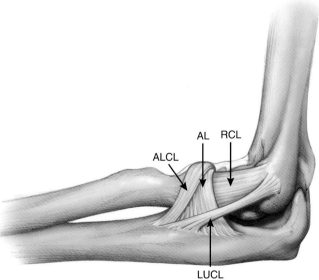

Figure 3-11 ■ Radial collateral ligaments. The radial collateral ligament is composed of four individual ligaments, the radial collateral ligament proper (RCL), the accessory lateral collateral ligament (ALCL), the lateral ulnar collateral ligament (LUCL), and portions of the annular ligament (AL).

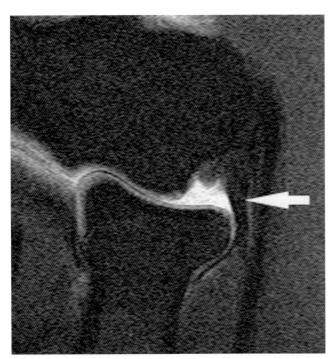

Figure 3-12 ■ Radial collateral ligament. The radial collateral ligament *(arrow)* provides resistance to varus stress and is composed of four individual ligaments, the radial collateral ligament proper, the accessory lateral collateral ligament, the lateral ulnar collateral ligament, and portions of the annular ligament.

complex can result in posterolateral rotatory instability of the elbow.[15] The annular ligament encircles the neck of the proximal radius and attaches to the anterior and posterior aspect of the radial notch of the ulna (Fig. 3-13).[9,10] The annular ligament is the primary stabilizer of the proximal radioulnar articulation.[9,10]

PATIENT SELECTION

Elbow injections and arthrography can be utilized to evaluate patients with elbow pain or dysfunction.[5] Elbow arthrography can precisely outline the articular cartilage and synovial margins of the elbow joint.[9,16] This can be helpful in patients with synovial proliferative processes or other synovial pathology such as synovial cysts.[2] Synovial proliferative disorders such as pigmented villonodular synovitis and synovial osteochondromatosis can be well delineated by elbow arthrography as filling defects in the opacified joint cavity (Fig. 3-14).[2,5] Intra-articular loose bodies can be demonstrated and their exact location confirmed with elbow arthrography (Fig. 3-15).[9] Capsular and ligamentous integrity of the elbow can be evaluated with elbow arthrography.[8,15] Joint aspiration can be performed in patients with joint effusions to evaluate for infection or crystal deposition disease.[1]

CT or MR examinations following arthrography add greatly to the value of elbow arthrography. Cross-sectional imaging following arthrography has the additional benefit over conventional arthrography of multiplanar imaging, which alleviates the difficulty of overlapping structures encountered with fluoroscopic evaluation alone. CT and MR arthrography can precisely depict the articular cartilage of the elbow joint and can aid in the evaluation of areas of abnormal articular cartilage wear or focal articular cartilaginous defects or tears (Fig. 3-16).[9,16] Osteochondral defects can be more precisely visualized with CT or MR elbow arthrography.[9,16] MR arthrography is useful for evaluation of full-thickness and articular surface partial-thickness tears of the ligamentous structures of the elbow, typically involving either the radial or ulnar collateral ligaments (Fig. 3-17).[8,15] MR arthrography combines the benefits of direct visualization of the ligament itself and arthrography can show the extravasation of contrast material from the joint cavity related to ligamentous disruption.[8,9,15]

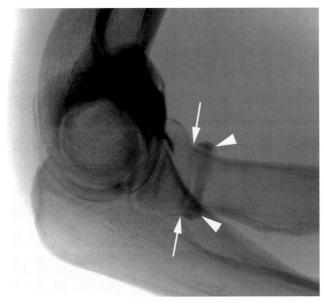

Figure 3-13 ■ Annular ligament. The annular ligament encircles the radial head and is the primary stabilizer of the proximal radioulnar articulation. Here we see the impression of the elbow joint by the annular ligament *(arrows)* forming the annular recess *(arrowheads)*.

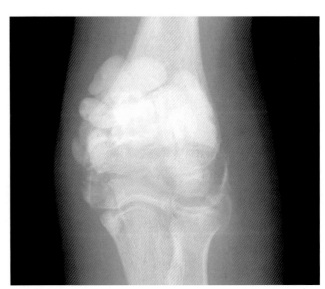

Figure 3-14 ■ Diffuse synovitis seen with conventional elbow arthrography. Young patient with severe synovitis involving the elbow articulation demonstrated by frond-like septations, nodular filling defects, and irregularity of the margins of the elbow joint.

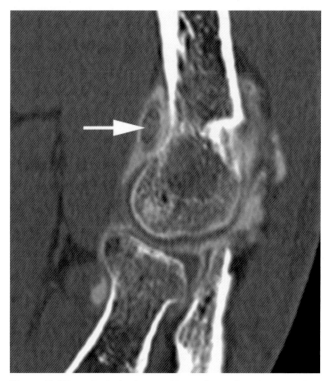

Figure 3-15 ■ Sagittal reformatted image from a CT arthrogram of the elbow depicts a loose body *(arrow)* within the anterior recess of the elbow joint surrounded by intra-articular contrast material.

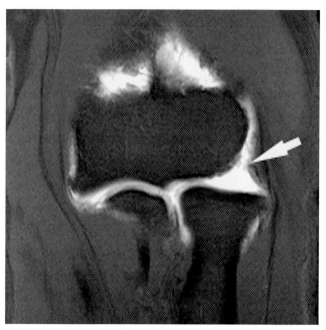

Figure 3-17 ■ Radial collateral ligament disruption. Coronal image from an MR arthrogram depicts disruption of the radial collateral ligament at its humeral attachment with associated widening of the radiocapitellar joint space *(arrow).*

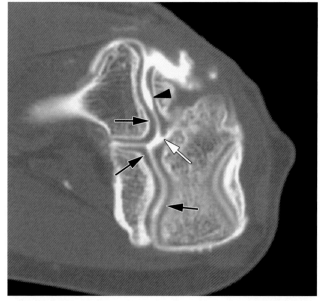

Figure 3-16 ■ Osseous and cartilaginous defects depicted with CT arthrography. Young patient with remote capitellar fracture. Axial image from a CT arthrogram depicts normal cartilage *(black arrows)* seen throughout the ulnar-trochlear articulation and radial head. Persistent osteocartilaginous defect seen at the old fracture site *(white arrow).* Thinning of the articular cartilage of the capitellum related to abnormal wear *(black arrowhead).*

CONTRAINDICATIONS[17]

- Coagulopathy (International Normalized Ratio [INR] >1.5 or platelets < 50,000/mm^3)
- Pregnancy (because of teratogenic effects of radiation)
- Systemic infection or skin infection over the puncture site
- Severe allergy to any component of the injectate
- The patient has received the maximum amount of steroid including systemic steroids allowed for a given time period unless the injection is to be performed without steroid

PROCEDURE

Equipment/Supplies

Procedural

- Spinal needle, 22-gauge, 3.5-inch (Quincke-type point, Becton Dickinson, Franklin Lakes, NJ)
- Luer-Lock (10-mL) syringe containing injection mixture
- Sterile tubing to connect injection solution to spinal needle
- Control 12-mL syringe with 25-gauge, 1.5-inch needle containing 8 mL 1% lidocaine for local anesthesia and 2 mL 8.4% sodium bicarbonate injectable (1 mEq/mL) to alleviate burning pain associated with anesthetic

- Sterile 4 × 4 gauze pads
- Povidone-iodine (Betadine) and alcohol for preparation
- Four sterile towels for draping
- Needle, 18-gauge, 1.5-inch, to draw up lidocaine and medication
- Surgical hat, mask, sterile gloves
- Adhesive bandages

Imaging

- Lead apron
- Multidirectional C-arm fluoroscopy with film archiving capability

Medications (Injection Mixtures)

Volume

The typical elbow joint volume is approximately 8 to 12 mL.[5,9] A 20-mL syringe is used for elbow joint injections. For conventional arthrography the joint should be maximally distended to allow contrast material to extend into small rents or tears, which may not fill if the joint is not adequately distended.[5] With conventional arthrography the joint should be injected until resistance is met because of fullness of the joint or the patient experiences discomfort related to fullness of the joint.[5] For CT or MR arthrography, less distention is necessary than for conventional arthrography. Overdistention of the articulation leads to leakage from the joint puncture site and possible capsular rupture prior to imaging, which markedly hinders image quality with both MR and CT.

Conventional Arthrography: Single Contrast

DIAGNOSTIC OR THERAPEUTIC

(8 to 12 mL total injected joint volume)
    20-mL syringe
    8 mL iodinated contrast (Reno-60, Omnipaque 300)
    8 to 10 mL anesthetic agent (bupivacaine hydrochloride 0.5%, lidocaine hydrochloride 1% MPF*)
    Optional: 0 to 2 mL steroid (Solu-Medrol, Kenalog, Celestone)

Conventional Arthrography: Double Contrast

(8 to 12 mL total injected joint volume)
    10- or 20-mL syringe
    4 mL iodinated contrast (Reno-60, Omnipaque 300)
    Optional: 0 to 2 mL anesthetic agent (bupivacaine 0.5%, lidocaine 1%)
    4 to 8 mL room air

CT Arthrography: Single Contrast

(6 to 10 mL total injected joint volume)
    20-mL syringe
    10 mL iodinated contrast (Reno-60, Omnipaque 300)

8 to 10 mL anesthetic agent (bupivacaine 0.5%, lidocaine 1%)
Optional: 0 to 2 mL steroid (Solu-Medrol, Kenalog, Celestone)

CT Arthrography: Double Contrast

(6 to 10 mL total injected joint volume)
    10- or 20-mL syringe
    4 mL iodinated contrast (Reno-60, Omnipaque 300)
    Optional: 0 to 2 mL anesthetic agent (bupivacaine 0.5%, lidocaine 1%)
    4 to 8 mL room air

MR Arthrography

(6 to 10 mL total injected joint volume)
    20-mL syringe
    4 to 6 mL iodinated contrast (Reno-60, Omnipaque 300)
    10 mL anesthetic agent (bupivacaine 0.5%, lidocaine 1%)
    0.1 mL gadolinium (Omniscan, Magnevist)

Methodology

Elbow Joint Injection

Before performing an elbow interventional procedure, routine radiographic images of the elbow are obtained and reviewed.[5] These should include anteroposterior (AP) views and lateral views (Fig. 3-18). The procedure should be explained to the patient and informed consent should be obtained.[5] The patient should be questioned regarding any preexisting drug allergies.[5] The patient can be positioned in either of two positions depending on the patient's physical condition and degree of comfort.[9] The patient can be placed on the fluoroscopy table in the prone position with the arm over the head (Fig. 3-19) or can be seated beside the fluoroscopy table with the arm abducted 90 degrees placed flat on the table (Fig. 3-20).[9] In either position, the elbow is flexed 90 degrees with the lateral elbow exposed upward. Under fluoroscopic monitoring, the patient should be positioned so that the radiocapitellar joint is parallel to the beam to facilitate entry into the elbow joint (Fig. 3-21). The fluoroscopic image should be collimated to minimize radiation exposure to the surrounding tissues.[5] A metallic object such as a Kelly clamp should be utilized to identify the precise location of the injection, and the patient's skin should be marked with an indelible marker (Fig. 3-22). The target site for elbow joint injection is the radiocapitellar articulation, the cavity between the capitellum and the proximal aspect of the radial head (Figs. 3-23 and 3-24).[5,9] Alternatively, a posterior puncture between the medial and lateral epicondyles just proximal to the olecranon can be utilized to enter the joint, although this is not recommended because the needle is not optimally seen along its axis and is therefore more difficult to control precisely (Fig. 3-25).[7] The field overlying the target should then be sterilely prepared and draped.

    The solution to be injected into the articulation should then be drawn up into a 10- or 20-mL syringe. Choice of agents to be included in the solution depends on the examination to be performed. Examples of solutions are listed in the medications section of the chapter. Flexible tubing

---

*Local anesthetics should be from single-use vials and be free of paraben (MPF) and phenol to prevent flocculation of the steroid.[18]

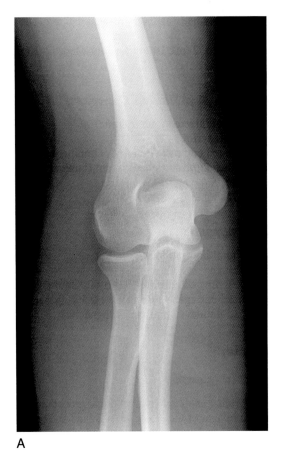

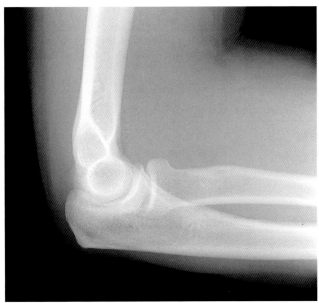

B

Figure 3-18 ■ AP and lateral radiographs of the elbow. Radiographs should be reviewed prior to performance of arthrography to evaluate for fractures, hardware, or other changes that may affect the performance of arthrography or positioning of the patient during the procedure.

A

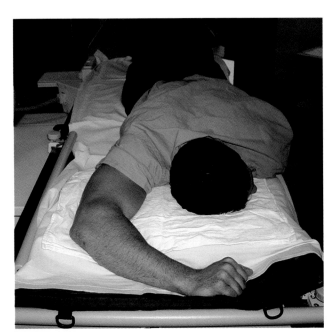

Figure 3-19 ■ Patient positioning. Placement of the patient on the fluoroscopy table in the prone position with the arm over the head. The elbow should be flexed 90 degrees with the lateral elbow exposed upward.

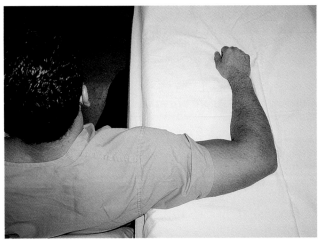

Figure 3-20 ■ Patient positioning. Patient is seated beside the fluoroscopy table with the arm abducted 90 degrees placed flat on the table. The elbow should be flexed 90 degrees with the lateral elbow exposed upward.

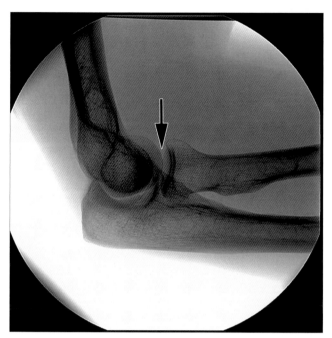

Figure 3-21 ■ Patient positioning. Under fluoroscopic monitoring, the patient should be positioned so that the radiocapitellar joint *(arrow)* is parallel to the fluoroscopic beam to facilitate needle entry into the elbow joint.

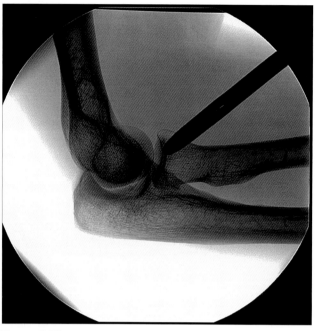

Figure 3-23 ■ The target site for elbow joint injection is the radiocapitellar articulation. The cavity between the capitellum and the proximal aspect of the radial head should be seen in profile and targeted.

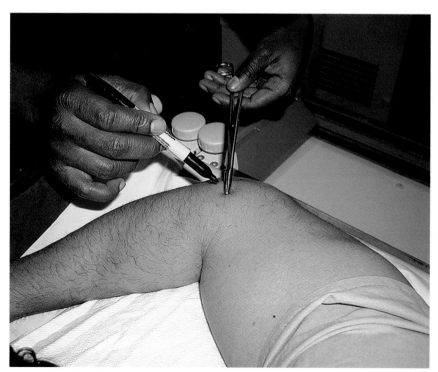

Figure 3-22 ■ A metallic object such as a Kelly clamp should be utilized to identify the precise location of the injection site, and the patient's overlying skin should be marked with an indelible marker.

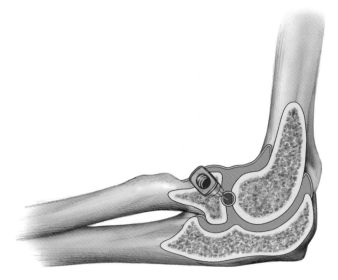

Figure 3-24 ■ Elbow joint injection—lateral approach. The target site for elbow joint injection is the radiocapitellar articulation, the cavity between the capitellum and the proximal aspect of the radial head.

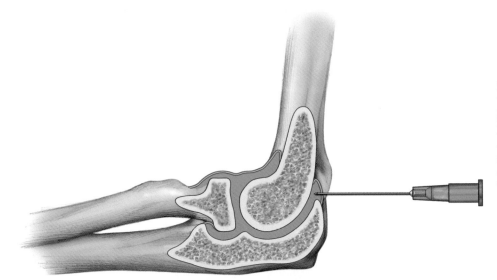

Figure 3-25 ■ Elbow joint injection—posterior approach. A posterior puncture site between the medial and lateral epicondyles just proximal to the olecranon can be utilized to enter the elbow joint, although this is not recommended as the needle is not seen along its axis and is therefore more difficult to control precisely.

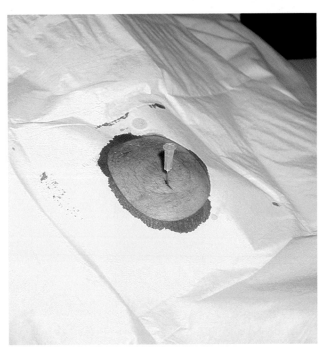

Figure 3-26 ■ The 0.5-inch or 1.5-inch, 25-gauge needle used to anesthetize the skin can be left at the puncture site and disconnected from the syringe to gauge the position of the planned puncture site relative to the target site.

should then be placed on the syringe and the solution should be advanced through the tubing to the tip. Any air bubbles should be expelled from the syringe and tubing. Local anesthesia of the skin and underlying subcutaneous tissue is obtained with 1% lidocaine with 8.4% sodium bicarbonate buffer. A 0.5-inch or 1.5-inch, 25-gauge needle can be used to anesthetize the skin and can be left at the puncture site and disconnected from the syringe (Fig. 3-26). This can be used to gauge the position of the planned puncture site relative to the target site. The needle should be vertically oriented, as seen end on, located directly over the radiocapitellar articulation. If this is not the case, a more appropriate puncture site should be chosen. This may require additional local anesthesia.

If the planned puncture site is concordant with the target site, the 25-gauge needle can be removed and exchanged for either a 25-gauge, 1.5-inch needle or a 22-gauge, 3.5-inch spinal needle. The needle is then advanced through the soft tissues overlying the elbow joint into the radiocapitellar joint. Fluoroscopy is used to verify the needle position (Fig. 3-27). If necessary, alterations in needle position can be made to ensure proper needle position. The target site between the radial head and capitellum can often be felt by the resistance of the bony structures to movement of the needle. Often the needle engages the articulation and allows further needle advancement, but this should be minimal and performed with care as damage to the articular cartilage can result from overaggressive insertion and manipulation of the needle within the radiocapitellar joint.

When the needle has been properly positioned, the syringe and tubing containing the solution to be injected into the elbow joint are connected to the indwelling needle. A small test injection should be performed to ensure appropriate intra-articular placement of the needle (Fig. 3-28). If resistance to injection is met, the needle may be embedded in

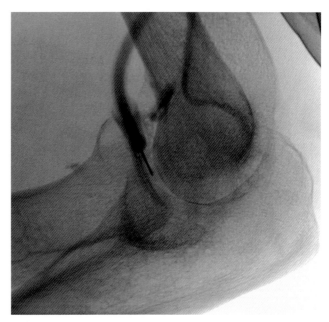

Figure 3-28 ■ A small test injection should be performed to ensure appropriate intra-articular placement of the needle. If contrast material collects at the needle tip, the needle is extra-articular and must be repositioned. If contrast *(arrow)* flows freely away from the needle tip as shown in this image, the injection solution can be instilled.

articular cartilage and the needle should be withdrawn slightly. If contrast material collects at the needle tip, the needle is extra-articular and must be repositioned. If contrast flows freely away from the needle tip, the injection solution can be instilled. The entire injection should be performed under continuous fluoroscopic monitoring (Fig. 3-29) because occasionally the needle withdraws and becomes extra-

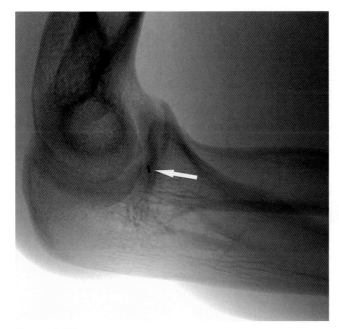

Figure 3-27 ■ The needle *(arrow)* can be advanced through the soft tissues overlying the elbow joint into the radiocapitellar articulation. Fluoroscopy is then utilized to check the needle position.

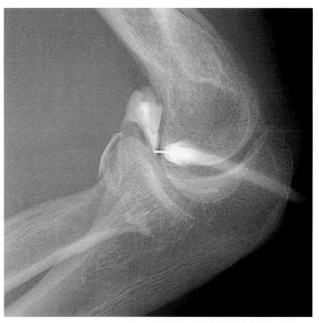

Figure 3-29 ■ The elbow joint injection should be performed under continuous fluoroscopic monitoring to ensure that the needle tip remains intra-articular throughout the entire injection.

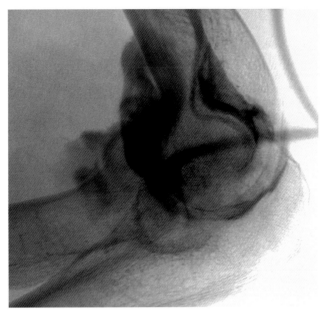

Figure 3-30 ■ With conventional arthrography, the joint should be injected until resistance is met when the joint is fully distended or the patient experiences discomfort related to fullness of the joint. This typically occurs when approximately 10 mL is injected for a normal-size patient.

articular during the injection. This is not problematic if detected early because the needle is then easily repositioned before a significant amount of contrast agent is injected into the extra-articular tissues.

The volume of the injection depends upon the indication for the injection. For evaluation of capsular or ligamentous integrity with conventional arthrography, the joint should be maximally distended to allow contrast material to extend into small rents or tears in the capsule or ligamentous structures, which may not fill if the joint is not adequately distended by the contrast agent. With conventional arthrography, the joint should be injected until resistance is felt or the patient experiences discomfort related to distention of the joint. This typically occurs when approximately 10 to 12 mL is injected into the joint for a normal-size patient (Fig. 3-30).[5,9] For CT or MR arthrography, less distention is necessary than for conventional arthrography. Overdistention of the joint leads to leakage from the puncture site along the needle or possible capsular rupture prior to imaging, which markedly hinders image quality with MR and CT. A volume of 6 to 10 mL is adequate to distend but not overdistend the elbow articulation in most patients.

Following the injection, the needle is withdrawn. For CT and MR arthrography, manipulation of the joint should be kept to a minimum to avoid extravasations from the joint prior to imaging. For conventional arthrography, vigorous exercise of the elbow should be performed followed by additional fluoroscopic evaluation.

Elbow Aspiration

Elbow joint aspiration is very similar to elbow joint injection; however, when the needle is in place a 60-mL syringe and tubing are connected to the needle and aspiration of the joint is performed. If no fluid is withdrawn, the needle is repositioned within the joint. If still no fluid can be aspirated, nonbacteriostatic saline is injected into the joint and reaspirated. Nonbacteriostatic saline is drawn up into a separate 10-mL syringe and tubing, and 10 mL is inserted into the joint through the indwelling needle. The syringe tubing is then exchanged for the 60-mL syringe and tubing and the nonbacteriostatic saline is reaspirated (Fig. 3-31). The aspirated fluid or nonbacteriostatic saline wash is then

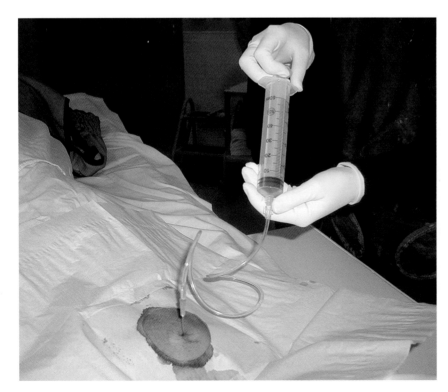

Figure 3-31 ■ Elbow joint aspiration. The technique is very similar to elbow joint injection. When the needle is in place, a 60-mL syringe and tubing are connected to the needle and aspiration of the joint is performed.

sent for aerobic and anaerobic culture. If enough fluid is present, Gram stain and additional analysis of the fluid can be performed depending upon the specific clinical situation.

POTENTIAL COMPLICATIONS

- Bleeding
- Infection (cellulitis, septic arthritis, or osteomyelitis)
- Drug-related allergic reactions
- Transient synovitis
- Transitory upper extremity weakness
- Transitory upper extremity paresthesia

POST-PROCEDURE CARE/FOLLOW-UP[17]

Immediate

1. The patient should be observed for 15 minutes after the injection.
2. Blood pressure, pulse, heart rate, and respiratory rate are monitored as necessary.

Discharge

1. An adhesive bandage may be placed on the puncture site. The bandage should remain dry for at least 24 hours, at which point it can be removed.
2. The patient is instructed to continue taking his or her prescription medication, although pain medication may be tapered as indicated.
3. A discharge sheet should be given to the patient outlining the following:
   a. Which procedure was performed
   b. Procedurally related symptoms that typically resolve in 7 to 10 days
      - Pain at the needle puncture site(s)
      - Mild increase in elbow stiffness with a feeling of fullness in the joint
      - Deep elbow pain
   c. Treatment for mild post-procedure symptoms
      - Rest the elbow for 1 to 2 days
      - Avoid movements that worsen the pain
      - Use cold compresses to the area that hurts
   d. Signs and symptoms of infection
      - Fever
      - Chills
      - Swelling or drainage from the puncture site(s)
      - New elbow pain that is different from the usual pain
   e. Signs and symptoms of possible more serious problems
      - Decreased range of motion of the elbow
      - Increasing pain
      - Motor dysfunction of the upper extremity
   f. Physician name and contact number if the patient has any concerns or if any problems were to arise as a result of the procedure
   g. Advice to schedule a follow-up appointment with the referring physician in 7 to 10 days.

SAMPLE DICTATIONS

After the procedure was explained to the patient and informed consent was obtained, the patient was placed on the table in the prone position. Preliminary fluoroscopic evaluation of the elbow was performed. The skin overlying the radiocapitellar articulation was sterilely prepared and draped in the usual fashion. Local anesthesia was obtained with 1% lidocaine with bicarbonate buffer. Under fluoroscopic guidance, a 25-gauge needle was advanced into the elbow articulation and an 8-mL solution containing iodinated contrast material, bupivacaine, and gadolinium was administered into the elbow articulation. The needle was withdrawn. Post-injection fluoroscopic evaluation was performed and appropriate spot films were obtained. The patient was sent to MR for additional imaging of the elbow after arthrography.

CASE REPORTS

CASE 1

Clinical Presentation

A 58-year-old male patient presented with a long history of osteoarthritis involving the left elbow joint. The patient had more recent complaints of occasional "catching" of the elbow joint with changes in position and an occasional "grinding" sensation. Physical examination demonstrated mild tenderness about the elbow with normal range of motion.

Imaging and Therapy

Conventional radiographs depicted osteoarthritis about the elbow joint with a small ossified focus anterior to the distal humerus in the region of the anterior recess of the elbow joint. CT arthrography of the elbow was requested to confirm this to be a loose body and not simply a focus of capsular calcification or heterotopic ossification. The elbow joint was entered with a 22-gauge needle by a lateral approach. A volume of 8 mL of a solution containing Omnipaque 300 and 0.5% bupivacaine was injected (Fig. 3-32). CT of the elbow was then obtained immediately following the injection, confirming the presence of a loose body within the anterior recess of the elbow joint (Fig. 3-33). Contrast material completely surrounded the ossified focus, confirming an intra-articular location. Elbow arthroscopy was performed with removal of an 8-mm loose body from the anterior recess. The patient reported complete resolution of the previously described symptoms following the arthroscopic removal of the loose body.

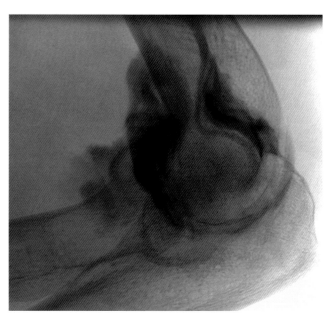

Figure 3-32 ■ Elbow joint injection. Typical radiographic appearance following elbow joint injection for CT arthrography.

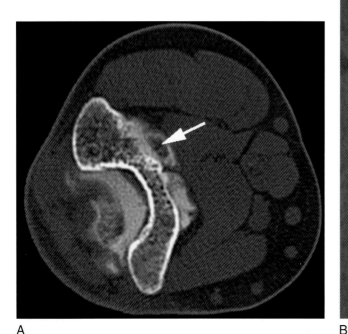

A

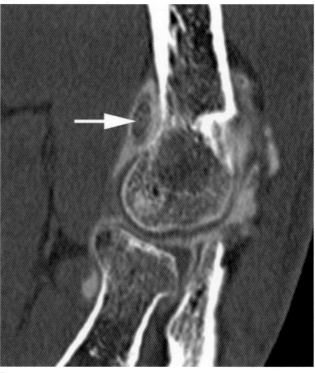

B

Figure 3-33 ■ Axial and coronal images from a CT arthrogram of the elbow depicting a small loose body. *A,* Axial image depicting a small ossified body *(arrow)* in the anterior recess of the elbow joint. *B,* Coronal image demonstrating contrast surrounding the ossification *(arrow)* confirming intra-articular position of the loose body.

CASE 2

Clinical Presentation

A 38-year-old patient presented with lateral instability of the elbow joint. The patient previously suffered from flexion contracture of the lateral elbow with prior surgical release. The patient presented to an outside institution for evaluation, and after failure of conservative methods, operative treatment was performed with surgical release of the lateral elbow joint capsule and release of the extensor tendon complex. Following the surgery, the patient developed marked lateral instability and subsequently presented to our institution for a second opinion. Physical examination confirmed significant instability of the lateral elbow, and it was suggested that the radial collateral ligament was severed in addition to release of the lateral extensor tendons.

Imaging and Therapy

MR arthrography of the elbow was performed. A 22-gauge needle was advanced under fluoroscopic guidance into the radiocapitellar articulation and a 6-mL solution containing Omnipaque 300, 0.5% bupivacaine, and gadodiamide (Omniscan) was injected (Fig. 3-34). MR imaging was then performed, confirming disruption of the radial collateral ligament with abnormal widening of the lateral aspect of the radiocapitellar articulation (Fig. 3-35).

The patient subsequently underwent surgical repair of the severed radial collateral ligament. Following the surgery, the patient was referred for physical therapy and strengthening. Postoperative follow-up evaluation demonstrated no residual instability of the elbow joint with resolution of the previously reported pain and sensation of instability.

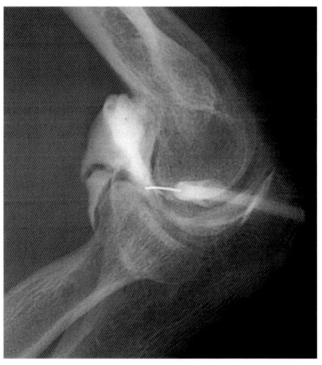

Figure 3-34 ■ Elbow joint injection. Image following elbow joint injection for the purposes of MR arthrography.

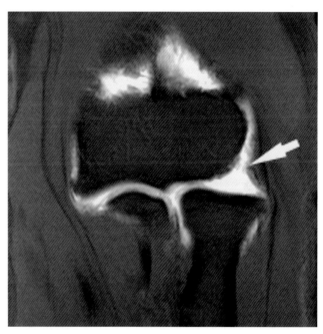

Figure 3-35 ■ Radial collateral ligament disruption. Coronal image from an MR arthrogram of the elbow demonstrates complete disruption of the radial collateral ligament with abnormal widening of the radiocapitellar joint space *(arrow)*.

CURRENT PROCEDURAL TERMINOLOGY (CPT) CODES[19]

CPT codes change often and sometimes are valid only for certain states or regions. It is best to consult with coding experts to make sure that coding for one's procedures is legitimate and complete. Below is a sample of codes that are being used for elbow injection procedures at this writing.

20605 Arthrocentesis, aspiration and/or injection; intermediate joint or bursa (e.g., temporomandibular, acromioclavicular, wrist, elbow or ankle, olecranon bursa)

(If imaging guidance is performed, see 76003, 76360, 76393, 76942)

24220 Injection procedure for elbow arthrography

(For radiologic supervision and interpretation, use 73085. Do not report 76003 in addition to 73085)

73070 Radiologic examination, elbow; two views

73080 complete, minimum of three views

73085 Radiologic examination, elbow, arthrography, radiologic supervision and interpretation

(Do not report 76003 in addition to 73085)

73200 Computed tomography, upper extremity; without contrast material

73201 with contrast material(s)

73202 without contrast material, followed by contrast material(s) and further sections

(To report three-dimensional [3D] rendering, see 76376, 76377)

73221 Magnetic resonance (e.g., proton) imaging, any joint of upper extremity; without contrast material(s)

73222 with contrast material(s)

73223 without contrast material(s), followed by contrast material(s) and further sequences

76003 Fluoroscopic guidance for needle placement (e.g., biopsy, aspiration, injection, localization device)

76360 Computed tomography guidance for needle placement (e.g., biopsy, aspiration, injection, or placement of localization device), radiologic supervision and interpretation

76376 3D rendering with interpretation and reporting of computed tomography, magnetic resonance imaging, ultrasound, or other tomographic modality; not requiring image postprocessing on an independent workstation

76377 requiring image postprocessing on an independent workstation

76393 Magnetic resonance guidance for needle placement (e.g., for biopsy, needle aspiration, injection, localization device), radiologic supervision and interpretation

76942 Ultrasonic guidance for needle placement (e.g., biopsy, aspiration, injection, localization device), imaging supervision and interpretation

References

1. Hodge JC. Musculoskeletal Imaging Diagnostic and Therapeutic Procedures. Montreal: Karger Landes Systems, 1997, pp 25–38.
2. Resnick D. Diagnosis of Bone and Joint Disorders, 4th ed. Philadelphia: WB Saunders, 2002, pp 193–318, 3054–3068.
3. Lindblom K. Arthrography. J Fac Radiol 1952; 3:151–163.
4. Arvidsson H, Johansson O. Arthrography of the elbow-joint. Acta Radiol 1955; 43:445–452.
5. Freiberger RH, Kaye JJ. Arthrography. Norwalk, CT: Appleton Century Crofts, 1979, pp xii, 1–3, 261–276.
6. Quinn SF, Haberman JJ, Fitzgerald SW, et al. Evaluation of loose bodies in the elbow with MR imaging. J Magn Reson Imaging 1994; 4:169–172.
7. Berquist TH. Diagnostic and therapeutic injections as an aid to musculoskeletal diagnosis. Semin Interv Radiol 1993; 10:326–344.
8. Katsuyuki N, Masatomi T, Ochi T, et al H. MR arthrography of elbow: Evaluation of the ulnar collateral ligament of elbow. Skeletal Radiol 1996; 25:629–634.
9. Steinbach LS, Schwartz M. Elbow arthrography. Radiol Clin North Am 1998; 36:635–649.
10. Berquist TH. MRI of the Musculoskeletal System, 5th ed. Philadelphia: Lippincott Williams & Wilkins, 2006, pp 686–772.
11. Rosenberg ZS, Beltran J, Cheung YY. Pseudodefect of the capitellum: Potential MR imaging pitfall. Radiology 1994; 191:821–823.
12. Rosenberg ZS, Beltran J, Cheung Y, Broker M. MR imaging of the elbow: Normal variant and potential diagnostic pitfalls of the trochlear groove and cubital tunnel. AJR Am J Roentgenol 1995; 164:415–418.
13. Munshi M, Pretterklieber ML, Chung CB, et al. Anterior bundle of ulnar collateral ligament: Evaluation of anatomic relationships by using MR imaging, MR arthrography, and gross anatomic and histologic analysis. Radiology 2004; 231:797–803.
14. Schwartz ML, Al-Zahrani S, Morwessel RM, Andrews JR. Ulnar collateral ligament injury in the throwing athlete: Evaluation with saline-enhanced MR arthrography. Radiology 1995; 197:297–299.
15. Carrino JA, Morrison WB, Zou KH, et al. Lateral ulnar collateral ligament of the elbow: Optimization of evaluation with two-dimensional MR imaging. Radiology 2001; 218:118–125.
16. Holland P, Davies AM, Cassar-Pullicino VN. Computed tomographic arthrography in the assessment of osteochondritis dissecans of the elbow. Clin Radiol 1994; 49:231–235.
17. Fenton DS, Czervionke LF. Image-Guided Spine Intervention. Philadelphia: WB Saunders, 2003.
18. Physician's Desk Reference, 60th ed. Montvale, NJ: Medical Economics, 2006.
19. CPT 2007, CPT Intellectual Property Services. Chicago: American Medical Association, 2007.

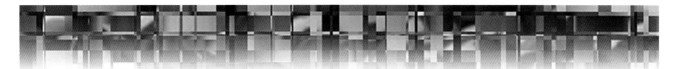

An Elbow Surgeon's Perspective

Elbow Injections

Peter M. Murray, MD

Injections of the elbow joint, in my practice, are more commonly performed for therapeutic benefit than as part of a diagnostic work-up, as conventional MR and CT are often adequate for diagnostic purposes. A notable exception to this would be aspiration for suspected intra-articular infection such as in the case of a loose, painful total elbow replacement. Therapeutic injections can be useful clinically to alleviate elbow joint pain and discomfort and can be helpful to confirm the site of the patient's symptoms. Diagnostic injections for conventional arthrography are not generally useful. However, CT or MR arthrography can be quite useful, particularly in patients with equivocal conventional nonarthrographic CT or MR imaging. These studies aid the surgeon in diagnosing a wide range of elbow internal derangements such as lateral collateral ligament disruptions, medial collateral ligament disruptions, and intra-articular loose bodies. CT or MR arthrography can be beneficial in patients with suspected loose bodies. Often calcifications or mineralization can be seen in or about the elbow joint. CT or MR arthrography can definitively determine whether the calcification is intra-articular, extra-articular, or capsular. MR arthrography can also be advantageous in baseball pitchers with suspected radial collateral ligamentous injuries related to chronic valgus stress. Intra-articular gadolinium allows precise visualization of the anterior band of the radial collateral ligament, providing valuable information to the surgeon.

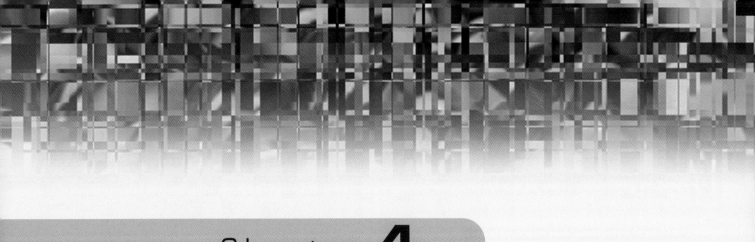

Chapter **4**

Wrist and Hand Injections

- Jeffrey J. Peterson, MD

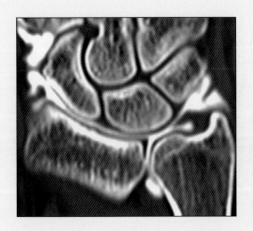

BACKGROUND

Wrist arthrography was introduced in 1961 as a minimally invasive technique for evaluating the integrity of the intercarpal ligaments.[1] For several decades, the examination continued to evolve and increase in utilization. Different techniques developed ranging from single-compartment injections to bilateral triple-compartment wrist arthrograms.[2-4] Today, conventional arthrography continues to be a useful tool for the evaluation of intercarpal ligamentous and triangular fibrocartilage complex (TFCC) pathology.[5]

The introduction of computed tomography (CT) and magnetic resonance (MR) imaging introduced additional alternatives to conventional triple-compartment wrist arthrography for certain indications.[6-8] CT and MR obtained after the performance of wrist arthrography can significantly increase the value of wrist arthrography in many instances.[8-10] CT and MR arthrography can reveal subtle pathology involving the intercarpal ligaments and precisely depict the articular cartilage about the various wrist compartments.[9-11] There still remains much controversy about which approach and technique is more accurate and appropriate for wrist arthrography. The goal of this chapter is to describe and delineate all of the common variations of wrist arthrography. The decision about the approach and technique utilized should be made by the reader, determined by the clinical presentation and the personal preference of the proceduralist and the referring clinician.

The other major focus of the chapter is on diagnostic and therapeutic injections of the small joints of the hand and wrist. Therapeutic injections can be utilized to treat a variety of painful conditions involving the hand and wrist and to identify and more precisely localize sites of symptoms.[12] Diagnostic injections can also be helpful for evaluation of the small joints of the hand and wrist, although these are less commonly performed as MR can often be used to evaluate for pathology in these joints in a noninvasive manner.

ANATOMIC CONSIDERATIONS

The anatomy of the wrist is quite complex; it is composed of a series of compartments and articulations rather than a single compartment as found in many other joints.[13] The wrist compartments include the radiocarpal compartment, the midcarpal compartment, the distal radioulnar joint, the common carpometacarpal compartment, the first carpometacarpal compartment, and the pisiform-triquetral joint.[13]

Although any of the joint compartments of the wrist can be injected, the three compartments that are most commonly injected are (1) the radiocarpal joint, (2) the distal radiocarpal compartment, and (3) the midcarpal compartment (Fig. 4-1). The most important compartment of the wrist is the radiocarpal compartment. The radiocarpal compartment is bounded proximally by the articular surface of the distal radius and the triangular fibrocartilage and distally by the proximal carpal row (Fig. 4-2).[13,14] The triangular fibrocartilage separates the radiocarpal articulation from the smaller, more proximal distal radioulnar articulation, which is bounded by the triangular fibrocartilage complex (TFCC) distally, the radius laterally, and the ulna medially (Fig. 4-3).[13,14] The proximal carpal row and the intervening intraosseous ligaments, the scapholunate and lunotriquetral ligaments, separate the radiocarpal articulation from the midcarpal articulation, which is distal to the radiocarpal articulation (Fig. 4-4).[13,14]

The TFCC acts as a fibrocartilaginous cushion between the distal ulna and the proximal carpal row (Fig. 4-5).[14] The TFCC is composed of several smaller fibrocartilaginous structures including the triangular fibrocartilage, the ulnomeniscal homologue, the ulnar collateral ligament, the dorsal and volar radioulnar ligaments, the ulnocarpal ligaments, and the extensor carpi ulnaris tendon and sheath.[13,15] The TFCC separates the radiocarpal articulation from the distal radioulnar articulation, and communication between the two indicates a tear or perforation of the TFCC (Fig. 4-6).[16–18]

Several ligaments course between the carpal bones and are referred to as the intraosseous ligaments of the wrist.[5,19] The most important intrinsic intraosseous ligaments are the

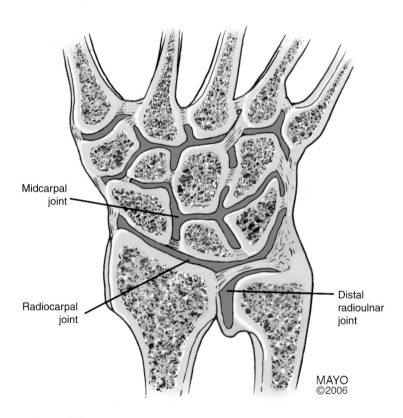

MAYO
©2006

Figure 4-1 ■ The wrist is composed of several joint compartments. The most important articulations for arthrography include the radiocarpal joint, the midcarpal joint, and the distal radioulnar joint.

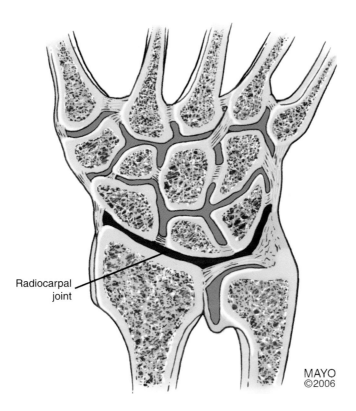

Radiocarpal
joint

MAYO
©2006

Figure 4-2 ■ The most important compartment of the wrist for arthrography is the radiocarpal joint. The radiocarpal articulation is bounded proximally by the articular surface of the distal radius and the triangular fibrocartilage and distally by the proximal carpal row.

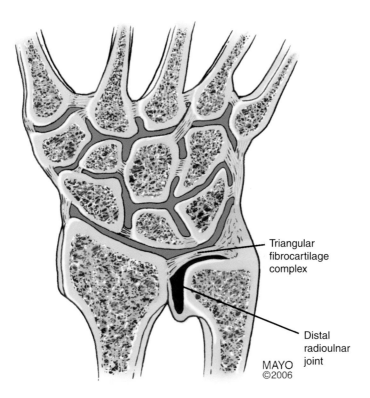

Triangular
fibrocartilage
complex

Distal
radioulnar
joint

MAYO
©2006

Figure 4-3 ■ The distal radioulnar joint is bounded by the triangular fibrocartilage complex distally, the radius laterally and the ulna medially.

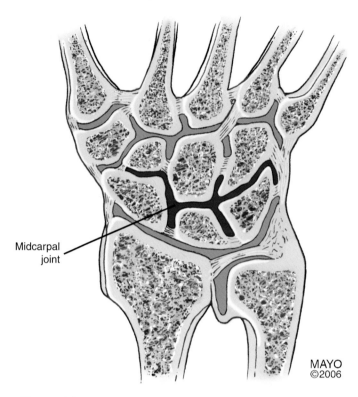

Figure 4-4 ■ The midcarpal articulation is bounded proximally by the proximal carpal row and the intercarpal ligaments. The distal margin of the midcarpal articulation varies but typically terminates at the level of the trapezium, trapezoid, and distal margins of the capitate and hamate. The midcarpal joint can communicate with the adjacent carpometacarpal articulations normally.

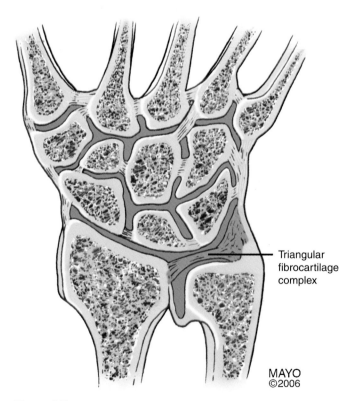

Figure 4-5 ■ The triangular fibrocartilage complex (TFCC) acts as a fibrocartilaginous cushion between the distal ulna and the proximal carpal row. The TFCC separates the radiocarpal articulation from the distal radioulnar articulation.

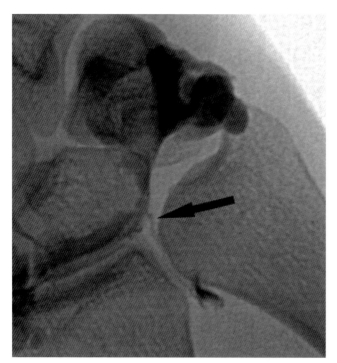

Figure 4-6 ■ The triangular fibrocartilage complex (TFCC) separates the radiocarpal articulation from the distal radioulnar articulation. Communication between the two indicates a tear or perforation of the TFCC *(arrow).*

scapholunate and the lunotriquetral ligaments.[5] These ligaments, along with the osseous structures of the proximal carpal row, effectively separate the radiocarpal articulation from the midcarpal articulation (Fig. 4-7).[15,19] Communication between the radiocarpal and midcarpal articulation is most commonly seen with tearing or perforation of either the scapholunate ligament or the lunotriquetral ligament.[15,17] Several extrinsic ligaments also aid in maintaining stability

about the wrist; they are often referred to as the radiocarpal ligaments and can be subdivided into the palmar and dorsal radiocarpal ligaments.[5,13,20,21]

The anatomy of the small joints of the hand, including the metacarpophalangeal and interphalangeal articulation, is fairly straightforward. The capsule surrounds the joints with strong palmar ligaments along the volar aspect of the joint and collateral ligaments present at each side of the articulation (Fig. 4-8).[19] The extensor tendons overlie the dorsum of the joints, and the larger flexor tendons extend superficial to the palmar aspect of the joints (see Fig. 4-8).[19]

PATIENT SELECTION

There are a number of indications for intra-articular injections about the wrist and hand.[12] Injections for wrist arthrography are most common. Arthrography is commonly performed to evaluate the integrity of the TFCC and the intraosseous ligaments of the wrist (Fig. 4-9).[15,22] Wrist arthrography is technically straightforward, minimally invasive, and provides functional and structural information, which can be difficult to ascertain from routine CT or MR of the wrist. Arthrography can also be used to evaluate or localize suspected loose bodies or demonstrate other synovial abnormalities such as synovitis, synovial cysts, or other synovial proliferative processes (Fig. 4-10).[14] CT or MR arthrography of the wrist can further evaluate the TFCC and intraosseous ligaments with even more precision as multiplanar thin-section images reveal a more detailed depiction of the wrist anatomy compared with conventional arthrography (Fig. 4-11). In addition, CT and MR arthrography can be used to evaluate the integrity of the hyaline articular cartilage of the osseous structures of the wrist.[11,22]

There has been debate over the optimal arthrographic technique to evaluate the wrist. Many have advocated triple-compartment arthrography, as this thoroughly evaluates the

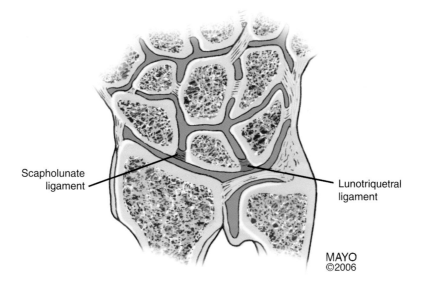

Figure 4-7 ■ The scapholunate ligament extends across the base of the scaphoid and lunate bones. The lunotriquetral ligament extends across the base of the lunate and triquetral bones. The scapholunate and lunotriquetral ligaments, along with the osseous structures of the proximal carpal row, separate the radiocarpal articulation from the midcarpal articulation.

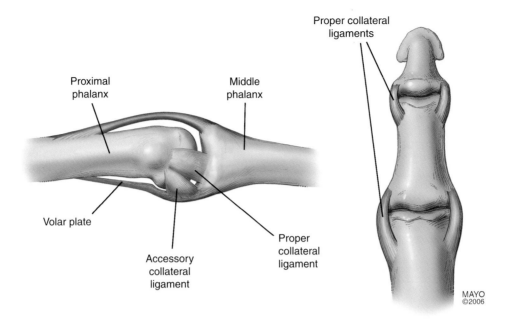

Figure 4-8 ■ The capsule of the first interphalangeal articulation surrounds the joint with the strong volar plate at the palmar aspect of the joint (*left*). The collateral ligaments are present at each side of the interphalangeal articulations (*right*).

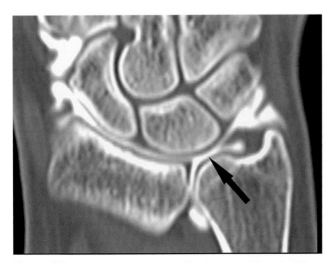

Figure 4-9 ■ Coronal image from a CT arthrogram of the wrist following a radiocarpal injection depicts a large tear of the central portion of the triangular fibrocartilage complex *(arrow)* with contrast spilling into the distal radioulnar articulation.

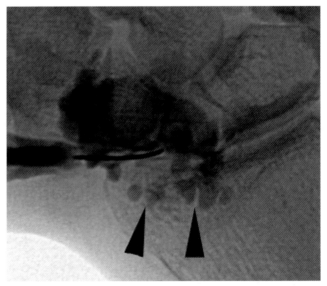

Figure 4-10 ■ Image obtained during a radiocarpal injection depicts irregularity and crenulations *(arrowheads)* of the radial aspect of the radiocarpal articulation compatible with synovitis with synovial proliferation.

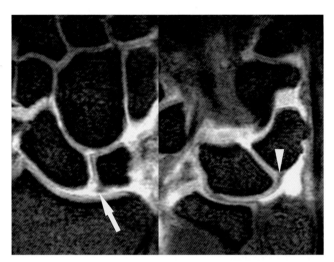

Figure 4-11 ■ Coronal images from an MR arthrogram of the wrist following a radiocarpal injection. The left image depicts complete disruption of the scapholunate ligament with contrast extending through the tear into the midcarpal articulation *(arrow)*. The right image precisely depicts the intact lunotriquetral ligament *(arrowhead)*.

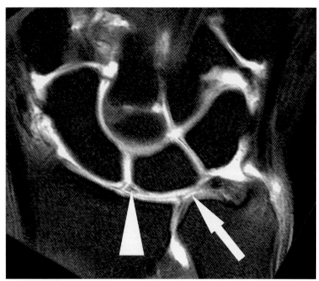

Figure 4-12 ■ Coronal image from an MR arthrogram of the wrist following a radiocarpal injection depicts tears of both the scapholunate ligament *(arrowhead)* and triangular fibrocartilage complex *(arrow)* allowing contrast to extend into the midcarpal and distal radioulnar articulations, respectively.

intraosseous ligaments and TFCC for full-thickness tears as well as partial tears and tears allowing one-way communication.[23] Triple-compartment arthrography can be performed with several techniques.[5] A commonly used approach is to inject the midcarpal and distal radioulnar joint (DRUJ) at one episode, then wait for a period of time, typically 2 to 3 hours, to allow resorption of the contrast material from the joints. After the contrast material within the midcarpal and DRUJ has dissipated, the radiocarpal joint injection is performed. Another method commonly used is digital subtraction imaging during the injection, which permits injection of all three compartments with no intervening waiting period.[24]

Injections of the radiocarpal articulation followed by CT and MR have gained increasing popularity. Radiocarpal injections can demonstrate the majority of defects in the intraosseous ligaments and TFCC, and multiplanar cross-sectional imaging with CT or MR following the injections provides additional delineation of these structures (Fig. 4-12).[25] In addition, CT and MR can provide better definition of cartilaginous defects in the wrist and can facilitate visualization of other pathology such as occult fractures, avascular necrosis, or extrinsic abnormalities such as tendon or ligamentous abnormalities, which cannot be adequately evaluated with conventional wrist arthrography (Fig. 4-13).[11] The technique utilized should be determined by personal preference, preference of the referring clinicians, and practice considerations including available physician and equipment time.[5]

Occasionally, diagnostic injections of the small joints of the hand are performed, but small joint injections are not as commonly performed as wrist arthrography.[12,26] The first metacarpal-phalangeal articulation may be injected to evaluate the integrity of the ulnar collateral ligament (Fig. 4-14).[27] Diagnostic injections of the metacarpal-phalangeal and interphalangeal joint can be performed to evaluate for synovial abnormalities such as synovial cysts or synovial prolifera-

tive processes, although such conditions are most commonly evaluated with conventional MR.[28]

Aspiration of the various wrist compartments and small articulations of the hand can be performed in cases of suspected infection or to obtain joint fluid in cases of suspected crystal deposition disease. The small joints of the hand are not uncommonly involved in septic arthritis. Therapeutic injections of anesthetic and steroid preparations can also be performed selectively in any of the joint compartments of the hand and wrist.[12]

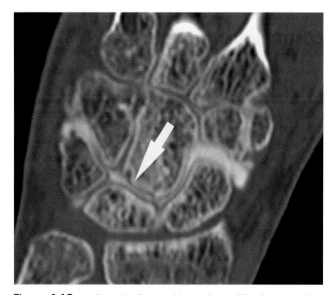

Figure 4-13 ■ Coronal reformatted image from a CT arthrogram of the wrist following a midcarpal injection reveals avascular necrosis of the proximal pole of the capitate with subtle impaction of the proximal articular surface *(arrow)*.

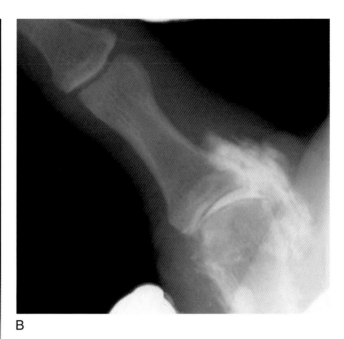

Figure 4-14 ■ Ulnar collateral ligament injury of the first metacarpophalangeal (MCP) joint. *A*, AP image of the thumb following a first MCP joint injection shows extravasation from the ulnar aspect of the MCP joint compatible with disruption of the ulnar collateral ligament. *B*, Stress views with abduction of the thumb reveal abnormal widening of the joint with angulation greater than 30 degrees confirming ulnar collateral ligament tear.

A

CONTRAINDICATIONS[29]

- Coagulopathy (International Normalized Ratio [INR] >1.5 or platelets < 50,000/mm^3)
- Pregnancy (because of the teratogenic effects of radiation)
- Systemic infection or skin infection over the puncture site
- Severe allergy to any component of the injectate
- The patient has received the maximum amount of steroid including systemic steroids allowed for a given time period unless the injection is to be performed without steroid

PROCEDURE

Equipment/Supplies

Procedural

- 25-gauge, 0.5-inch or 1.5-inch needle
- 10-mL Luer-Lock syringe containing injection mixture

- Sterile tubing to connect injection solution to needle
- Control 12-mL syringe with 25-gauge, 1.5-inch needle containing 8 mL 1% lidocaine for local anesthesia and 2 mL 8.4% sodium bicarbonate injectable (1 mEq/mL) to alleviate burning pain associated with anesthetic
- Sterile 4 × 4 gauze pads
- Povidone-iodine (Betadine) and alcohol for preparation
- Sterile towels or fenestrated drapes for sterile draping
- Needle, 18-gauge, 1.5-inch, to draw up lidocaine and medication
- Sterile gloves
- Adhesive bandages

Injection Volume

The typical radiocarpal and midcarpal joint volume is approximately 3 to 5 mL. The DRUJ and other smaller joints about the hand and wrist have a volume of approximately 1 mL. A 10-mL syringe is utilized for hand and wrist injections. A 20-mL syringe can be used if multiple injections are planned. For conventional arthrography, the joint should be maximally distended to allow contrast material to extend into small rents or tears, which may not fill if the joint is not adequately distended. With conventional arthrography the joint should be injected until resistance is met because of fullness of the joint or the patient experiences discomfort related to fullness of the joint. For CT or MR arthrography, less joint distention is necessary than for conventional arthrography. Overdistention of the articulation leads to leakage from the joint puncture site and possible capsular rupture prior to imaging, which markedly hinders image quality with both MR and CT.

Radiocarpal Compartment Injection

CONVENTIONAL ARTHROGRAPHY

DIAGNOSTIC OR THERAPEUTIC
(3 to 5 mL total joint injected volume)
  10-mL syringe
  5 mL iodinated contrast (Reno-60, Omnipaque 300)
  4 to 5 mL anesthetic agent (bupivacaine hydrochloride 0.5%, lidocaine hydrochloride 1% MPF*)
  Optional: 0 to 1 mL steroid methylprednisolone sodium succinate (Solu-Medrol 40 mg/mL, Depo-Medrol 40 mg/mL), triamcinolone (Kenalog-40), betamethasone sodium phosphate and betamethasone acetate (Celestone Soluspan 6 mg/mL)

CT ARTHROGRAPHY

(3 to 5 mL total injected joint volume)
  10-mL syringe
  5 mL iodinated contrast (Reno-60, Omnipaque 300)
  4 to 5 mL anesthetic agent (bupivacaine 0.5%, lidocaine 1% MPF*)
  Optional: 0 to 1 mL steroid (Solu-Medrol, Kenalog, Celestone)

MR ARTHROGRAPHY

(3 to 5 mL total injected joint volume)
  10-mL syringe
  4 to 5 mL iodinated contrast (Reno-60, Omnipaque 300)
  5 mL anesthetic agent (bupivacaine hydrochloride 0.5%*, lidocaine hydrochloride 1% MPF*)
  0.1 to 0.2 mL gadopentetate dimeglumine MR contrast (Omniscan, Magnevist)

Midcarpal Compartment Injection

Common Carpometacarpal Compartment Injection

DIAGNOSTIC OR THERAPEUTIC
(3 to 5 mL total injected joint volume)
  10-mL syringe
  5 mL iodinated contrast (Reno-60, Omnipaque 300)
  4 to 5 mL anesthetic agent (bupivacaine hydrochloride 0.5%, lidocaine hydrochloride 1% MPF*)
  Optional: 0 to 1 mL steroid (Solu-Medrol, Kenalog, Celestone)

---

*Local anesthetics should be from single-use vials and be free of paraben (MPF) and phenol to prevent flocculation of the steroid.[30]

Distal Radioulnar Articulation Injection

Pisiform Triquetral Articulation Injection

First Carpometacarpal Articulation Injection

Metacarpal-Phalangeal Articulation Injection

Interphalangeal Articulation Injection

(1 mL total injected joint volume)
  10-mL syringe
  5 mL iodinated contrast (Reno-60, Omnipaque 300)
  4 to 5 mL anesthetic agent (bupivacaine hydrochloride 0.5%, lidocaine hydrochloride 1% MPF*)
  Optional: 0 to 1 mL steroid (Solu-Medrol, Kenalog, or Celestone)

Methodology

Radiocarpal Joint Injection

Routine radiographic images of the wrist are obtained and reviewed prior to wrist interventions. A four-view examination of the wrist is suggested including the posteroanterior, lateral, and oblique lateral projections in semisupination and semipronation. The procedure should be explained to the patient, and informed consent should be obtained. A directed history of the presenting complaint and symptoms should be ascertained. Questioning the patient and physical examination should be performed to identify the site or sites of symptoms. The patient should be questioned regarding any preexisting drug allergies. The patient is then placed on the fluoroscopy table. The patient can be placed on the table in the prone position with the wrist above the head (Fig. 4-15) or can be sat next to the table with the arm abducted and the elbow flexed to allow placement of the wrist flat on the table with the palm down (Fig. 4-16). Preliminary fluoroscopic

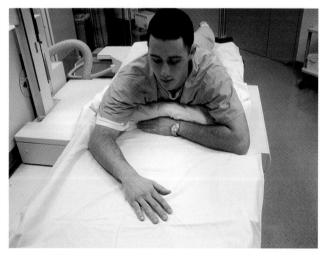

Figure 4-15 ■ For wrist arthrography the patient can be placed on the fluoroscopy table in the prone position with the wrist above the head and the palm down. This position allows mobility about the table for the physician but can be uncomfortable for certain patients.

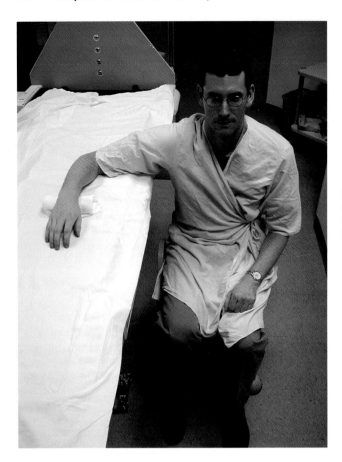

Figure 4-16 ■ For wrist injections the patient can alternatively be sat in the erect position next to the fluoroscopy table with the arm abducted and the elbow flexed to allow placement of the wrist flat on the table with the palm down.

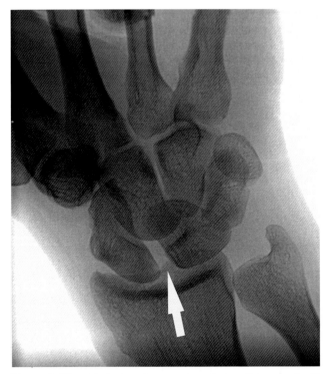

Figure 4-17 ■ Preliminary fluoroscopic evaluation of the wrist should also be performed before proceeding with the arthrogram. Fluoroscopic evaluation of the wrist with clenched fist maneuver depicts abnormal widening of the scapholunate space *(arrow)* compatible with scapholunate dissociation.

evaluation of the wrist should also be performed before proceeding with the arthrogram. Fluoroscopic evaluation of the wrist with clenched fist maneuvers and ulnar translation can be useful to identify scapholunate dissociation (Fig. 4-17).

Radiocarpal injections are facilitated by flexing the wrist and placing a triangular sponge beneath the wrist to maintain this position passively (Fig. 4-18). This serves to open the radiocarpal articulation anteriorly and facilitate passage of the needle into the joint over the overhanging dorsal lip of the distal radius. The fluoroscopic image should be collimated to minimize radiation exposure to the surrounding tissues.

The solution to be injected into the articulation should then be drawn up into a 10-mL syringe. Choice of agents to be included in the solution depends on the examination to be performed. Examples of solutions are listed in the solutions section of the chapter. Flexible tubing should be placed on the syringe and the solution should be advanced through the tubing to the tip. Any air bubbles should be expelled from the syringe and tubing. The target site for a radiocarpal joint injection is the dorsal aspect of the radioscaphoid joint (Figs. 4-19 and 4-20). A metallic object such as a Kelly clamp placed on the skin surface should be used to define the precise location of the injection, and the patient's skin should be marked with an indelible marker (Fig. 4-21).

The field should then be sterilely prepared and draped. Local anesthesia of the skin and underlying subcutaneous tissue is obtained with 1% lidocaine with 8.4% sodium bicarbonate buffer. The 0.5- or 1.5-inch, 25-gauge needle

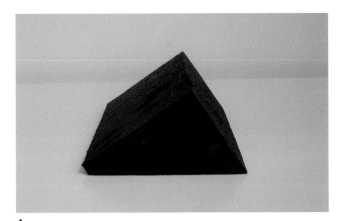

A

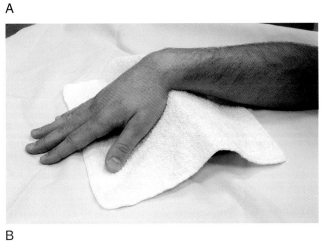

B

Figure 4-18 ■ A triangular sponge (*A*) is useful to place under the wrist to flex the wrist passively for radiocarpal injections. The triangular sponge is placed under the wrist (*B* and *C*) to flex the wrist passively. This opens the joint dorsally and facilitates needle placement.

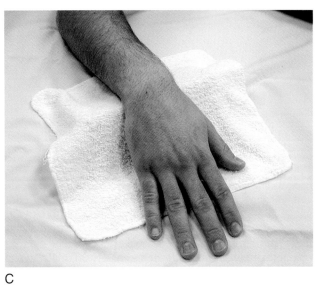

C

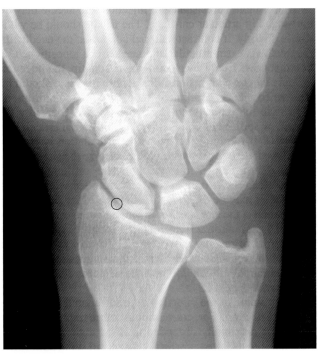

Figure 4-19 ■ The target site for a radiocarpal joint injection is the dorsal aspect of the radioscaphoid joint *(open circle)*.

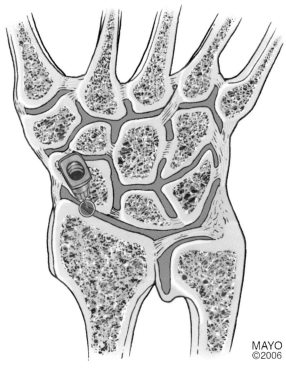

Figure 4-20 ■ The target site for a radiocarpal joint injection is the dorsal aspect of the space between the distal radius and the scaphoid.

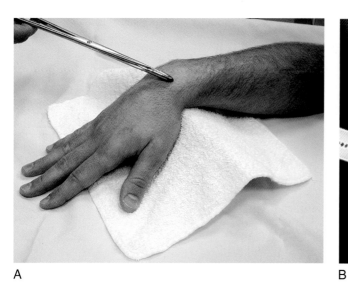

A

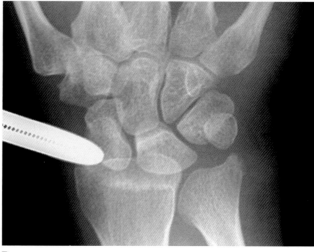

B

Figure 4-21 ■ A metallic object such as a Kelly clamp can be placed on the skin surface to define the precise location of the injection. The site should then be marked with an indelible marker.

used to anesthetize the skin can be left at the puncture site and disconnected from the syringe. This can then be used to gauge the position of the planned puncture site relative to the target site (Fig. 4-22). Entry into the radiocarpal articulation is often facilitated by a needle puncture site over the scaphoid or triquetrum with approximately 30 to 45 degrees of cephalad angulation of the needle tip.

If the initial puncture site does not allow optimal needle positioning, another puncture site should be chosen. This may require additional local anesthesia. If the planned puncture site is concordant with the target site, the needle can then be advanced through the soft tissues overlying the

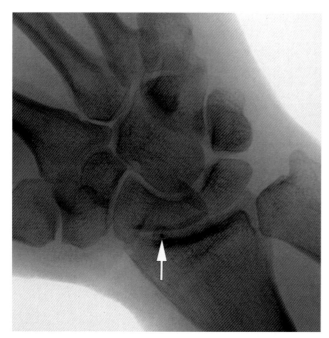

Figure 4-22 ■ The 0.5- or 1.5-inch, 25-gauge needle used to anesthetize the skin can be left in place to gauge the position (*arrow*) of the planned puncture site relative to the target site.

radiocarpal articulation until the needle is placed into the joint or contact is made with bone. Advancement should be performed with care as damage to the articular cartilage can result from overaggressive placement and manipulation of the needle. It is not uncommon for the patient to experience discomfort when the needle enters the joint or makes contact with the periosteum of the bone. Fluoroscopy is utilized to confirm the needle position. Adjustments to needle position can be made if necessary. When the needle is placed in a satisfactory position, the syringe and tubing containing the solution to be injected into the joint are connected to the indwelling needle. A small test injection should be performed to ensure appropriate intra-articular placement of the needle. If there is resistance to injection, the needle may be embedded in articular cartilage. The needle should be withdrawn slightly. If contrast material collects at the needle tip, the needle is extra-articular and needs to be repositioned. If contrast flows freely away from the needle tip, the injection mixture can be administered. The entire injection should be performed under continuous fluoroscopic monitoring as defects in the intraosseous ligaments or TFCC rapidly fill and allow spillage of contrast into the midcarpal articulation or DRUJ. If filling of the midcarpal articulation is present, the immediate images are helpful to localize the site of communication in either the scapholunate or lunotriquetral space. When the two compartments are filled with contrast material, it may be difficult to define the exact site of communication if the site was not identified at the time of injection. Digital subtraction imaging while injecting the radiocarpal articulation is often helpful to evaluate more precisely exact sites of abnormal communication between the radiocarpal articulation and the adjacent compartments of the wrist (Fig. 4-23).[24]

The volume of the injection depends upon the indication for the injection. For conventional arthrography, the joint should be maximally distended to allow contrast to extend into small rents or tears, which may not fill if the joint is not adequately distended. With conventional arthrography the joint should be injected until resistance is met related to full-

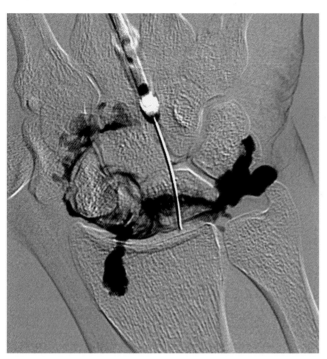

Figure 4-23 ■ Digital subtraction image from a radiocarpal injection depicts early abnormal communication between the radiocarpal articulation and the midcarpal joint through the scapholunate space indicative of a scapholunate ligament tear.

ness of the joint or the patient experiences discomfort related to fullness of the joint. This typically occurs at approximately 3 mL in a normal-size patient. Less distention is necessary with CT or MR arthrography than conventional arthrography. Overdistention of the articulation leads to

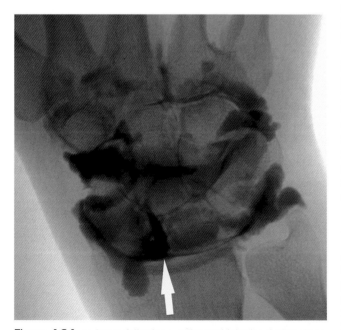

Figure 4-24 ■ Image following a radiocarpal injection depicts abnormal communication between the radiocarpal joint and the midcarpal articulation through the torn and disrupted scapholunate ligament *(arrow)*.

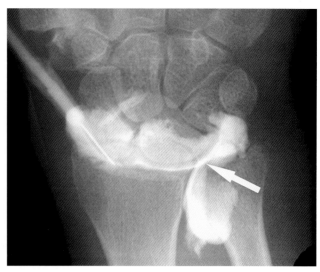

Figure 4-25 ■ Triangular fibrocartilage complex (TFCC) tear. Image from a radiocarpal joint injection reveals contrast material spilling into the adjacent distal radioulnar articulation through a tear in the TFCC *(arrow)*.

leakage from the joint puncture site and possible capsular rupture prior to imaging, which markedly hinders image quality with both MR and CT.

The needle is withdrawn following the injection. Fluoroscopic evaluation of the joint should then be performed in various positions including ulnar translation and in the clenched fist position. Spot films should be obtained in each of these positions. For CT and MR arthrography, manipulation of the joint should be kept to a minimum to avoid extravasation from the joint prior to imaging. For conventional arthrography, vigorous exercise of the wrist or hand should be performed followed by additional fluoroscopic evaluation, as many small tears become evident after increased intra-articular pressure related to exercise and positional changes force contrast material into small defects.

Communication between the radiocarpal space and the midcarpal space typically indicates perforation of the scapholunate or lunotriquetral ligaments. Imaging should be performed to identify the site of communication (Fig. 4-24). Communication with the radiocarpal articulation and the adjacent distal radioulnar articulation most often results from perforation of the TFCC (Fig. 4-25). Perforation of the intraosseous ligaments and TFCC does not always indicate acute injury or the site of the patient's symptoms. Assessment of the site of symptomatology must take in to consideration both the imaging findings and clinical information.

Midcarpal Joint Injection

A similar technique is utilized for injection of the midcarpal compartment as for the radiocarpal compartment. The patient should be placed on the fluoroscopy table as with radiocarpal injection. The patient can be placed on the table in the prone position with the wrist above the head (see Fig. 4-15) or can be sat next to the table with the arm abducted and the elbow flexed to allow placement of the wrist flat on the table with the palm down (see Fig. 4-16). Preliminary

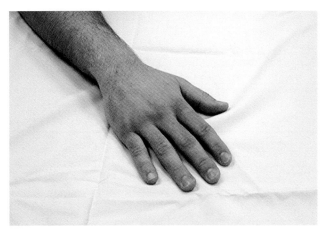

Figure 4-26 ■ Positioning for midcarpal injection. Unlike the position for radiocarpal injection, the hand is placed flat on the table with the palm down for midcarpal joint injection.

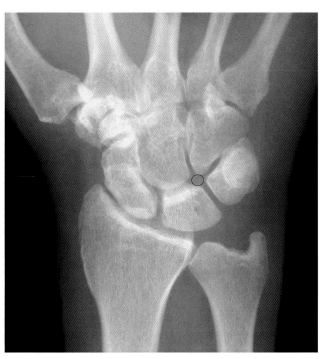

Figure 4-28 ■ The preferred target site for the midcarpal injection is the triquetrolunohamate space at the intersection of the triquetrum, lunate hamate, and capitate *(open circle)*.

fluoroscopic evaluation of the wrist should also be performed before proceeding. Fluoroscopic evaluation of the wrist with clenched fist maneuvers and ulnar translation can be useful to identify scapholunate dissociation.

With midcarpal injections, the wrist should be placed flat on the table as opposed to the flexed wrist utilized for radiocarpal injections (Fig. 4-26). The preferred target site for the midcarpal injection is the triquetrolunohamate space at the intersection of the triquetrum, lunate hamate, and capitate (Figs. 4-27 and 4-28). The target site should be identified and marked (Fig. 4-29). A 0.5- or 1.5-inch, 25-gauge needle

is utilized for the injection. The volume is similar to that utilized with radiocarpal injections, with typical injections consisting of approximately 3 mL.

Continuous fluoroscopic evaluation is necessary during injection to identify the site of communication as evaluation for the site of perforation may be difficult when both the midcarpal and radiocarpal articulations are opacified. Digital subtraction imaging may be useful to delineate more precisely sites of abnormal communication.[24] Following the injection, fluoroscopic evaluation and appropriate spot films of the

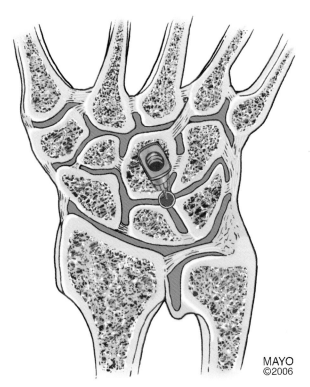

Figure 4-27 ■ The preferred target site for a midcarpal injection is the triquetrolunohamate space at the intersection of the triquetrum, lunate hamate, and capitate.

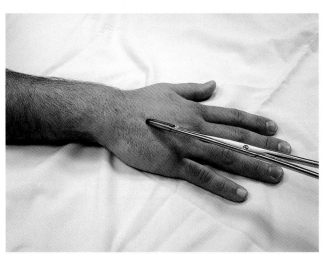

Figure 4-29 ■ A metallic object such as a Kelly clamp can be utilized to define the target site for the midcarpal joint injection. The patient's skin should then be marked.

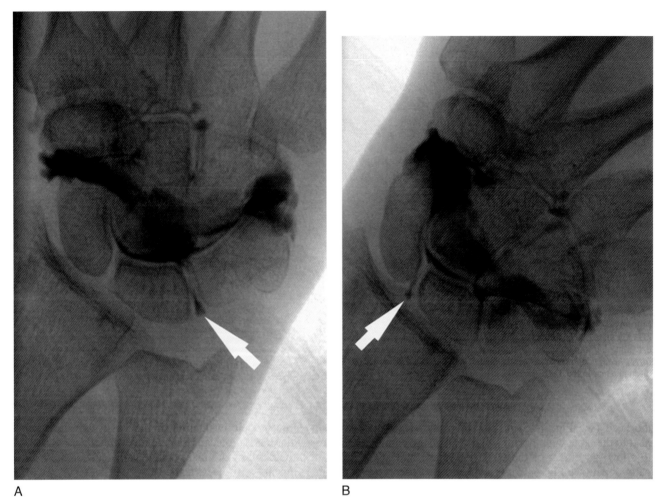

A   B

Figure 4-30 ■ Fluoroscopic spot images obtained with radial (*A*) and ulnar (*B*) deviation of the wrist depict the lunotriquetral (*A*) and scapholunate (*B*) ligaments, respectively *(arrows)*. Contrast can extend into the scapholunate and lunotriquetral spaces, as shown here, but should not extend into the adjacent radiocarpal articulation.

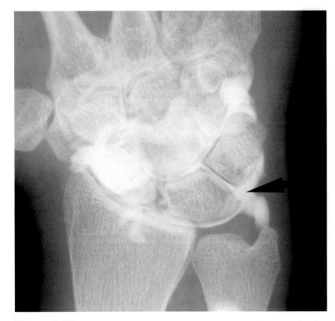

Figure 4-31 ■ Lunotriquetral ligament tear. Abnormal communication between the midcarpal compartment and the radiocarpal compartment through the torn lunotriquetral ligament *(arrow)*.

scapholunate and lunotriquetral ligaments in profile are obtained (Fig. 4-30). Provocative maneuvers such as ulnar translation and clenched fist positioning are also performed. Contrast material injected into the midcarpal articulation may communicate with the common carpometacarpal articulations but should not communicate with the first carpometacarpal articulation or, more important, should not communicate with the radiocarpal articulation (Fig. 4-31). Communication between the midcarpal compartment and the radiocarpal compartment is most often due to disruption of either the scapholunate or lunotriquetral ligaments (Fig. 4-32). Again, correlation of the patient's symptoms with the imaging findings is necessary as asymptomatic degenerative perforations of the intraosseous ligaments can be seen.

Distal Radioulnar Joint Injection

DRUJ injections can be more challenging than midcarpal or radiocarpal articulation injections. The DRUJ is small with a typical volume of 1 mL and variable in morphology, posing a slightly more challenging target than other injections about the wrist. The patient should be placed on the fluoroscopy table as with midcarpal injection. The patient can be placed on the table in the prone position with the wrist above

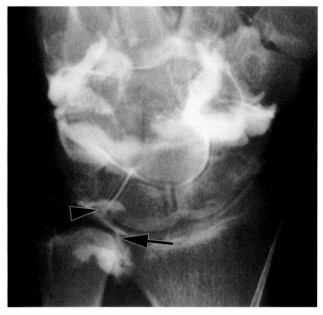

Figure 4-32 ■ Lunotriquetral and triangular fibrocartilage complex (TFCC) tear. Image following midcarpal joint injection depicts contrast extending into the radiocarpal joint through a lunotriquetral ligament tear *(arrowhead)*. Contrast subsequently extends into the distal radioulnar joint through a tear in the TFCC *(arrow)*.

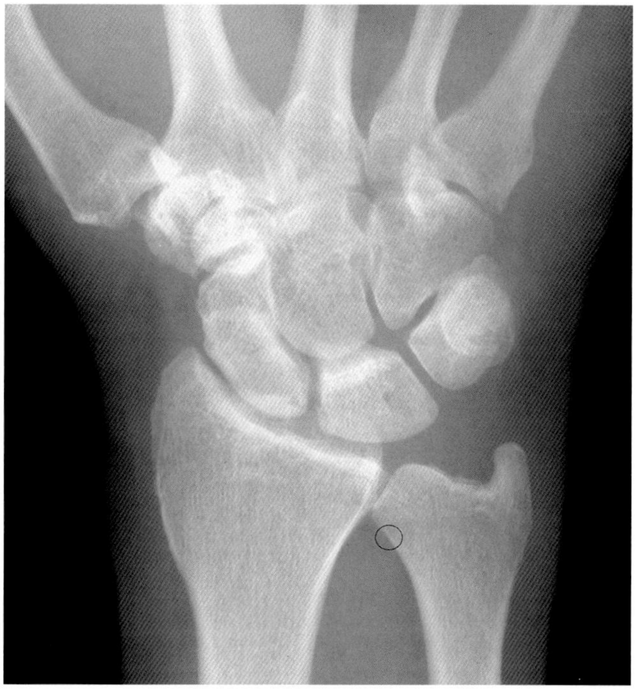

Figure 4-34 ■ The target site for the injection is the ulnar aspect of the space between the distal radius and ulna *(open circle)*.

the head (see Fig. 4-15) or placed in the sitting position next to the table with the arm abducted and the elbow flexed to allow placement of the wrist flat on the table with the palm down (see Fig. 4-16). Preliminary fluoroscopic evaluation of the wrist should also be performed before proceeding. Fluoroscopic evaluation of the wrist with both radial and ulnar translation can be useful to evaluate for ulnar abutment morphology or ulnar positive variance, conditions that can predispose to TFCC tears.

The target site for the injection is the ulnar aspect of the space between the distal radius and ulna (Figs. 4-33 and 4-34). The target site should be identified and the patient's skin should be marked with an indelible marker (Fig. 4-35). The field should then be sterilely prepared and draped. A 0.5- or 1.5-inch, 25-gauge needle is utilized for the injection. The needle should be advanced onto the most radial aspect of the distal ulnar head and then directed radially and advanced further to access the joint. The vol-

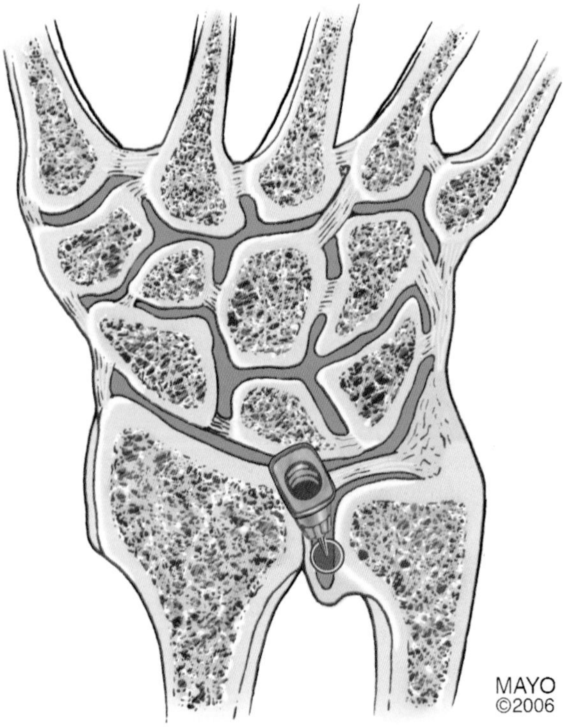

MAYO
©2006

Figure 4-33 ■ The target site for the distal radioulnar joint injection is the ulnar aspect of the space between the distal radius and ulna.

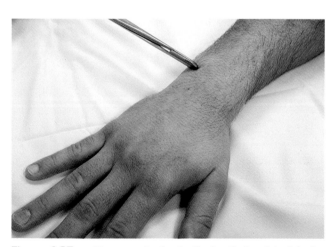

Figure 4-35 ■ The target site for the distal radioulnar joint injection should be identified under fluoroscopy and the patient's skin should be marked with an indelible marker.

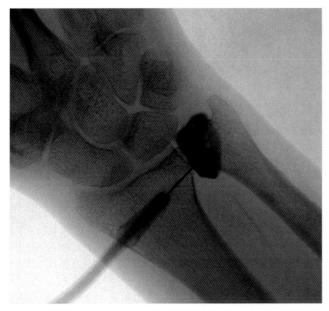

Figure 4-36 ▪ Normal distal radioulnar joint (DRUJ) injection. The volume of a typical injection is small, consisting of approximately 1 mL. Contrast material injected into the DRUJ should not communicate with the adjacent radiocarpal articulation.

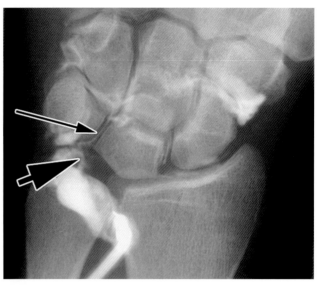

Figure 4-38 ▪ Triangular fibrocartilage complex (TFCC) and lunotriquetral ligament tears. Image following a distal radioulnar joint injection depicts contrast extending into the radiocarpal joint through the torn TFCC *(large arrow)*. Contrast subsequently extends into the midcarpal articulation through a defect in the lunotriquetral ligament *(small arrow)*.

ume of the DRUJ is very small, with a typical injection consisting of 1 mL. Contrast material injected into the DRUJ should not communicate with the adjacent radiocarpal articulation (Fig. 4-36). Communication with the radiocarpal compartment indicates disruption of the TFCC (Figs. 4-37 and 4-38).

Wrist Compartment Aspiration

Aspiration of the various compartments of the wrist is very similar to injections; however, it is often helpful to use a larger gauge needle such as a 22- or 20-gauge needle as this

Figure 4-37 ▪ Triangular fibrocartilage complex (TFCC) tear. Abnormal communication with the radiocarpal compartment following a distal radioulnar joint injection indicates disruption of the TFCC *(arrow)*.

facilitates aspiration of more viscous fluid. When the needle is in place, a 60-mL syringe and tubing are connected to the needle, and aspiration of the joint is performed. If no fluid can be withdrawn, repositioning within the joint may be helpful. If no fluid can be aspirated, the joint can be washed with nonbacteriostatic saline and reaspirated. Nonbacteriostatic saline is drawn up into a separate 10-mL syringe and tubing and a small amount is injected into the joint through the indwelling needle. The syringe tubing is then exchanged for the 60-mL syringe and tubing and the nonbacteriostatic saline is reaspirated. The aspirated fluid or nonbacteriostatic saline wash is then sent for aerobic and anaerobic culture. If enough fluid is present, Gram stain and additional analysis of the fluid can be performed, depending upon the specific clinical situation.

First Carpometacarpal Joint Injection
Metacarpal-Phalangeal Joint Injection
Interphalangeal Joint Injection

Radiographs should be obtained and reviewed prior to injection of the small joints of the hand. The patient should be placed on the fluoroscopy table as with a midcarpal injection. The patient can be placed on the table in the prone position with the wrist above the head (see Fig. 4-15) or can be sat next to the table with the arm abducted and the elbow flexed to allow placement of the wrist flat on the table with the palm down (see Fig. 4-16). Additional preliminary fluoroscopic evaluation of the joint should be performed, noting any abnormal motion or instability at the articulation.

The solution to be injected into the articulation should then be drawn up into a 10-mL syringe. The target site of the injection and the patient's skin should be marked with an indelible marker. A dorsal approach is utilized for the first

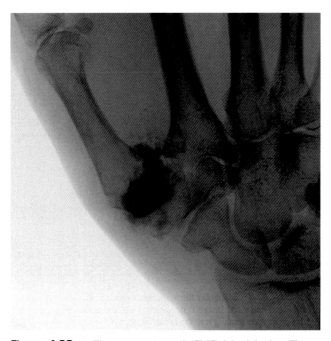

Figure 4-39 ■ First carpometacarpal (CMC) joint injection. Fluoroscopic image following therapeutic injection of the first CMC joint in a patient with chronic pain and osteoarthritis at the base of the thumb.

carpometacarpal articulation, the metacarpal-phalangeal articulations, or the interphalangeal articulations with care taken to avoid the extensor tendons of the thumb and fingers.

The field should be sterilely prepared and draped. A 0.5-inch, 25-gauge needle can be advanced through the soft tissues into the joint. Fluoroscopy is utilized to check the needle position. Alterations in needle position can then be made. When the needle has been properly positioned, the syringe and tubing containing the solution to be injected are connected to the indwelling 25-gauge needle. A small test injection should be performed to ensure appropriate intra-articular placement of the needle. The joint is very small and low in volume and resistance to injection is normal. Imaging must be used to confirm proper position. If contrast material collects at the needle tip, the needle is extra-articular and needs to be repositioned. If contrast flows away from the needle tip in a linear fashion along the joint line, the remainder of the injection is made (Figs. 4-39 and 4-40). The first carpometacarpal joint and the metacarpophalangeal (MCP) and interphalangeal (IP) joints are very small in volume and typically accept only a 1-mL injection volume. The entire injection should be performed under continuous fluoroscopic monitoring. Following the injection, the needle is withdrawn. Fluoroscopic evaluation of the joint should then be performed with a spot film obtained to document the injection.

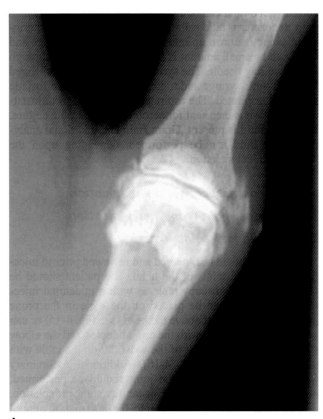

A

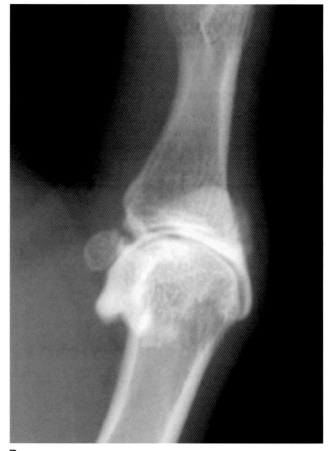

B

Figure 4-40 ■ First metacarpophalangeal (MCP) joint injection. Fluoroscopic images following diagnostic and therapeutic injection of bupivacaine into the first MCP joint.

POTENTIAL COMPLICATIONS[29]

- Bleeding
- Infection (cellulitis, septic arthritis, or osteomyelitis)
- Drug-related allergic reactions
- Transient synovitis
- Transitory hand weakness
- Transitory hand paresthesia
- Vascular injury (radial or ulnar artery or vein)

POST-PROCEDURE CARE/FOLLOW-UP[29]

Immediate

1. The patient should be observed for 15 minutes following injection.
2. Blood pressure, pulse, heart rate, and respiratory rate are monitored as necessary.

Discharge

1. An adhesive bandage may be placed on the puncture site. The bandage should remain dry for at least 24 hours, at which point it can be removed.
2. The patient is instructed to continue taking his or her prescription medication, although pain medication may be tapered as indicated.
3. A discharge sheet should be given to the patient outlining the following:
   a. Which procedure was performed
   b. Procedure-related symptoms that typically resolve in 7 to 10 days
      - Pain at the needle puncture site(s)
      - Mild increase in joint stiffness with a feeling of fullness in the joint
      - Deep hand or wrist pain
   c. Treatment for mild post-procedure symptoms
      - Rest the hand and wrist for 1 to 2 days
      - Avoid movements that worsen the pain
      - Use cold compresses to the area that hurts
   d. Signs and symptoms of infection
      - Fever
      - Chills
      - Swelling or drainage from the puncture site(s)
      - New pain that is different from the usual pain
   e. Signs and symptoms of possible more serious problems
      - Decreased range of motion
      - Increasing pain
      - Motor dysfunction of the upper extremity
   f. Physician name and contact number if the patient has any concerns or if any problem were to arise as a result of the procedure
   g. Advice to schedule a follow-up appointment with the referring physician in 7 to 10 days.

SAMPLE DICTATIONS

Radiocarpal Injection

The procedure and potential complications were explained to the patient, and voluntary informed, signed consent was obtained. The patient was placed on the table in the supine position. Preliminary fluoroscopic evaluation of the wrist was performed with both ulnar translation and clenched fist maneuvers. The skin overlying the radiocarpal articulation was prepared and draped in a sterile fashion. Local anesthesia was obtained with 1% lidocaine with bicarbonate buffer. Under fluoroscopic guidance, a 25-gauge, 1.5-inch needle was advanced into the radiocarpal articulation and a 4-mL solution containing 2 mL iodinated contrast material (iohexol, 300 mg I/mL), 2 mL bupivacaine (0.5%), and 0.1 mL gadolinium was administered into the radiocarpal articulation. The needle was withdrawn. Post-injection fluoroscopic evaluation was performed and appropriate spot films were obtained. The patient was sent to MR for additional imaging of the wrist following arthrography.

Triple-Compartment Wrist Arthrogram

The procedure and potential complications were explained to the patient, and voluntary informed, signed consent was obtained. The patient was placed on the table in the supine position. Preliminary fluoroscopic evaluation of the wrist was performed with both ulnar translation and clenched fist maneuvers. (1) Midcarpal joint injection: The skin overlying the midcarpal articulation was prepared and draped in a sterile fashion. Local anesthesia was obtained with 1% lidocaine with bicarbonate buffer. Under fluoroscopic guidance a 25-gauge, 0.5-inch needle was advanced into the midcarpal articulation and a 4-mL solution containing 2 mL iodinated contrast material (iohexol, 300 mg I/mL), and 2 mL bupivacaine (0.5%) was administered into the midcarpal articulation. Post-injection fluoroscopic evaluation was performed and appropriate spot films were obtained. (2) Distal radioulnar joint injection: Local anesthesia was obtained with 1% lidocaine with bicarbonate buffer. Under fluoroscopic guidance, a 25-gauge, 0.5-inch needle was advanced into the distal radioulnar articulation and a 2-mL solution containing 1 mL iodinated contrast material (iohexol, 300 mg I/mL), and 1 mL bupivacaine (0.5%) was administered into the DRUJ. Post-injection fluoroscopic evaluation was performed and appropriate spot films were obtained. (3) Radiocarpal injection: After 3 hours, the patient returned to the department and the skin overlying the radiocarpal articulation was prepared and draped in a sterile fashion. Local anesthesia was obtained with 1% lidocaine with bicarbonate buffer. Under fluoroscopic guidance, a 25-gauge, 1.5-inch needle, was advanced into the radiocarpal articulation and a 4-mL solution containing 2 mL iodinated contrast material (iohexol, 300 mg I/mL), and 2 mL bupivacaine (0.5%) was administered into the radiocarpal articulation. Post-injection fluoroscopic evaluation was performed and appropriate spot films were obtained.

Findings: No foci of abnormal communication are seen between the radiocarpal and midcarpal articulations, indicating intact scapholunate and lunotriquetral ligaments. No foci of abnormal communication are seen between the radiocarpal articulation and the DRUJ, indicating an intact TFCC. No filling defects were identified to suggest loose bodies or synovitis.

CASE REPORTS

CASE 1

Clinical Presentation

A 36-year-old male patient presented with right ulnar-sided wrist pain and swelling for 3 months. The symptoms were mostly centered about the distal aspect of the ulna on physical examination. The patient reported working as a laboratory assistant and utilized a pipette, performing a repetitive maneuver with his wrist that exacerbated the pain. The patient denied any trauma or injury and reported no numbness or loss of sensation of the wrist and hand.

Imaging and Therapy

The patient was referred for an MR arthrogram of the right wrist to evaluate the integrity of the TFCC and the lunotriquetral ligament. The patient was placed on the table in the prone position with the wrist above the head. Under fluoroscopic guidance, a 25-gauge, 0.5-inch needle was advanced into the radioscaphoid portion of the radiocarpal articulation and a 4-mL injection containing iodinated contrast material,

gadolinium, and bupivacaine was injected. Imaging immediately demonstrated spilling of contrast from the radiocarpal articulation into the DRUJ compatible with a tear of the TFCC (Fig. 4-41). MR imaging of the wrist was performed immediately following the procedure. MR arthrography precisely depicted the tear in the central portion of the triangular fibrocartilage that allowed the abnormal communication between the radiocarpal articulation and the DRUJ (Fig. 4-42).

The patient subsequently underwent arthroscopy of the right wrist. Arthroscopy confirmed the presence of a focal tear in the midportion of the triangular fibrocartilage. The tear was repaired arthroscopically.

Results

The wrist was splinted with no range of motion for 4 weeks, followed by a formal range-of-motion and strengthening regimen. The patient recovered fully following arthroscopic repair of the TFCC tear with no residual discomfort or disability.

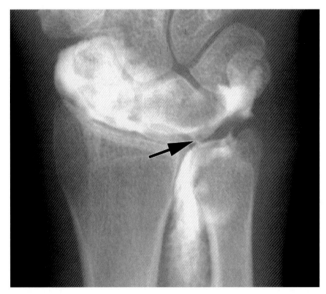

Figure 4-41 ■ Image following radiocarpal joint injection depicts extension of contrast from the radiocarpal articulation into the distal radioulnar joint *(arrow)* compatible with a tear of the triangular fibrocartilage complex.

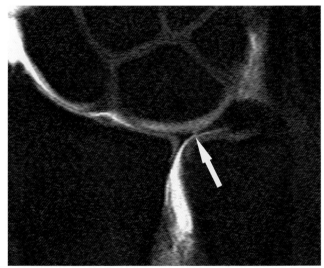

Figure 4-42 ■ MR arthrography following radiocarpal joint injection precisely demonstrates the tear in the central portion of the triangular fibrocartilage *(arrow)* that allows abnormal communication between the radiocarpal articulation and the distal radioulnar joint.

CASE 2

Clinical Presentation

An 18-year-old male patient presented to the emergency room with marked pain and swelling of the right thumb following an acute injury playing flag football. The mechanism of injury included both abduction and hyperextension of the thumb. Physical examination demonstrated overall diminished range of motion of the first MCP joint related to soft tissue swelling but did reveal laxity of the ulnar collateral ligament with stress.

Imaging and Therapy

An MR arthrogram of the right first MCP joint was performed. The patient was seated beside the fluoroscopy table with the palm of the hand placed flat on the table surface. Utilizing a dorsal approach and avoiding the extensor mechanism of the first digit, a 25-gauge, 0.5-inch needle was advanced into the first MCP joint under fluoroscopic guidance. A 2-mL solution containing iodinated contrast material, gadolinium, and bupivacaine was administered into the joint. Imaging immediately revealed extravasation from the ulnar aspect of the joint indicative of an ulnar collateral ligament injury (Fig. 4-43). MR imaging was performed

immediately following the injection. MR arthrography revealed a small avulsion fracture of the ulnar aspect of the base of the first proximal phalanx with associated thickening of the ulnar collateral ligament compatible with partial tearing (Fig. 4-44).

The patient subsequently underwent operative repair of the ulnar collateral ligament. At surgery, the ulnar collateral ligament was indeed fully avulsed from the base of the first proximal phalanx with small bone fragments avulsed with the ligament. The bone fragments were removed from the ligament and then the distal portion of the ulnar collateral ligament was reattached to the base of the first proximal phalanx with a Mitek suture anchor.

Results

The thumb was placed in a cast for 2 weeks followed by a splint for 4 additional weeks. A formal range-of-motion and strengthening regimen was then completed. Postoperative results were good with complete healing of the ulnar collateral ligament and no residual instability or pain.

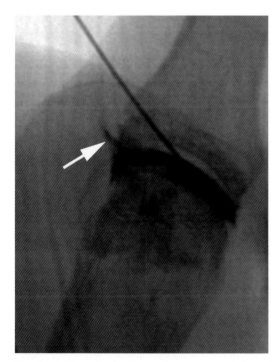

Figure 4-43 ■ Image from a first metacarpophalangeal joint injection shows extravasation from the ulnar aspect of the joint *(arrow)* indicative of an ulnar collateral ligament tear.

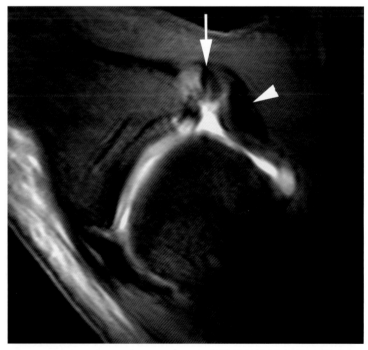

Figure 4-44 ■ MR arthrography following first metacarpophalangeal joint injection reveals a small avulsion fracture *(arrow)* at the ulnar aspect of the base of the first proximal phalanx with associated thickening of the ulnar collateral ligament *(arrowhead)* compatible with partial tearing.

CURRENT PROCEDURAL TERMINOLOGY (CPT) CODES[31]

CPT codes change often and sometimes are valid only for certain states or regions. It is best to consult with coding experts to make sure that coding for one's procedures is legitimate and complete. Below is a sample of codes that are being used for elbow injection procedures at this writing.

20605 Arthrocentesis, aspiration and/or injection; intermediate joint or bursa (e.g., temporomandibular, acromioclavicular, wrist, elbow or ankle, olecranon bursa)

(If imaging guidance is performed, see 76942, 77002, 77012, 77021)

25246 Injection procedure for wrist arthrography

(For radiologic supervision and interpretation, use 73115. Do not report 77002 in addition to 73115)

73100 Radiologic examination, wrist; two views
73110 complete, minimum of three views
73115 Radiologic examination, wrist, arthrography, radiologic supervision and interpretation

(Do not report 77002 in addition to 73115)

73120 Radiologic examination, hand; two views
73130 minimum of three views
73140 Radiologic examination, finger(s); minimum of two views
73200 Computed tomography, upper extremity; without contrast material
73201 with contrast material(s)
73202 without contrast material, followed by contrast material(s) and further sections

(To report 3D rendering, see 76376, 76377)

73221 Magnetic resonance (e.g., proton) imaging, any joint of upper extremity; without contrast material(s)
73222 with contrast material(s)
73223 without contrast material, followed by contrast material(s) and further sequences
76376 3D rendering with interpretation and reporting of computed tomography, magnetic resonance imaging, ultrasound, or other tomographic modality; not requiring image postprocessing on an independent workstation

(Use 76376 in conjunction with code(s) for base imaging procedure(s))

76377 requiring image postprocessing on an independent workstation

(Use 76376 in conjunction with code(s) for base imaging procedure(s))

76942 Ultrasonic guidance for needle placement (eg, biopsy, aspiration, injection, localization device), imaging supervision and interpretation

(Do not report 76942 in conjunction with 43232, 43237, 43242, 45341, 45342, or 76975)

77002 Fluoroscopic guidance for needle placement (eg, biopsy, aspiration, injection, localization device)

(See appropriate surgical code for procedure and anatomic location)

(77002 includes all radiographic arthrography with the exception of supervision and interpretation for CT and MR arthrography)

(Do not report 77002 in addition to 70332, 73040, 73085, 73115, 73525, 73580, 73615)

77012 Computed tomography guidance for needle placement (e.g., biopsy, aspiration, injection, localization device), radiologic supervision and interpretation

77021 Magnetic resonance guidance for needle placement (e.g., for biopsy, needle aspiration, injection, or placement of localization device), radiologic supervision and interpretation

References

1. Kessler I, Silberman Z. An experimental study of the radiocarpal joint by arthrography. Surg Gynecol Obstet 1961; 112:33–44.
2. Conway WF, Hayes CW. Three compartment wrist arthrography: Use of a low-iodine-concentration contrast agent to decrease study time. Radiology 1989; 173:569–570.
3. Dalinka MK, Turner ML, Osterman AL, Batra P. Wrist arthrography. Radiol Clin North Am 1981; 19:217–226.
4. Herbert TJ, Faithfull RG, McCann DJ. Bilateral arthrography of the wrist. J Hand Surg [Br] 1990; 15:233–235.
5. Linkous DM, Gilula LA. Wrist arthrography today. Radiol Clin North Am 1998; 36:651–672.
6. Cerofolini E, Luchetti R, Pederzini L, et al. MR evaluation of triangular fibrocartilage complex tears in the wrist: Comparison with arthrography and arthroscopy. J Comput Assist Tomogr 1990; 14:963–967.
7. Quinn SF, Belsole RS, Greene TL, Rayhack JM. Work in progress: Postarthrography computed tomography of the wrist: Evaluation of the triangular fibrocartilage complex. Skeletal Radiol 1989; 17:565–569.
8. Zanetti M, Bram J, Hodler J. Triangular fibrocartilage and intercarpal ligaments of the wrist: Does MR arthrography improve standard MRI. J Magn Reson Imaging 1997; 7:590–594.
9. Steinbach LS, Smith DK. MRI of the wrist. Clin Imaging 2000; 24:298–322.
10. Theumann N, Favarger N, Schnyder P, Meuli R. Wrist ligament injuries: Value of post-arthrography computed tomography. Skeletal Radiol 2001; 30:88–93.
11. Cerezal L, Abascal F, Garcia-Valtuille R, del Pinal F. Wrist MR arthrography: How, why, when. Radiol Clin North Am 2005; 43:709–731.
12. Berquist TH. Diagnostic and therapeutic injections as an aid to musculoskeletal diagnosis. Semin Interv Radiol 1993; 10:326–344.
13. Berquist TH. MRI of the Hand and Wrist. Philadelphia: Lippincott Williams & Wilkins, 2003.
14. Resnick D. Diagnosis of Bone and Joint Disorders, 4th ed. Philadelphia: WB Saunders, 2002, pp 193–318, 3021–3053.
15. Gilula LA, Hardy DC, Totty WG, Reinus WR. Fluoroscopic identification of torn intercarpal ligaments after injection of contrast material. AJR Am J Roentgenol 1987; 149:761–764.
16. Arons MS, Fishbone G, Arons JA. Communicating defects of the triangular fibrocartilage complex without disruption of the triangular fibrocartilage: A report of two cases. J Hand Surg [Am] 1999; 24:148–151.
17. Freiberger RH, Kaye JJ. Arthrography. Norwalk, CT: Appleton Century Crofts, 1979, pp 1–3, 277–290.
18. Shionoya K, Nakamura R, Imaeda T, Makino N. Arthrography is superior to magnetic resonance imaging for diagnosing injuries of the triangular fibrocartilage. J Hand Surg [Br] 1998; 23:402–405.
19. Berquist TH. MRI of the Musculoskeletal System, 5th ed. Philadelphia: Lippincott Williams & Wilkins, 2006, pp 719–801.

20. Brown RR, Fliszar E, Cotton A, et al. Extrinsic and intrinsic ligaments of the wrist: Normal and pathologic anatomy at MR arthrography with three-compartment enhancement. Radiographics 1998; 18:667–674.

21. Zdravkovic V, Sennwald GR, Fischer M, Jacob HAC. The palmar wrist ligaments revisited, clinical relevance. Ann Chir Main Memb Super 1994; 13:378–382.

22. Hodge JC. Musculoskeletal Imaging: Diagnostic and Therapeutic Procedures. Montreal: Karger Landes Systems, 1997, pp 39–54.

23. Levinsohn EM, Rosen ID, Palmer AK. Wrist arthrography: Value of the three-compartment injection method. Radiology 1991; 179:231–239.

24. Yin Y, Wilson AJ, Gilula LA. Three-compartment wrist arthrography: Direct comparison of digital subtraction with nonsubtraction images. Radiology 1995; 197:287–290.

25. Scheck RJ, Romagnolo A, Hierner R, et al. The carpal ligaments in MR arthrography of the wrist: Correlation with standard MRI and wrist arthroscopy. J Magn Reson Imaging 1999; 9:468–474.

26. Theumann NH, Pfirrman CW, Drape JL, et al. MR imaging of the metacarpophalangeal joints of the fingers: Part I. Conventional MR imaging and MR arthrographic findings in cadavers. Radiology 2002; 222:437–445.

27. Harper MT, Chandnani VP, Spaeth J, et al. Gamekeeper thumb: Diagnosis of ulnar collateral ligament injury using magnetic resonance imaging, magnetic resonance arthrography and stress radiography. J Magn Reson Imaging 1996; 6:322–328.

28. Pfirrman CW, Theumann NH, Botte MJ, et al. MR imaging of the metacarpophalangeal joints of the fingers: Part II. Detection of simulated injuries in cadavers. Radiology 2002; 222:447–452.

29. Fenton DS, Czervionke LF. Image-Guided Spine Intervention. Philadelphia: WB Saunders, 2003.

30. Physicians' Desk Reference, 60th ed. Montvale, NJ: Medical Economics Company, 2006.

31. Derived from CPT 2007, CPT Intellectual Property Services. Chicago: American Medical Association, 2007.

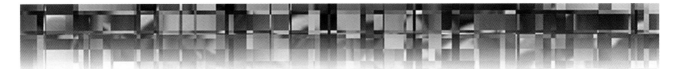

A Hand Surgeon's Perspective

Wrist and Hand Injections

Peter M. Murray, MD

To the hand surgeon, hand and wrist injections are the cornerstone of diagnosis and treatment of many conditions. Under some circumstances, it is the most important diagnostic tool and the information gained is used to delineate the type and scope of surgical intervention. Often, pain in the hand and wrist area is difficult to localize clinically. Selective diagnostic and therapeutic injections can help solve the puzzle or at least narrow down the possibilities. Lidocaine or bupivacaine is mixed with a steroid suspension and delivered directly into the target site. Immediately after delivery, the patient can be questioned for symptom resolution. Immediate improvement provides extremely useful data. In many disorders involving the hand and wrist, the first line of treatment involves therapeutic injection. Many injections can be performed in the office by an experienced clinician without image guidance. These include injections for carpal tunnel syndrome, trigger finger, and de Quervain's tenosynovitis. Other injections, including injections of the various compartments of the wrist as well as the metacarpophalangeal and interphalangeal articulations, are often best performed under image guidance to ensure adequate placement of the anesthetic and steroid preparations.

In addition to therapeutic injections, diagnostic injections can be useful to evaluate the integrity of the ligamentous structures about the hand and wrist. The integrity of the scapholunate and lunotriquetral ligaments can be evaluated with wrist injections. Triangular fibrocartilage complex pathology can be delineated. Wrist injections can also be helpful for CT or MR arthrography of the wrist, which can precisely depict all forms of pathology about the hand and wrist. Articular cartilage abnormalities are often well demonstrated with CT or MR arthrography of the wrist. The imaging findings from diagnostic wrist injections can be very helpful in guiding therapy and can determine whether surgery is warranted in many cases.

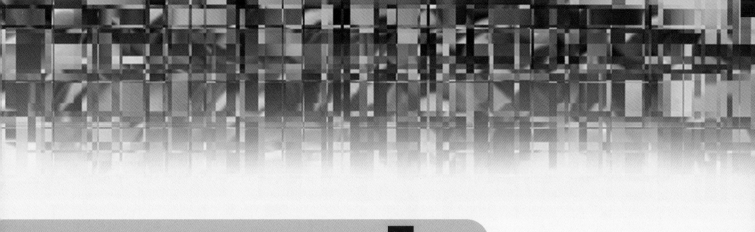

Chapter 5

Hip Injections

- Jeffrey J. Peterson, MD

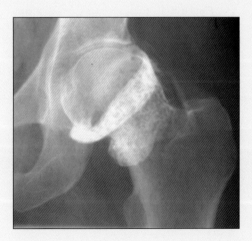

BACKGROUND

The first report of hip arthrography in the English literature was presented by Severin in 1939 describing the utility of hip arthrography in children.[1,2] Ozonoff, in 1973, first described the modern technique for hip arthrography utilizing fluoroscopic guidance in children,[1,3] and Razzano and colleagues in 1974 first described this method for adult hip arthrography.[1,4] Later in the 1970s, variations of the technique for hip aspiration and anesthetic arthrography or hip block were developed.[1,5] In the 1990s, techniques for CT and MR arthrography of the hip were introduced and evolved.[1] Today, many variations on hip arthrography and hip injections exist, and are covered in this chapter. There is still an important role for hip arthrography for both diagnostic and therapeutic purposes. Therapeutic injections continue to have an important clinical role in evaluation of hip pain, helping to differentiate radicular pain from symptoms arising from pathology relating to the hip articulation.[1,5,6] Today, conventional arthrography is rarely indicated; however, hip arthrography followed by cross-sectional imaging such as CT or MR plays an important role in the evaluation of internal derangement of the hip joint.[7-9] CT and MR arthrography can precisely delineate pathology involving the acetabular labrum as well as defects involving the articular hyaline cartilage of the hip joint.[7-9]

ANATOMIC CONSIDERATIONS

The hip joint is a ball-and-socket synovium-lined articulation that exists between the spherical femoral head and the cup-shaped acetabulum.[5,10] The femoral head is completely covered by hyaline articular cartilage apart from the fovea capitis, which is the site of insertion of the ligament of the head of the femur, also known as the ligamentum teres (Fig. 5-1).[5,11] The articular surface of the acetabulum is horseshoe shaped with a central depression termed the acetabular fossa that contains pulvinar (intra-articular fat).[5,11,12] The acetabular articular surface is open inferiorly, which is referred to as the acetabular notch (see Fig. 5-1).[5,12] Compared with the shoulder joint, the hip has less range of motion but has significantly greater stability.[10,11] This stability is conferred by the shape and morphology of the hip in addition to the acetabular labrum and surrounding ligaments, tendons, and musculature.[10,11]

The acetabular labrum is a fibrocartilaginous structure that is firmly adherent to the margins of the bony acetabulum and effectively serves to deepen the acetabular articular surface (Fig. 5-2).[11,13] The labrum is triangular shaped in cross section extending about the rim of the acetabulum, adding several millimeters to the circumference of the articular surface of the hip.[11,13] The acetabular labrum blends inferiorly with the transverse acetabular ligament, which traverses the acetabular notch (see Fig. 5-2).[8,9] The acetabular labrum contributes to joint stability and is densely innervated; therefore, the labrum plays an important role in proprioception and the potential for pain production.[8,9]

Other notable ligaments about the hip joint include the iliofemoral ligament, the pubofemoral ligament, the ischiofemoral ligament, and the ligament of the head of the femur (Fig. 5-3).[10,11] The iliofemoral ligament is thought to be the strongest of the supporting ligaments of the hip.[10–12] The ligament has a shape similar to an inverted Y and overlies the anterior surface of the hip joint capsule.[10] The diverging portions of the ligament inferiorly attach to the anterior surface of the intertrochanteric line (see Fig. 5-3).[10,11] This ligament is taut in hip extension and is often injured in hip dislocations.[11]

The pubofemoral and ischiofemoral ligaments are additional stabilizing ligaments of the hip but are relatively weak in comparison with the iliofemoral ligament (see Fig. 5-3).[10,11] The pubofemoral ligament is a weak ligament medial to the

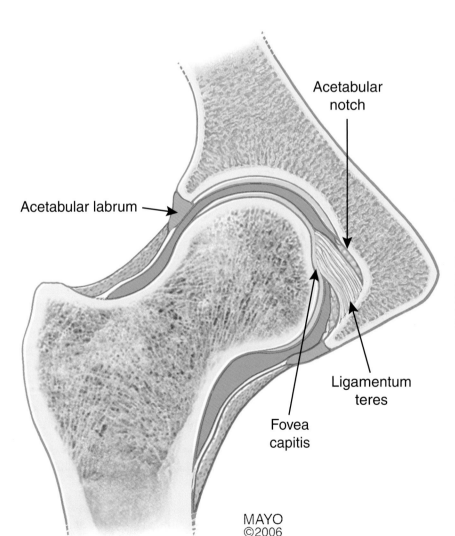

Acetabular notch

Acetabular labrum

Ligamentum teres

Fovea capitis

MAYO
©2006

Figure 5-1 ■ Ligamentum teres and acetabular notch. The fovea capitis is the site of insertion of the ligamentum teres. The acetabulum is horseshoe shaped with a central depression termed the acetabular fossa that contains pulvinar (intra-articular fat).

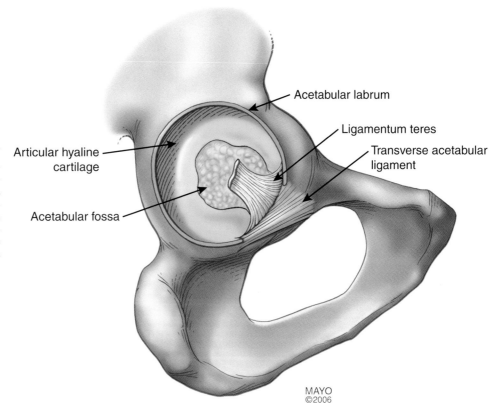

Figure 5-2 ■ Acetabular labrum and transverse acetabular ligament. The acetabular labrum is firmly adherent to the margins of the bony acetabulum and effectively serves to deepen the acetabular articular surface. The acetabular labrum blends inferiorly with the transverse acetabular ligament, which traverses the acetabular notch. The ligamentum teres is seen centrally.

iliofemoral ligament extending along the medial inferior aspect of the hip joint capsule.[10,11] The pubofemoral ligament arises from the medial acetabulum and pubis, extending inferiorly to attach to the undersurface of the femoral neck.[10,11] The ischiofemoral ligament extends along the posterior aspect of the hip capsule, arising from the ischium and extending laterally and superiorly to insert on the superior and posterior aspect of the femoral neck (see Fig. 5-3).[10,11]

The ligament for the head of the femur, also known as the ligamentum teres, is an intra-articular ligament that extends from the fovea capitis of the femoral head to the margin of the acetabular notch medially.[10,11] The artery of the fovea capitis, which supplies portions of the femoral head, runs along with the ligament of the head of the femur.[10,11] These structures, tethered to the femoral head, are well seen with MR or CT arthrography within the hip joint (Fig. 5-4).

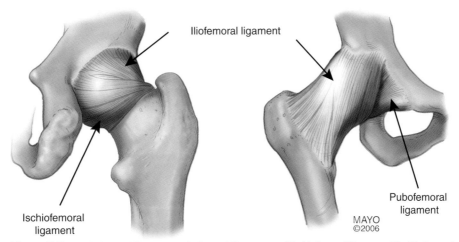

Figure 5-3 ■ Iliofemoral ligament, pubofemoral ligament, and ischiofemoral ligament. The iliofemoral ligament is thought to be the strongest of the supporting ligaments of the hip and overlies the anterior surface of the hip joint capsule. The pubofemoral ligament is medial to the iliofemoral ligament, extending along the medial inferior aspect of the hip joint capsule. The ischiofemoral ligament extends along the posterior aspect of the hip capsule.

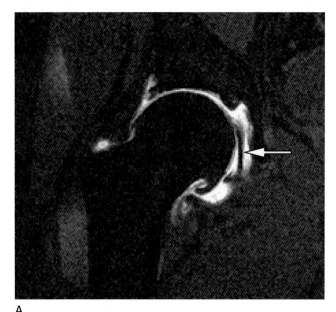

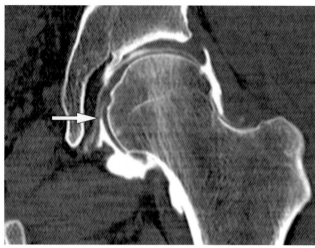

A   B

Figure 5-4 ■ Ligamentum teres. Coronal image from an MR arthrogram of the hip (*A*) and coronal reformatted image from a CT arthrogram (*B*) depict the ligamentum teres *(arrows)* extending from the fovea capitis of the femoral head to the margin of the acetabular notch medially. The artery of the fovea capitis, which supplies portions of the femoral head, runs with the ligamentum teres.

The external ligamentous structures include the ilio-femoral, pubofemoral, and ischiofemoral ligaments and extend along the capsule of the hip joint.[10,11] The capsule is lined by synovial tissue that extends around the hip joint, attaching to the margin of the bony acetabulum and labrum.[11] Synovial tissue extends into the acetabular notch, where it surrounds the pulvinar and ligament of the head of the femur.[10] The capsule extends inferiorly, becoming more capacious about the femoral neck, and includes several collar-like recesses where joint fluid may collect (Fig. 5-5).[11] A circumferential band extends about the femoral neck, termed the zona orbicularis, which separates the superior articular recesses from the more inferior collicular recesses (see Fig. 5-5).[11] The superior articular recess extends superiorly and laterally about the acetabular margin and labrum.[11] The inferior articular recess is seen just above the zona orbicularis medially.[11] The superior (lateral) and inferior (medial) collicular recesses form a circumferential collar around the femoral neck, just inferior to the zona orbicularis (see Fig. 5-5).[11]

There are more than 20 muscles that arise and extend about the hip. These are best categorized by their function.[10] The extensors of the hip include the gluteus maximus and adductor magnus muscles.[10] Variable contributions are also provided by the gluteus minimus, gluteus medius, biceps femoris, semimembranosus, and semitendinosus muscles.[10] The gluteus minimus and gluteus medius muscles also aid in hip abduction.[10]

The primary hip flexor is the iliopsoas muscle located anteriorly; however, the sartorius, adductor brevis, and pectineus muscles, as well as the tensor fasciae latae, also contribute to hip flexion.[10] The gluteus minimus, gracilis, and adductor longus muscles also contribute to a lesser extent to hip flexion.[10] The iliopsoas muscle and tendon at the level of the hip and thigh represent a combination of the

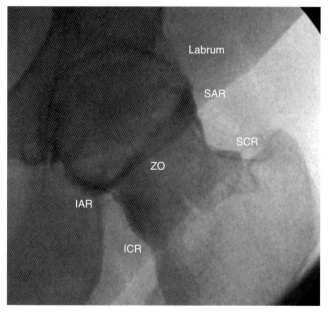

Figure 5-5 ■ Anatomic recesses of the hip joint. The hip joint capsule extends inferiorly about the femoral neck and includes several collar-like recesses where joint fluid collects. A circumferential band extends about the femoral neck, termed the zona orbicularis (ZO), which separates the articular recesses superiorly from the collicular recesses inferiorly. The superior articular recess (SAR) extends superiorly and laterally about the acetabular margin and labrum. The inferior articular recess (IAR) is seen just above the zona orbicularis medially. The superior collicular recess (SCR) and the inferior collicular recess (ICR) form a circumferential collar around the femoral neck, just inferior to the zona orbicularis.

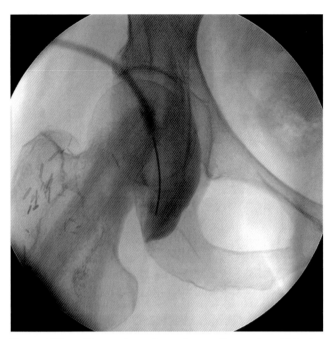

Figure 5-6 ■ Iliopsoas bursa. Image from an iliopsoas bursal injection shows the bursa located just anterior to the hip joint extending vertically along the iliopsoas muscle and tendon.

iliacus and psoas major muscles.[10,11] The psoas muscle arises in the retroperitoneum along the lateral margin of the T12-L5 vertebrae and extends inferiorly and laterally, where it joins the iliacus muscle to insert on the lesser trochanter.[10,11] The iliacus muscle arises from the internal surface of the ilium and passes obliquely, anterior to the hip, to join with the psoas muscle, inserting upon the lesser trochanter.[10,11] Occasionally, anatomic variations occur that result in friction between the iliopsoas muscle and tendon and the iliopectineal eminence just anterior and superior to the hip joint or the lesser trochanteric ridge, which is often accompanied by an audible snap. This is typically referred to as snapping iliopsoas tendon syndrome.[11]

The gracilis and adductor musculature, including the adductor magnus, adductor longus, and adductor brevis muscles, provide most of the necessary force for hip adduction.[10] Adduction is also aided by the gluteus maximus, pectineus, and obturator externus muscles.[10]

Several prominent bursae are seen about the hip.[10,11] The largest is the iliopsoas bursa located just anterior to the hip joint extending vertically, which is closely associated with the iliopsoas muscle and tendon (Fig. 5-6).[11] The bursae are present in 98% of the population and communicate with the hip joint in approximately 15% of patients (Fig. 5-7).[11] When present, this communication occurs between the iliofemoral and pubofemoral ligaments.[11]

Additional bursae in close proximity to the hip joint include the trochanteric bursae.[14] The three gluteal tendons

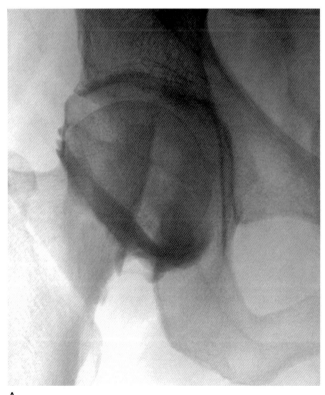

A

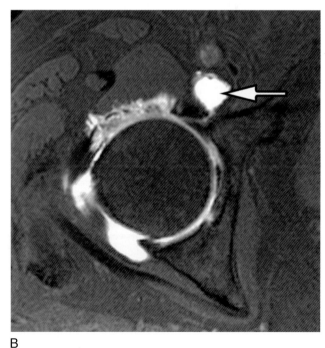

B

Figure 5-7 ■ Communication between the hip joint and the iliopsoas bursa. *A,* Image from a hip injection depicting communication between the hip joint and the iliopsoas bursa. This occurs in up to 15% of patients. *B,* Axial image from an MR arthrogram of the hip depicts intra-articular contrast extending into the iliopsoas bursa *(arrow).* Communication occurs between the iliofemoral and pubofemoral ligaments.

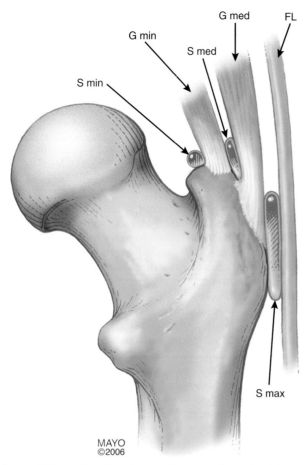

Figure 5-8 ■ Gluteal tendon attachments and associated bursae. G Med = gluteus medius tendon; G min = gluteus minimus tendon; FL = fascia lata; S max = subgluteus maximus bursa; S med = subgluteus medius bursa; S min = subgluteus minimus bursa.

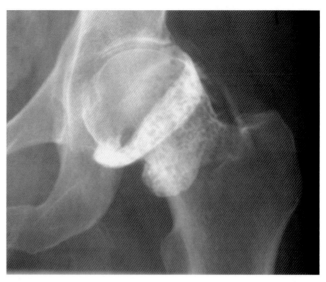

Figure 5-9 ■ Synovial chondromatosis. Image from a conventional arthrogram of the hip depicting innumerable small radiolucent filling defects throughout the hip joint consistent with synovial chondromatosis.

pain related to pathology in the spine.[6] Hip arthrography can be used to diagnose intra-articular pathology.[5] Conventional arthrography has been used previously to evaluate synovial processes and intra-articular loose bodies (Fig. 5-9).[5,11] Today, most hip arthrograms are performed with post-arthrography CT or MR not only to allow more precise identification of synovial pathology including loose bodies but also to demonstrate the cartilaginous structures adjacent to the hip.[7,9] CT or MR arthrography of the hip can be used to reliably evaluate the articular cartilage of the femoral head

attach upon the proximal femur and are associated with bursa juxtaposed between the tendons and the underlying femur (Fig. 5-8).[14,15] The gluteus maximus tendon attaches distally to the gluteal tuberosity of the proximal posterior femur.[14,15] The subgluteus maximus bursa, also referred to as the trochanteric bursa, is a large bursa found beneath the broad distal tendon of the gluteus maximus muscle and the fascia lata.[14,15] The gluteus medius tendon inserts on the superoposterior and lateral facet of the greater trochanter.[14,15] The small subgluteus medius bursa is found deep to the gluteus medius tendon covering portions of the superior facet of the greater trochanter. The gluteus minimus tendon inserts distally on the anterior facet of the greater trochanter of the femur and is associated with a small subgluteus minimus bursa just deep to the tendon.[14,15] The subgluteus minimus bursa covers portions of the anterior facet of the greater trochanter and extends medially, covering the portions of the anterior aspect of the hip joint capsule (see Fig. 5-8).[14,15]

PATIENT SELECTION

There are numerous indications for hip injections and arthrography. Therapeutic hip injections are widely used to alleviate joint pain and to differentiate hip pain from radiating

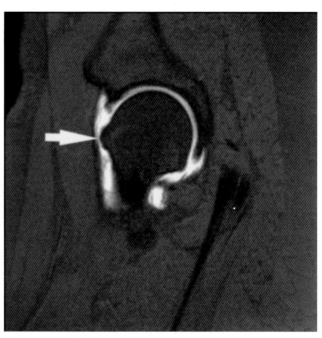

Figure 5-10 ■ Sagittal image from an MR arthrogram of the hip depicting a small osseous protrusion *(arrow)* from the femoral neck in a patient with cam-type femoroacetabular impingement.

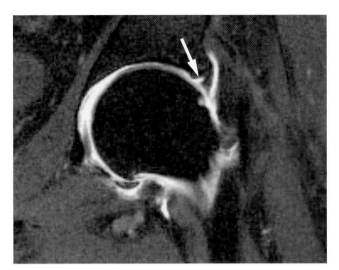

Figure 5-11 ▪ Coronal image from an MR arthrogram of the hip depicting contrast material extending into a rent in the superior acetabular labrum compatible with a superior acetabular labral tear *(arrow)*.

and acetabulum as well as the integrity of the acetabular labrum (Fig. 5-10).[7,8] CT or MR arthrography can also be used to evaluate for findings suggestive of femoroacetabular impingement syndrome (Fig. 5-11).[16,17] In addition to injections, hip aspiration can be performed to evaluate hip joint fluid for crystal deposition disease and to assess for hip joint infection.[5,18] Image-guided interventions play an important role in evaluation of painful hip arthroplasties. Aspiration and conventional arthrography can be performed to evaluate

for infection or loosening of the prosthetic components.[19] Three other diagnostic and therapeutic injections are included in this chapter: trochanteric bursal injections, iliopsoas bursal injections, and pubic symphysis injections.

Therapeutic Hip Injection

Therapeutic hip injections are commonly performed for hip pain.[1,6] Injections typically contain anesthetic agents such as bupivacaine or lidocaine, often in combination with long-acting corticosteroids. Substantial relief can often be obtained with therapeutic hip injections. The duration of pain relief is variable, but occasionally lasting relief can be achieved.

In addition to pain relief, these injections play an important diagnostic role in the evaluation of hip pain. Intra-articular injections of anesthetic agents aid in determining the location of origin of the patient's symptoms.[6] Significant pain relief from an anesthetic injection suggests an intra-capsular origin of the symptoms. Lack of response to diagnostic hip injection suggests an extracapsular etiology of pain such as radicular pain originating from the spine.[6]

MR Arthrography

MR arthrography has proved to be an excellent means for evaluating the articular hyaline and acetabular labral fibro-cartilage of the hip joint (Fig. 5-12).[9,20] Patients with acetabular labral pathology often present with clicking or locking of the hip and mechanical hip pain.[9,21] MR arthrography is most helpful in young and middle-aged patients as most

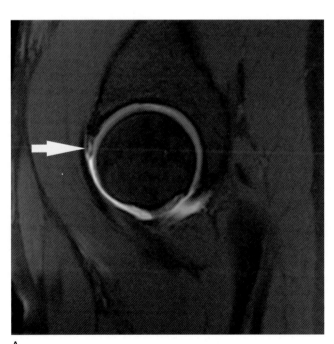

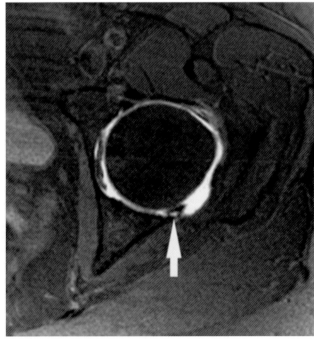

A   B

Figure 5-12 ▪ Acetabular labral tears. Sagittal (*A*) and coronal (*B*) images from MR arthrograms of the hip depicting acetabular labral tears *(arrows)* anteriorly (*A*) and posteriorly (*B*) in two different patients.

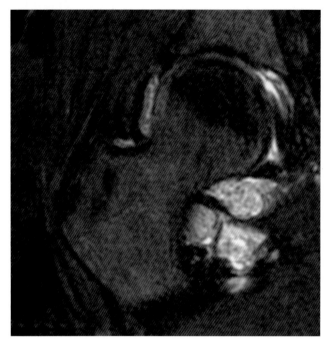

Figure 5-13 ■ Coronal image from an MR arthrogram of the hip in a patient with synovial chondromatosis with innumerable small cartilaginous loose bodies filling the hip joint.

symptomatic labral tears that are surgical candidates occur in this age group (younger than 40 to 50 years of age). Acetabular labral degenerative tearing is common in older patients and is frequently seen in advanced osteoarthritis. Surgical repair is rarely indicated in older individuals, in whom hip pain is often multifactorial and related to osteoarthritis. Articular cartilage wear or focal cartilage defects are well delineated with MR arthrography, which can provide valuable information to the orthopedic surgeon who is contemplating treatment options.[8,20]

MR arthrography can also precisely evaluate and characterize synovial disorders and synovial proliferative processes.[11,22] Synovial proliferative disorders, such as pigmented villonodular synovitis or synovial osteochondromatosis, are well demonstrated with MR arthrography (Fig. 5-13).[11,22] In addition, articular loose bodies can be precisely localized within the joint with post-arthrogram MR. Occasionally, the osseous or chondral donor sites from which the loose body originated can be identified as well.

CT Arthrography

CT arthrography can be substituted for MR arthrography in patients with contraindications to MR imaging or in patients who cannot tolerate the examination. CT arthrography, like MR arthrography, can precisely depict the acetabular labrum.[23] CT arthrography can also characterize the articular cartilage of the femoral head and acetabulum.[24] Synovial proliferative disorders and loose bodies are also well characterized with CT arthrography (Fig. 5-14).[23]

Prosthesis Evaluation

Image-guided interventions play an important role in the evaluation of the painful hip prosthesis. Percutaneous

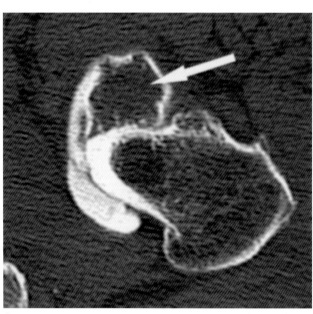

A

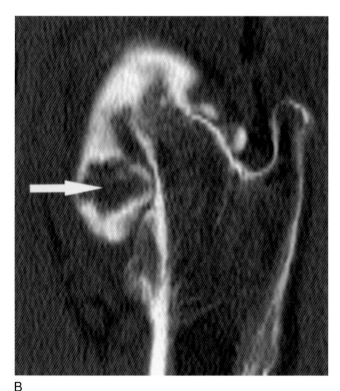

B

Figure 5-14 ■ Axial (*A*) and sagittal (*B*) images from a CT arthrogram of the left hip depicting a large osteocartilaginous loose body within the anterior aspect of the inferior collicular recess of the left hip joint.

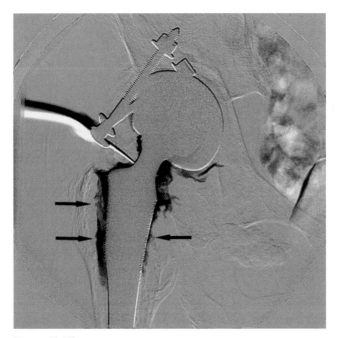

Figure 5-15 ■ Loose femoral component of a hip prosthesis. Digital subtraction image from an arthrogram in a patient with a total hip arthroplasty depicts contrast material *(arrows)* extending about the proximal femoral component compatible with loosening of the prosthesis.

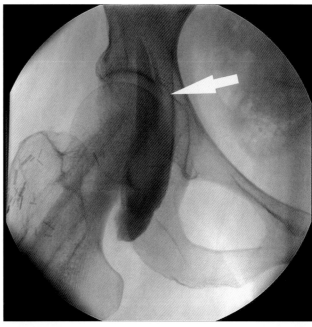

Figure 5-16 ■ Diagnostic and therapeutic injection of the iliopsoas bursa. Patient with snapping iliopsoas tendon syndrome with audible and visual snapping of the iliopsoas tendon during provocative maneuvers as it crosses over the iliopectineal eminence *(arrow)*.

image-guided hip aspiration allows sampling of the joint fluid to evaluate for joint infection.[5,19] Conventional hip arthrography in patients with hip arthroplasties allows evaluation of component loosening by identifying contrast extension about the loose components (Fig. 5-15). Arthrography also allows depiction of bursa formation or sinus tract extension, which can occasionally be seen with an infected prosthesis.[5]

Iliopsoas Bursal Injection

Iliopsoas bursal injections and aspirations can be used for both diagnostic and therapeutic purposes.[11] Diagnostic injections of the iliopsoas bursa can be helpful to identify the etiology of anterior groin and hip pain (Fig. 5-16). Relief following the injection confirms the iliopsoas bursa as the cause, whereas continued symptoms despite the injection suggest another etiology such as the hip or spine. Diagnostic injections can also evaluate snapping iliopsoas tendon syndrome (see Fig. 5-16). Patients with snapping iliopsoas tendon syndrome note pain and audible snapping over the region of the hip related to catching of the iliopsoas tendon as it crosses either the iliopectineal eminence or lesser trochanteric ridge. Following injection of the bursa, with provocative maneuvers, the tendon can often be seen catching, corresponding to the audible and palpable snap.

Aspiration of the iliopsoas bursa can be performed in patients with iliopsoas bursal fluid identified with other imaging modalities.[1,11] This can either be therapeutic, to relieve the tension associated with a distended bursa, or diagnostic, to identify the constituents of the fluid.

Trochanteric Bursal Injection

As with the hip and iliopsoas bursa, the trochanteric bursa can be injected for diagnostic and therapeutic purposes (Fig. 5-17). Trochanteric bursitis is a common source of hip pain.[15] Often this condition is associated with pathology of

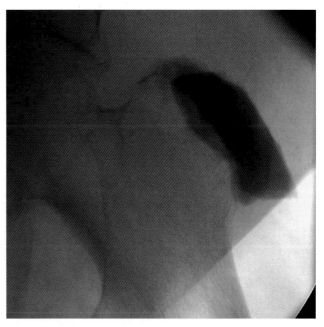

Figure 5-17 ■ Trochanteric bursa injection. Fluoroscopic image following therapeutic injection of the trochanteric bursa.

the distal gluteal tendons at their insertion upon the greater trochanter. Pain relief following trochanteric injections confirms that the bursa is the site of origin for the symptoms, whereas lack of improvement in symptoms suggests an alternative cause of pain, such as hip or iliopsoas bursa pathology. Fluoroscope-guided injections confirm appropriate injection sites and adequate localization of the injection.[18]

Pubic Symphysis Injection

Therapeutic injections can be made into the pubic symphysis for relief of symptoms referable to this articulation (Fig. 5-18).[25] Pubic pain is a common complaint and can be attributed to many causes. Disorders affecting the pubic symphysis include osteitis pubis, degenerative or inflammatory arthropathy, chronic post-traumatic symphysial injury, postpartum symphyseal injury, and parasymphysial insufficiency fractures (Fig. 5-19).[26] Therapeutic injections can relieve pain and confirm the origin of the symptoms in cases of suspected infection or osteomyelitis.[25] Aspiration of the pubic symphysis is performed to evaluate for septic arthritis.

CONTRAINDICATIONS[27]

* Coagulopathy (caution in patients with International Normalized Ratio [INR] >1.5 or platelets < 50,000/mm^3)
* Pregnancy (because of teratogenic effects of radiation)
* Systemic infection or skin infection over the puncture site
* Severe allergy to any component of the injectate
* The patient has received the maximum amount of steroid including systemic steroids allowed for a given time period unless the injection is to be performed without steroid

PROCEDURE

Equipment/Supplies

Procedural

* Spinal needle, 22- or 25-gauge, 3.5-inch (Quincke-type point, Becton Dickinson, Franklin Lakes, NJ)
* Luer-Lock (10- or 20-mL) syringe containing injection mixture
* Sterile tubing to connect injection solution to spinal needle
* Control 12-mL syringe with 25-gauge, 1.5-inch needle containing 8 mL 1% lidocaine for local anesthesia and 2 mL 8.4% sodium bicarbonate injectable (1 mEq/mL) to alleviate burning pain associated with anesthetic
* Sterile 4 × 4 gauze pads
* Povidone-iodine (Betadine) and alcohol for preparation

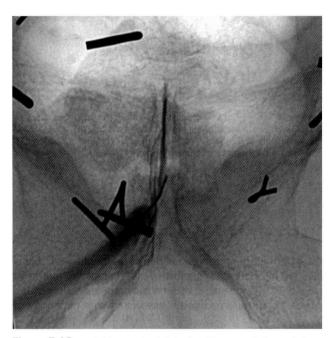

Figure 5-18 ■ Pubic symphysis injection. Fluoroscopic image following a diagnostic and therapeutic injection of the pubic symphysis in a patient with pain following prostatectomy and radiation therapy.

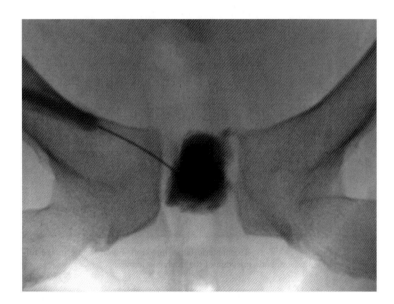

Figure 5-19 ■ Pubic symphysis injection. Therapeutic injection of the pubic symphysis in a patient with diastasis of the pubic symphysis following birth trauma.

- Sterile towels or fenestrated drape for draping
- Needle, 18-gauge, 1.5-inch, to draw up lidocaine and medication
- Sterile gloves
- Adhesive bandage

Medications (Injection Mixtures)

Volume

The typical hip joint total volume is approximately 15 mL.[5,11] A 20-mL syringe is utilized for hip injections.[11] For diagnostic hip injections, 10 to 15 mL is typically injected into the hip.[5,11] For CT or MR arthrography, overdistention of the articulation can lead to leakage from the joint puncture site and possible capsular rupture prior to imaging, which markedly hinders image quality. A volume of 10 to 12 mL is adequate to distend but not overdistend the hip articulation in most patients. The iliopsoas bursa is much more variable in volume. Typically, 5 to 10 mL is utilized for iliopsoas injections.[11] Trochanteric bursal injections require a smaller joint volume, typically about 5 to 10 mL.[18] The pubic symphysis is a very small joint with a volume of approximately 1 mL.[25]

Diagnostic and Therapeutic Hip Injection (Hip Block)

    20-mL syringe
    10 to 15 mL total injected joint volume
    10 mL iodinated contrast (Reno-60, Omnipaque 300)
    8 to 10 mL anesthetic agent (bupivacaine hydrochloride 0.5%,* lidocaine hydrochloride 1% MPF*)
    Optional: 0 to 2 mL steroid (methylprednisolone sodium succinate (Solu-Medrol 40 mg/mL, Depo-Medrol 40 mg/mL), triamcinolone (Kenalog-40), betamethasone sodium phosphate and betamethasone acetate (Celestone Soluspan 6 mg/mL)

CT Arthrography

    20-mL syringe
    10 to 12 mL total injected joint volume
    10 mL iodinated contrast (Reno-60, Omnipaque 300)
    8 to 10 mL anesthetic agent (bupivacaine 0.5%, lidocaine 1%)
    Optional: 0 to 2 mL steroid (Solu-Medrol, Kenalog, Celestone)

MR Arthrography

    20-mL syringe
    10 to 12 mL total injected joint volume
    5 mL iodinated contrast (Reno-60, Omnipaque 300)
    10 mL anesthetic agent (bupivacaine 0.5%, lidocaine 1%)
    5 mL normal saline
    0.1 to 0.2 mL gadopentetate dimeglumine MR contrast (Omniscan, Magnevist)

*Local anesthetics should be from single-use vials and be free of paraben (MPF) and phenol to prevent flocculation of the steroid.[27]

Iliopsoas Bursal Injection

    20-mL syringe
    5 to 10 mL total injected bursal volume
    10 mL iodinated contrast (Reno-60, Omnipaque 300)
    8 to 10 mL anesthetic agent (bupivacaine 0.5%, lidocaine 1%)
    Optional: 0 to 2 mL steroid (Solu-Medrol, Kenalog, Celestone)

Trochanteric Bursal Injection

    20-mL syringe
    5 to 10 mL total injected bursal volume
    10 mL iodinated contrast (Reno-60, Omnipaque 300)
    8 to 10 mL anesthetic agent (bupivacaine 0.5%, lidocaine 1%)
    Optional: 0 to 2 mL steroid (Solu-Medrol, Kenalog, Celestone)

Pubic Symphysis Injection

    10-mL syringe
    1 mL total injected bursal volume
    5 mL iodinated contrast (Reno-60, Omnipaque 300)
    4 to 5 mL anesthetic agent (bupivacaine 0.5%, lidocaine 1%)
    Optional: 0 to 1 mL steroid (Solu-Medrol, Kenalog, Celestone)

Methodology

Hip Joint Injection

Prior to hip joint interventions, routine radiographic images of the hip should be obtained and reviewed.[5] The patient is placed on the fluoroscopy table in the supine position. The fluoroscopic image is collimated to minimize radiation exposure to the surrounding tissues.[5] The solution to be injected into the articulation is then drawn up in a 20-mL syringe.

The hip joint can be entered by one of three approaches.[18] A direct vertical approach can be utilized that targets the lateral aspect of the femoral head-neck junction (Figs. 5-20 and 5-21). Alternatively, a slightly oblique (lateral to medial) vertical approach can be used (see Fig. 5-20).[18] This approach targets the middle to lateral aspect of the femoral head-neck junction (Fig. 5-22). A third lateral approach can be utilized but is not recommended as the needle is placed perpendicular to the fluoroscopic beam, which does not allow as precise needle control. The lateral approach targets the lateral aspect of the femoral head with the needle passing over the greater trochanter (see Fig. 5-20).[18] The direct vertical and oblique vertical approaches are most commonly utilized. The advantage of the vertical approach is that the needle remains parallel to the x-ray fluoroscopic beam. A simple, straight, end-on approach is used to enter the joint. The oblique vertical approach is slightly more challenging; however, this approach is easily mastered. The advantage of the oblique lateral approach is that the femoral neurovascular bundle and lateral femoral cutaneous nerve are

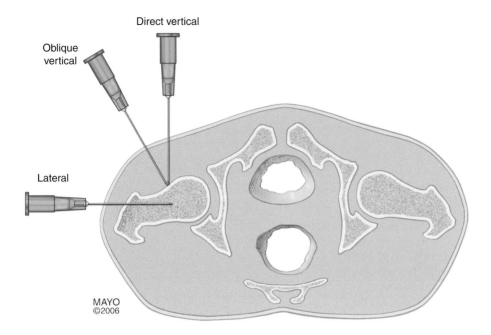

Figure 5-20 ■ Various approaches for access to the hip joint: direct vertical, oblique vertical, and lateral.

avoided, which can occasionally be an issue with direct vertical approaches.

A metallic object such as a set of Kelly clamps should be used to identify the precise location of the injection, and the patient's skin should be marked with an indelible marker. The target site for a hip joint injection is the middle to lateral aspect of the junction of the head and neck of the femur (Fig. 5-23).[18] The anatomy of the hip joint is advantageous for hip injections because the target area suitable for injection is large. Contact anywhere on the head or neck of the proximal femur should result in an intra-articular position of the needle. The middle or lateral aspect of the femur should be targeted to avoid the femoral neurovascular bundle, which is located medially.

The field overlying the target site should then be sterilely prepared and draped. Local anesthesia of the skin and underlying subcutaneous tissue is obtained with 1% lidocaine with 8.4% sodium bicarbonate buffer. A 22-gauge, 3.5-inch spinal needle can then be advanced through the soft tissues overlying the hip articulation until contact is made with the femur. It is not uncommon for the patient to experience discomfort when the needle enters the joint or makes contact with the periosteum of the bone. Fluoroscopy is used to check the needle position. Alterations in needle position can then be made to place the needle at the target site.

When the needle has been properly positioned, the stylet of the spinal needle is withdrawn. The syringe and tubing containing the solution to be injected into the hip joint are

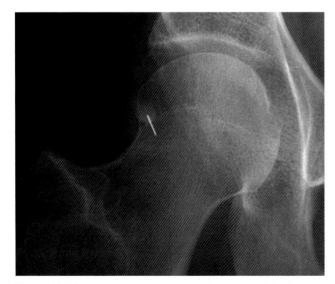

Figure 5-21 ■ Direct vertical approach for hip joint injection. The direct vertical approach targets the lateral aspect of the femoral head-neck junction. The needle is nearly parallel to the fluoroscopic beam, allowing a simple, straight, end-on approach to enter the joint.

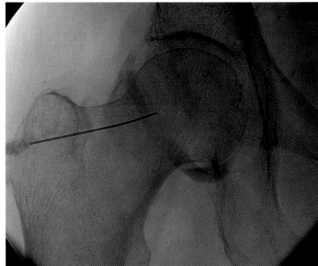

Figure 5-22 ■ Oblique vertical approach for hip joint injection. The needle is oblique (lateral to medial) to the fluoroscopic beam. The target is the middle to lateral aspect of the femoral head-neck junction. The femoral neurovascular bundle and lateral femoral cutaneous nerve are avoided with the oblique vertical approach.

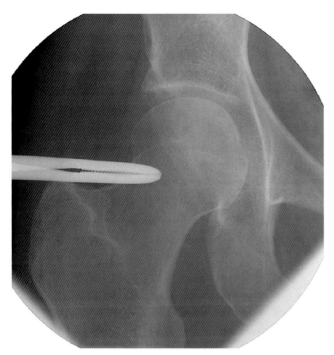

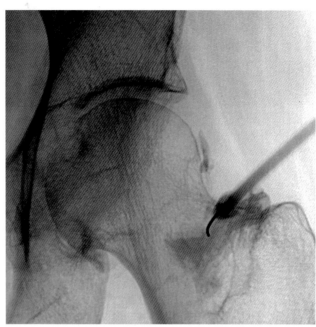

Figure 5-23 ▪ Target site for hip injection. A metallic object such as a Kelly clamp is used to identify the precise location of the injection. The target site for a hip joint injection is the middle to lateral aspect of the junction of the head and neck of the femur.

Figure 5-25 ▪ Extra-articular injection. If contrast material collects at the needle tip, the needle is extra-articular and needs to be repositioned.

then connected to the indwelling needle (Fig. 5-24). A small test injection should be performed to ensure appropriate intra-articular placement of the needle. If resistance to the injection is met, the needle may be embedded in the bone or the capsule may be tented over the needle. Rotating the needle may facilitate penetration of the capsule if it is tented over the needle, and slight withdrawal of the needle may be

helpful if the needle is embedded in the bone. If contrast material collects at the needle tip, the needle is extra-articular and needs to be repositioned (Fig. 5-25). If contrast flows freely away from the needle tip (Fig. 5-26), the injection can be administered. The entire injection should be performed under continuous or intermittent fluoroscopic monitoring to ensure continued intra-articular placement of the needle

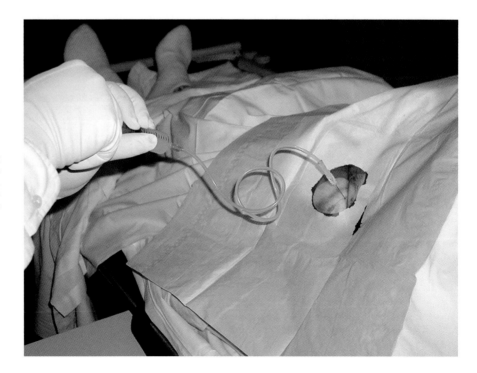

Figure 5-24 ▪ The syringe and tubing containing the solution to be injected are connected to the indwelling needle. A small test injection should be performed to ensure intra-articular placement of the needle.

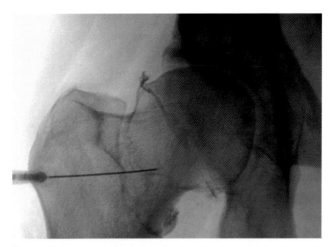

Figure 5-26 ■ If contrast material flows freely away from the needle tip as in this image, the injection can proceed. The entire injection should be performed under continuous or intermittent fluoroscopic monitoring to ensure continued intra-articular placement of the needle throughout the injection and avoid inadvertent extra-articular injection.

throughout the injection and avoid inadvertent extra-articular injection.

The volume of the injection depends upon the indication for the injection. For therapeutic hip injections, 10 to 15 mL is an adequate volume. For CT or MR arthrography, care should be taken to avoid overdistention of the articulation, which could lead to leakage from the joint puncture site or possible capsular rupture prior to imaging, which markedly hinders image quality with both MR and CT (Fig. 5-27). A volume of 10 to 12 mL is adequate to distend but not overly distend the hip joint. For CT and MR arthrography, movement of the joint should be kept to a minimum to avoid

extravasation from the joint prior to imaging. The patient should be transferred to the CT or MR scanner with an MR-compatible wheelchair.

Hip Joint Aspiration

Hip joint aspiration is very similar to hip joint injection; however, when the needle is in place, a 60-mL syringe and tubing are connected to the needle and aspiration of the joint is performed. Most hip aspirations in adults are performed in patients with hip arthroplasties for the evaluation of joint infection.[19] The target site for a prosthesis aspiration is just posterolateral to the junction of the head and neck of the femoral component (Fig. 5-28). For aspiration of hip arthroplasties, an oblique vertical approach facilitates entry into the pseudocapsule posteriorly (Fig. 5-29). Often the needle strikes the anterior or lateral aspects of the neck first. Attempts can be made to aspirate as soon as contact is made with the prosthesis. If they are unsuccessful, placement of the needle toward the posterolateral aspect of the femoral prosthetic component is often necessary because fluid tends to collect posteriorly with the patient supine. If no fluid can be withdrawn, repositioning of the needle along the lateral aspect of the femoral head and neck can be helpful. If still no fluid can be aspirated, nonbacteriostatic saline is injected into the joint and then reaspirated. Nonbacteriostatic saline is drawn up into a separate 20-mL syringe and tubing, and 10 mL is administered into the joint through the indwelling needle. The syringe and connecting tube are then exchanged for the 60-mL syringe and new connecting tube and the nonbacteriostatic saline is reaspirated.

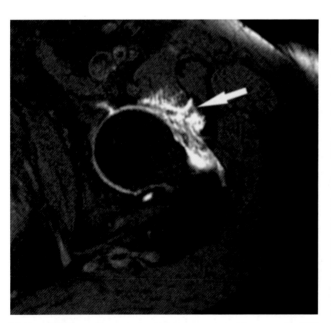

Figure 5-27 ■ Extravasation of contrast material seen with MR arthrography. Care should be taken to avoid overdistention of the joint for MR or CT arthrography as this can lead to leakage from the joint puncture site *(arrow)* or possible capsular rupture, which markedly hinders image quality with both MR and CT.

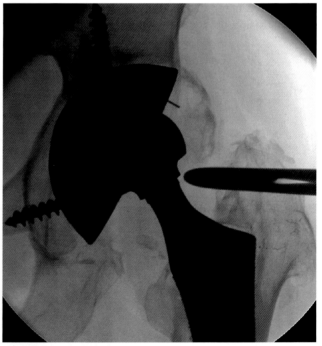

Figure 5-28 ■ Target site for aspiration and injection of hip prosthesis. The target site for a hip prosthesis is the posterolateral aspect of the junction of the head and neck of the femoral component (indicated by tip of Kelly clamp), which is where fluid tends to pool in the pseudocapsule with the patient in the supine position.

subtraction imaging subtracts the cement, allowing better visualization of the injection solution and more precise evaluation of loosening of the prosthesis (Fig. 5-31).

Volume of the injection varies. Typically, 10 to 15 mL is adequate; however, if a bursal formation is present, a greater volume may be necessary. Following the injection, the needle is withdrawn. Additional fluoroscopic evaluation and spot images of the joint may be useful with positioning of the leg in both internal and external rotation as well as abduction to evaluate the prosthesis completely.

Iliopsoas Bursal Injection

Prior to injection, examination of the patient is often helpful to evaluate for snapping of the iliopsoas tendon or to identify specific positions that exacerbate the patient's symptoms. The patient is placed on the fluoroscopy table in the supine position with the leg in neutral position.

The target site for entering the iliopsoas bursa is the superomedial aspect of the femoral head (Fig. 5-32). Care

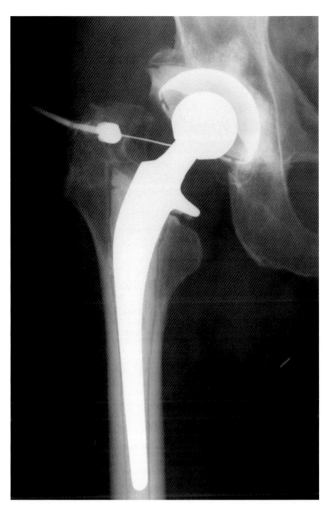

Figure 5-29 ■ An oblique vertical approach facilitates entry into the pseudocapsule for hip prosthesis injections or aspirations. The target is the posterolateral aspect of the head-neck junction of the femoral component, which is where fluid tends to pool with the patient supine.

The aspirated fluid or nonbacteriostatic saline wash is sent for aerobic and anaerobic culture. If enough fluid is present, Gram stain and additional analysis of the fluid can be performed, depending upon the specific clinical situation.

Conventional Hip Arthrography

Conventional hip arthrography is most useful for evaluation of a suspected loosened hip prosthesis. Arthrography is typically performed following hip aspiration as described previously. Before placing the needle, the injection solution should be drawn up into a 20-mL syringe and connected to sterile extension tubing. The same solution used for hip injection is sufficient for hip arthrography.

For hip prosthesis evaluation, an injection using digital subtraction imaging may be helpful. With standard fluoroscopic imaging, the dense contrast material is often difficult to differentiate from the dense cement about the components (Fig. 5-30). This can result in difficulty distinguishing areas of subtle loosening from normal radiopaque cement. Digital

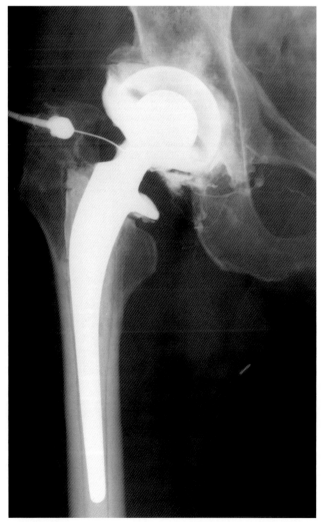

Figure 5-30 ■ Hip prosthesis joint injection. With standard fluoroscopic imaging, the dense contrast material is often difficult to differentiate from the dense cement about the components, which can result in difficulty distinguishing areas of subtle loosening from normal radiopaque cement.

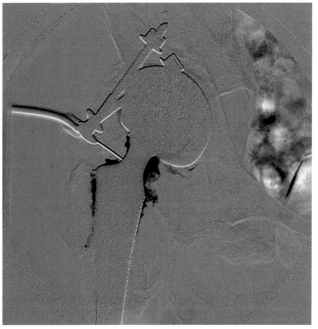

A

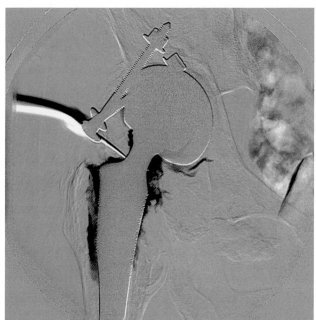

B

Figure 5-31 ■ Sequential digital subtraction imaging during hip prosthesis injection (*A*, *B*, and *C*). Digital subtraction technique subtracts the cement, allowing better visualization of the injection solution and more precise evaluation of loosening of the prosthesis. Note the widened contrast-filled space indicative of loosening of the proximal femoral component.

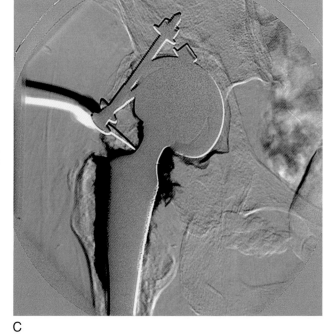

C

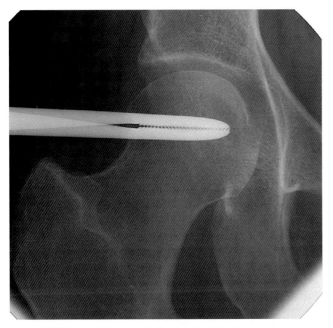

Figure 5-32 ▪ The target site for entering the iliopsoas bursa is the superomedial aspect of the femoral head, indicated by the tip of the clamp.

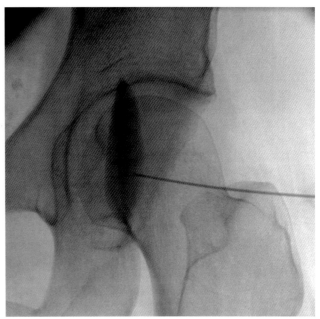

Figure 5-34 ▪ Iliopsoas bursa injection. Contrast material should flow away from the needle tip in a vertical fashion as in this image if the needle is within the bursa. The bursa volume is variable but is typically 5 to 10 mL.

should be taken to palpate and locate the femoral neurovascular bundle to avoid inadvertent puncture of these structures. A slight oblique vertical approach may be helpful to avoid the femoral neurovascular bundle.

The field should then be prepared and draped in the usual sterile fashion. Local anesthesia of the skin and underlying subcutaneous tissue is obtained with 1% lidocaine with 8.4% sodium bicarbonate buffer. A 0.5- or 1.5-inch, 25-gauge needle is used to anesthetize the skin and entry site. A 22-gauge, 3.5-inch spinal needle is advanced through the soft tissues until contact is made with the surface of the femur (Fig. 5-33). Withdrawal of the needle approximately 5 mm usually places the needle in the region of the bursa.

The syringe and tubing containing the solution to be injected are connected to the indwelling needle. A small test injection should be performed to ensure appropriate intrabursal placement of the needle. Repositioning of the needle is often needed to locate the bursa precisely. If contrast material collects at the needle tip, the needle is extrabursal and needs to be repositioned. Contrast should flow away from the needle tip in a vertical fashion if the bursa is penetrated (Fig. 5-34).[1] The bursal volume is variable, but typically an injection of about 5 to 10 mL should be adequate to distend and visualize the bursa. The entire injection should be performed under continuous fluoroscopic monitoring (Fig. 5-35). The iliopsoas bursa reportedly communicates

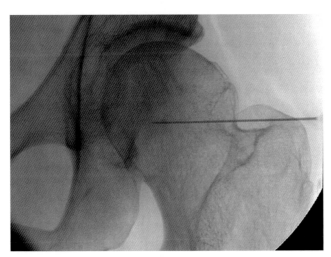

Figure 5-33 ▪ A 22-gauge spinal needle inserted using an oblique vertical approach to the region of the iliopsoas bursa anterior to the medial aspect of the femoral head.

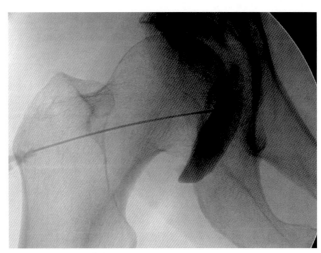

Figure 5-35 ▪ Iliopsoas bursa injection. The iliopsoas bursa is vertically oriented anterior to the hip joint along the iliopsoas muscle and tendon.

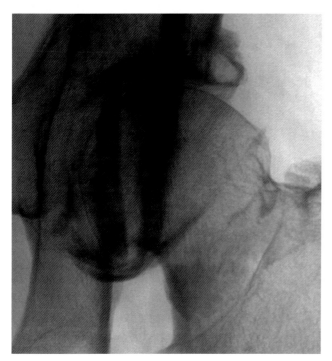

Figure 5-36 ■ Communication of the iliopsoas bursa with the hip joint following an iliopsoas bursa injection.

with the hip joint in approximately 15% of cases,[11] although we observe this communication less commonly in our experience (Fig. 5-36).

Following the injection, the needle is withdrawn. Fluoroscopic evaluation of the bursa should then be per-

formed with a spot film obtained when appropriate. Video fluoroscopy may also be useful. Provocative maneuvers such as external rotation or flexion and abduction should be performed to evaluate for catching of the iliopsoas on the iliopectineal eminence or lesser trochanteric ridge.

Greater Trochanteric Bursal Injection

The patient should be placed on the fluoroscopy table in the supine position. The solution to be injected into the articulation should then be drawn up into a 10-mL syringe. A direct lateral approach or oblique lateral (anterior to posterior) approach should be utilized. The target is the lateral aspect of the greater trochanter (Fig. 5-37).[10]

The field should then be prepared and draped in the usual fashion. Local anesthesia of the skin and underlying subcutaneous tissue is obtained with 1% lidocaine with 8.4% sodium bicarbonate buffer. A 1.5-inch, 25-gauge needle is used to anesthetize the skin. A 3.5-inch, 22-gauge spinal needle can be advanced through the soft tissues lateral to the greater trochanter until contact is made with bone (Fig. 5-38). It is not uncommon for the patient to experience discomfort when the needle enters the joint or makes contact with the periosteum of the bone. Fluoroscopy is then used to check the needle position and alterations in needle position can be made. When contact is made with the bone, the needle is withdrawn 1 to 2 cm and the syringe and tubing containing the solution to be injected are connected to the needle. A small test injection should be performed to ensure appropriate intra-articular placement of the needle (Fig. 5-39). The volume of the trochanteric bursa is variable; however, a 5- to 10-mL injection volume is typically adequate (Fig. 5-40). Following the injection, the needle is withdrawn.

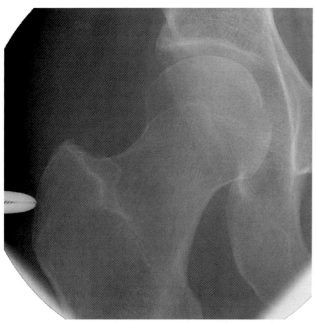

Figure 5-37 ■ The target site for trochanteric bursa injection is the lateral aspect of the greater trochanter, as indicated by the tip of the clamp.

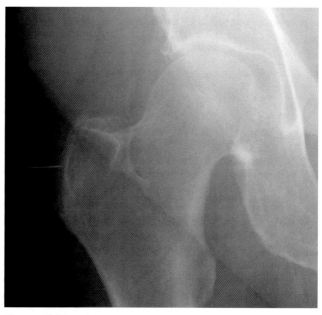

Figure 5-38 ■ Trochanteric bursa injection. A 3.5-inch, 22-gauge spinal needle is inserted into the soft tissues lateral to the greater trochanter until contact is made with bone.

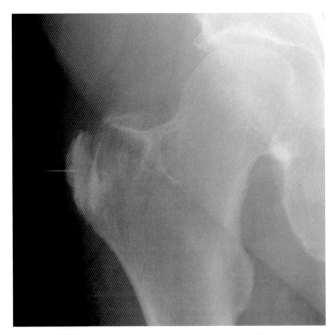

Figure 5-39 ■ Trochanteric bursa injection. A small test injection should be performed to ensure appropriate placement of the needle within the trochanteric bursa.

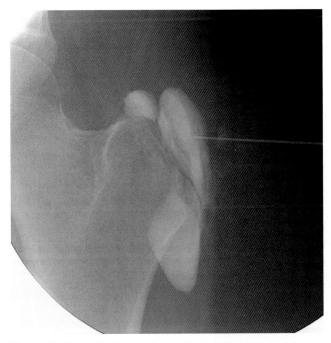

Figure 5-40 ■ Trochanteric bursa injection. The volume of the trochanteric bursa is variable, although 5 to 10 mL is typical.

Pubic Symphysis Injection

The patient should be placed on the fluoroscopy table in the supine position. Additional preliminary fluoroscopic evaluation of the pubic symphysis should be performed, and the fluoroscopic image should be collimated to minimize radiation exposure to the surrounding tissues. The solution to be injected into the articulation should then be drawn up into a 10-mL syringe. An anterior approach is utilized for the pubic symphysis injection.[25] It is often beneficial to angle the x-ray tube, above the patient, slightly cephalad to caudad to facilitate the injection.

The field should then be prepared and draped in a sterile fashion. Local anesthesia of the skin and underlying subcutaneous tissue is obtained with 1% lidocaine with 8.4% sodium bicarbonate buffer. A 1.5-inch, 25-gauge needle used to anesthetize the skin can be left at the puncture site and disconnected from the syringe. This can then be utilized to gauge the position of the planned puncture site relative to the target site (Fig. 5-41). If the planned puncture site is concordant with the target site, the 1.5-inch, 25-gauge needle can be advanced through the soft tissues overlying the pubic symphysis into the symphyseal space. Fluoroscopy is utilized to check the needle position. Alterations in needle position can then be made. The articulation between the pubic bones is usually very narrow. If the pubic symphysis is significantly widened, it is helpful to advance the needle down onto the margin of the pubic bone to judge the depth of the articulation. The needle can be advanced slightly medially to enter the joint just deep to the anterior margin of the pubic bones. When the needle has been properly positioned, the syringe and tubing containing the solution to be injected are connected to the indwelling 25-gauge needle (Fig. 5-42). A small test injection should be performed to ensure appropriate intra-articular placement of the needle (Fig. 5-43). Typically, the joint is very small in volume and

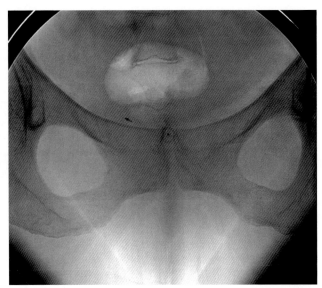

Figure 5-41 ■ Pubic symphysis injection. A 1.5-inch, 25-gauge needle is used to anesthetize the skin and can be left in place to gauge the position of the planned puncture site relative to the target.

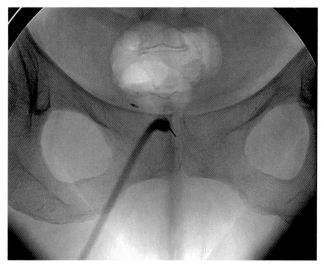

Figure 5-42 ■ Pubic symphysis injection. The 1.5-inch, 25-gauge needle is advanced into the symphyseal space and the syringe and tubing containing the injection solution are connected to the needle.

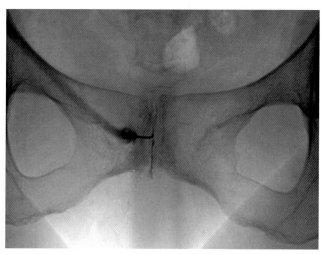

Figure 5-44 ■ Pubic symphysis injection. The pubic symphysis is typically very low in volume, requiring only a 1- to 2-mL injection.

resistance to injection is encountered. Imaging must be used to confirm proper position. If contrast material collects at the needle tip, the needle is extra-articular and needs to be repositioned. If contrast flows away from the needle tip in a linear fashion along the joint line, the remainder of the injection is made (Fig. 5-44). The pubic symphysis is typically very low in volume, requiring only a 1-mL injection.[25] The entire injection should be performed under continuous fluoroscopic monitoring. Following the injection, the needle is withdrawn.

POTENTIAL COMPLICATIONS[27]

- Bleeding
- Infection (cellulitis, septic arthritis, or osteomyelitis)
- Drug-related allergic reactions
- Transient synovitis
- Transitory lower extremity weakness
- Transitory lower extremity paresthesia
- Femoral artery or vein injury

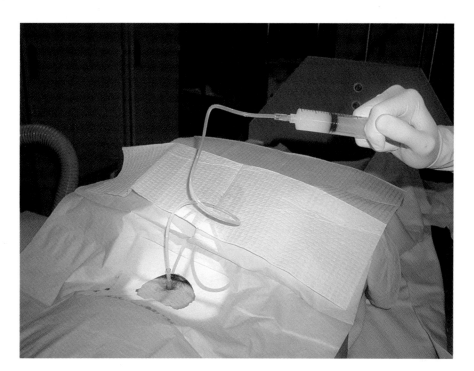

Figure 5-43 ■ Pubic symphysis injection. A small test injection is performed to ensure appropriate intra-articular placement of the needle. Typically, the joint is very small in volume and resistance to injection is encountered.

POST-PROCEDURE CARE/FOLLOW-UP[27]

Immediate

1. The patient should be observed for 15 minutes following the injection.
2. Blood pressure, pulse, heart rate, and respiratory rate are monitored as necessary.

Discharge

1. An adhesive bandage may be placed on the puncture site. The bandage should remain dry for at least 24 hours, at which point it can be removed.
2. The patient is instructed to continue taking his or her prescription medication, although pain medication may be tapered as indicated.
3. A discharge sheet should be given to the patient outlining the following:
   a. The procedure performed
   b. Procedure-related symptoms that typically resolve in 7 to 10 days
      * Pain at the needle puncture site(s)
      * Mild increase in stiffness with a feeling of fullness in the joint
      * Deep hip pain
   c. Treatment for mild post-procedure symptoms
      * Rest the hip for 1 to 2 days
      * Avoid movements that worsen the pain
      * Use cold compresses to the area that hurts
   d. Signs and symptoms of infection
      * Fever
      * Chills
      * Swelling or drainage from the puncture site(s)
      * New hip pain that is different from the usual pain
   e. Signs and symptoms of possible more serious problems
      * Decreased range of motion of the hip
      * Increasing pain
      * Motor dysfunction of the upper extremity
   f. Physician name and contact number if the patient has any concerns or if any problems were to arise as a result of the procedure
   g. Advice to schedule a follow-up appointment with the referring physician in 7 to 10 days.

SAMPLE DICTATIONS

Hip MR Arthrogram

After the procedure was explained to the patient and informed consent was obtained, the patient was placed on the table in the supine position. The skin overlying the hip joint was prepared and draped in the usual sterile fashion. Local anesthesia was obtained with 1% lidocaine with bicarbonate buffer. Under fluoroscopic guidance, a 22-gauge, 3.5-inch spinal needle was advanced into the hip joint and a 12-mL solution containing bupivacaine, Omnipaque 300, saline, and 0.1 mL Omniscan was administered into the hip joint. The needle was withdrawn. The patient was sent to MR for additional imaging of the hip after arthrography.

Trochanteric Bursal Injection

After the procedure was explained to the patient and informed consent was obtained, the patient was placed on the table in the supine position. The skin overlying the trochanteric bursa was sterilely prepared and draped in the usual fashion. Local anesthesia was obtained with 1% lidocaine with bicarbonate buffer. Under fluoroscopic guidance, a 22-gauge, 3.5-inch spinal needle was advanced into the trochanteric bursa and a 9-mL solution containing Omnipaque 300, bupivacaine, and Kenalog was administered into the bursa. The needle was withdrawn. The patient reported moderate relief of symptoms immediately following the injection.

Pubic Symphysis Injection

After the procedure was explained to the patient and informed consent was obtained, the patient was placed on the table in the supine position. The skin overlying the pubic symphysis was sterilely prepared and draped in the usual fashion. Local anesthesia was obtained with 1% lidocaine with bicarbonate buffer. Under fluoroscopic guidance, a 25-gauge, 3.5-inch spinal needle was advanced into the pubic symphysis and a 5-mL solution containing Omnipaque 300, bupivacaine, and Kenalog was administered. The needle was withdrawn. Post-injection fluoroscopic evaluation was performed and a spot film was obtained.

CASE REPORTS

CASE 1

Clinical Presentation

A 16-year-old female presented with chronic left hip pain. The pain was described as a dull ache. The patient also complained of clicking or popping in the left hip with provocative maneuvers and felt that the hip was "catching." Physical examination demonstrated slightly decreased range of motion with a positive impingement test with sharp pain evoked with flexion, adduction, and internal rotation of the hip.

Imaging and Therapy

Routine radiographs depicted no abnormalities and no evidence of dysplasia of the hip. MR arthrography revealed a complex tear of the anterosuperior aspect of the acetabular labrum (Fig. 5-45). This was associated with a small bony prominence on the anterior neck of the femur (see Fig. 5-45). Findings were compatible with cam-type femoroacetabular impingement with resultant anterosuperior acetabular labral tear.

 The patient was taken to surgery. During intraoperative provocative maneuvering of the hip, the bony prominence on the anterior femoral neck clearly impinged upon the anterosuperior acetabular labrum in the exact area where the labrum was torn. The bony prominence was subsequently removed using osteotomes and the bed was contoured with a burr. The anterosuperior labrum was then resected and debrided. Following these steps, the hip demonstrated no evidence of impingement even with maximum provocative maneuvers.

Results

The patient did very well following surgery with complete relief of the previously noted hip pain and no recurrence of the previously experienced mechanical symptoms.

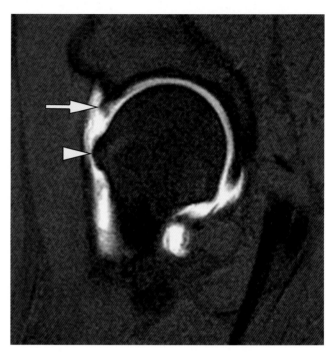

Figure 5-45 ■ Coronal image from an MR arthrogram depicting a complex macerated tear of the anterosuperior acetabular labrum *(arrow)*. This resulted from cam-type femoroacetabular impingement related to a small bony prominence on the anterior neck of the femur *(arrowhead)*.

CASE 2

Clinical Presentation

A 32-year-old woman presented with pubic pain and incontinence following a difficult childbirth 1 year previously. Physical examination of the pubic region revealed palpable separation of the pubic symphysis with pain upon provocative pelvic motion. Urodynamic testing revealed stress incontinence with disordered voiding.

Imaging and Therapy

Radiographs demonstrated widening of the pubic symphysis. To confirm the origin of pain, a diagnostic and therapeutic injection of the pubic symphysis was performed. A 25-gauge needle was advanced into the pubic symphyseal cleft, which was abnormally widened. A volume of 2 mL of a mixture containing iodinated contrast material, bupivacaine, and corticosteroid was injected (Fig. 5-46). The patient reported approximately 3 weeks of near-complete relief of pain following the injection.

The patient subsequently underwent open reduction and internal fixation of the pubic symphysis diastasis with malleable plate and screws and bone graft placement. A pelvic sling procedure was performed at the same time to correct the patient's urinary incontinence.

Results

The patient's pain and pelvic instability completely resolved following operative fixation of the pubic symphysis diastasis. Urinary stress incontinence also resolved after the sling procedure.

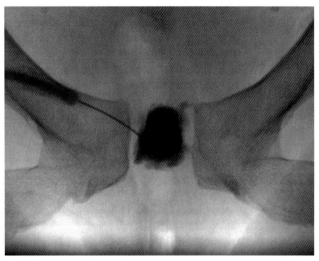

Figure 5-46 ■ Diagnostic and therapeutic injection of the pubic symphysis in a young female patient with diastasis of the pubic symphysis following birth trauma.

CURRENT PROCEDURAL TERMINOLOGY (CPT) CODES[28]

CPT codes change often and sometimes are valid only for certain states or regions. It is best to consult with coding experts to make sure that coding for one's procedures is legitimate and complete. Below is a sample of codes that are being used for hip injection procedures at this writing.

20610 Arthrocentesis, aspiration and/or injection; major joint or bursa (e.g., shoulder, hip, knee joint, subacromial bursa)

(If imaging guidance is performed, see 76942, 77002, 77012, 77021)

27093 Injection procedure for hip arthrography; without anesthesia

(For radiologic supervision and interpretation, use 73525. Do not report 77002 in addition to 73525)

27095 with anesthesia

(For radiologic supervision and interpretation, use 73525. Do not report 77002 in addition to 73525)

27599 Unlisted procedure, femur or knee

73500 Radiologic examination, hip, unilateral; one view

73510 complete, minimum of two views

73520 Radiologic examination, hips, bilateral, minimum of two views of each hip, including anteroposterior view of pelvis

73525 Radiologic examination, hip, arthrography, radiologic supervision and interpretation

(Do not report 73525 in conjunction with 77002)

73700 Computed tomography, lower extremity; without contrast material

73701 with contrast material(s)

73702 without contrast material, followed by contrast material(s) and further sections

(To report 3D rendering, see 76376, 76377

76376 3D rendering with interpretation and reporting of computed tomography, magnetic resonance imaging, ultrasound, or other tomographic modality; not requiring image postprocessing on an independent workstation

(Use 76376 in conjunction with code(s) for base imaging procedure(s))

(Do not report 76376 in conjunction with 70496, 70498, 70544-70549, 71275, 71555, 72159, 72191, 72198, 73206, 73225, 73706, 73725, 74175, 74185, 75635, 76377, 78000–78999, 0066T, 0067T, 0144T–0151T)

76377 requiring image postprocessing on an independent workstation

(Use 76377 in conjunction with code(s) for base imaging procedure(s))

Do not report 76377 in conjunction with 70496, 70498, 70544–70549, 71275, 71555, 72159, 72191, 72198, 73206, 73225, 73706, 73725,

74175, 74185, 75635, 76376, 78000-78999, 0066T, 0067T, 0144T-0151T)

76942 Ultrasonic guidance for needle placement (e.g., biopsy, aspiration, injection, localization device), imaging supervision and interpretation

(Do not report 76942 in conjunction with 43232, 43237, 43242, 45341, 45342, or 76975)

77002 Fluoroscopic guidance for needle placement (e.g., biopsy, aspiration, injection, localization device)

(See appropriate surgical code for procedure and anatomic location)

(77002 includes all radiographic arthrography with the exception of supervision and interpretation for CT and MR arthrography)

(Do not report 77002 in addition to 70332, 73040, 73085, 73115, 73525, 73580, 73615)

77012 Computed tomography guidance for needle placement (e.g., biopsy, aspiration, injection, localization device), radiological supervision and interpretation

77021 Magnetic resonance guidance for needle placement (e.g., for biopsy, needle aspiration, injection, or placement of localization device) radiologic supervision and interpretation

References

1. Aliabadi P, Baker ND, Jaramillo D. Hip arthrography, aspiration, block, and bursography. Radiol Clin North Am 1998; 36:673–690.
2. Severin E. Arthrography in congenital dislocation of the hip. J Bone Joint Surg Am 1939; 21:304.
3. Ozonoff MB. Controlled arthrography of the hip: A technique of fluoroscopic monitoring and recording. Clin Orthop Relat Res 1973; 93:260–264.
4. Razzano CD, Nelson CL, Wilde AH. Arthrography of the adult hip. Clin Orthop Relat Res 1974; 99:86–94.
5. Freiberger RH, Kaye JJ. Arthrography. Norwalk, CT: Appleton Century Crofts, 1979, pp 1–3, 189–235.
6. Kleiner JB, Thorne RP, Curd JG. The value of bupivacaine hip injection in the differentiation of coxarthrosis from lower extremity neuropathy. J Rheumatol 1991; 18:422–427.
7. Klein A, Sumner TE, Volberg FM. Combined CT-arthrography in recurrent traumatic hip dislocation. AJR Am J Roentgenol 1982; 138:963–964.
8. Petersilge CA. Chronic adult hip pain: MR arthrography of the hip. Radiographics 2000; 20:S43–S52.
9. Petersilge CA. MR arthrography for evaluation of the acetabular labrum. Skeletal Radiol 2001; 30:423–430.
10. Berquist TH. MRI of the Musculoskeletal System, 5th ed. Philadelphia: Lippincott Williams & Wilkins, 2006, pp 195-291.
11. Resnick D. Diagnosis of Bone and Joint Disorders, 4th ed. Philadelphia: WB Saunders, 2002, pp 193–318, 3146–3166.
12. Haims A, Katz LD, Busconi B. MR arthrography of the hip. Radiol Clin North Am 1998; 36:691–702.
13. Steinbach LS, Palmer WE, Schweitzer ME. MR arthrography. Radiographics 2002; 22:1223–1246.
14. Kingzett-Taylor A, Tirman PFJ, Feller J, et al. Tendinosis and tears of gluteus medius and minimus muscles as a cause of hip pain: MR imaging findings. AJR Am J Roentgenol 1999; 173:1123–1126.
15. Pfirrmann CWA, Chung CB, Theumann NH, et al. Greater trochanter of the hip: Attachment of the abductor mechanism and complex of three bursae—MR imaging and MR bursography in cadavers and MR imaging in asymptomatic volunteers. Radiology 2001; 221:469–477.
16. Kassarjian A, Yoon LS, Belzile E, et al. Triad of MR arthrographic findings in patients with cam-type femoroacetabular impingement. Radiology 2005; 236:588–592.
17. Leunig M, Bec M, Kim YJ, et al. Fibrocystic changes at anterosuperior femoral neck: Prevalence in hips with femoroacetabular impingement. Radiology 2005; 236:237–246.
18. Berquist TH. Diagnostic and therapeutic injections as an aid to musculoskeletal diagnosis. Semin Interv Radiol 1993; 10:326–344.
19. Barrack RL, Harris WH. The value of aspiration of the hip joint before revision total hip arthroplasty. J Bone Joint Surg Am 1993; 75:66–76.
20. Schmid MR, Notzli HP, Zanetti M, et al. Cartilage lesions in the hip: Diagnostic effectiveness of MR arthrography. Radiology 2003; 226:382–386.
21. Farjo LA, Glick JM, Sampson TG. Hip arthroscopy for acetabular labral tears. Arthroscopy 1999; 15:132–137.
22. Ghebontni L, Roger B, El-Khoury J, et al. MR arthrography of the hip: Normal intra-articular structures and common disorders. Eur Radiol 2000; 10:83–88.
23. Hodge JC. Musculoskeletal Imaging: Diagnostic and Therapeutic Procedures. Montreal: Karger Landes Systems, 1997, pp 55-71.
24. Nishii T, Tanaka H, Nakanishi K, et al. Fat-suppressed 3D spoiled gradient-echo MRI and MDCT arthrography of articular cartilage in patients with hip dysplasia. AJR Am J Roentgenol 2005; 185:379–385.
25. O'Connell MJ, Powell T, McCaffrey NM, et al. Symphyseal cleft injection in the diagnosis and treatment of osteitis pubis in athletes. AJR Am J Roentgenol 2002; 179:955-959.
26. Gibbon WW, Hession PR. Diseases of the pubis and pubic symphysis: MR imaging appearances. AJR Am J Roentgenol 1997; 169:849–853.
27. Fenton DS, Czervionke LF. Image Guided Spine Intervention. Philadelphia: WB Saunders, 2003.
28. CPT 2007, CPT Intellectual Property Services. Chicago: American Medical Association, 2007.

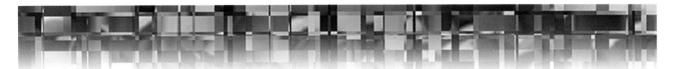

A Hip Surgeon's Perspective

Hip Injections

Gavan P. Duffy, MD

As a hip surgeon, I frequently utilize hip injections both to diagnose disorders involving the hip joint and for therapeutic relief of symptoms related to the hip. In the young patient with unremarkable hip radiographs, MR arthrography is useful to diagnose intra-articular hip pathology such as synovial diseases or loose bodies. MR arthrography is also excellent for the diagnosis of labral tears. These disease processes can be surgically treated with hip arthroscopy. Surgical treatment of femoroacetabular impingement is also more common now as this disorder is becoming more recognized. MR arthrography is often very helpful in diagnosing femoroacetabular impingement and delineating the area of impingement usually associated with an acetabular labral tear.

In the older patient with more advanced arthritic conditions of the hip, hip injections with anesthetic agents combined with long-acting corticosteroids are very helpful as both a therapeutic and diagnostic procedure. In older medically compromised patients, pain relief can be substantial and long-lasting. From a diagnostic side, useful information can be obtained to help distinguish back pain with radicular symptoms from true hip pain. The patient needs to document the pain relief clearly and evaluate the effect of the injection.

All patients undergoing revision total hip arthroplasty in my practice have a preoperative hip aspiration for culture and sensitivity. In diagnosing a painful total hip, hip arthrography can be helpful in looking at a loose prosthesis or extent of osteolytic bursal sac around the hip. Iliopsoas bursal injections can localize pain to that bursa in both the natural hip and a total hip arthroplasty. With a malpositioned acetabular component, the anterior lip of the component can impinge on the iliopsoas tendon, causing pain.

Good communication and a team approach between the surgeon and the proceduralist are critical to ensure that the correct procedure is performed for each patient and the maximum benefit from hip joint interventions is achieved.

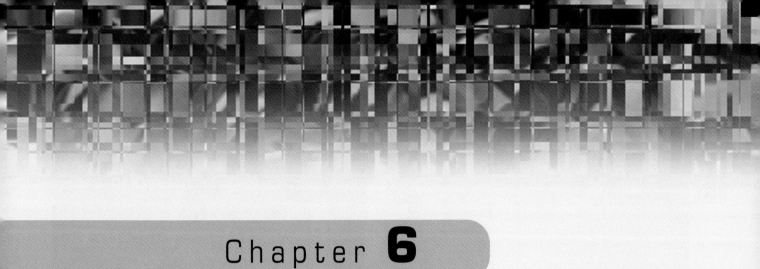

Chapter 6

Knee Injections

- Jeffrey J. Peterson, MD

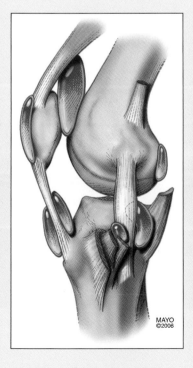

MAYO
©2006

BACKGROUND

Reports describing arthrography of the knee joint date back to 1905.[1,2] Initially, single-contrast techniques were utilized for conventional knee arthrography. However, double-contrast knee arthrographic techniques proved to be superior for evaluation of the menisci and articular cartilage.[1,3] For several decades, double-contrast conventional knee arthrography was the standard procedure for detection of internal derangement of the knee (Fig. 6-1).[1,3] Although conventional double-contrast knee arthrography proved examiner dependent and labor intensive, diagnostic accuracy of greater than 90% was reported for detection of meniscal pathology when performed by experienced radiologists (Fig. 6-2).[1,4]

The introduction of cross-sectional imaging in the 1970s and 1980s had a dramatic effect on knee arthrography. This began with the introduction of computed tomography (CT); however, preliminary evaluation of unenhanced CT of the knee met with mixed results.[1,5] It was not until the introduction of magnetic resonance (MR) in the 1980s that cross-sectional imaging could rival conventional knee arthrography.[6] Soon thereafter, indications for conventional knee arthrography rapidly diminished as MR produced multiplanar images with excellent spatial resolution and soft tissue contrast.[1,6] At present, conventional MR imaging of the knee has completely replaced conventional arthrography for the evaluation of internal derangement of the knee.

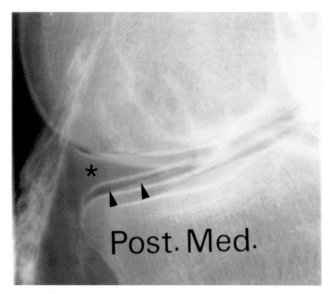

Figure 6-1 ■ Double-contrast conventional knee arthrogram depicting the intact posterior horn of the medial meniscus *(asterisk)* and underlying tibial articular hyaline cartilage *(arrowheads)*.

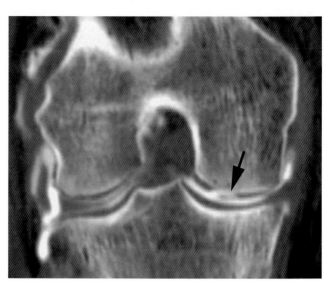

Figure 6-3 ■ CT arthrography of the knee. Coronal reformatted image depicts a focal flap tear of the articular hyaline cartilage of the medial femoral condyle *(arrow)*.

In the 1990s, knee arthrography followed by CT or MR was introduced for specific clinical circumstances. For patients with contraindications to MR imaging such as pacemakers, intraorbital metal, or patients who cannot tolerate MR imaging because of claustrophobia, CT arthrography provides a suitable alternative. CT arthrography of the knee with multiplanar reformatted images provides an effective technique for evaluation of the menisci and articular cartilage of the knee (Fig. 6-3).[7,8] MR arthrography of the knee has proved very useful for evaluation of the postoperative meniscus (Fig. 6-4).[9,10] MR arthrography is considered by many to be preferable to conventional MR imaging for

detection of recurrent tears of the meniscus in patients with prior meniscectomy.[9–12] CT and MR arthrography can also be helpful in assessing the integrity of articular cartilage of the knee and in assessing stability of osteochondral defects (Fig. 6-5).[7,13–16]

In addition to diagnostic arthrography, a variety of image-guided techniques can be performed to evaluate the

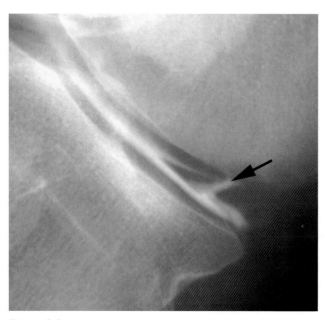

Figure 6-2 ■ Double-contrast conventional knee arthrogram depicting an oblique tear of the posterior horn of the medial meniscus *(arrow)*.

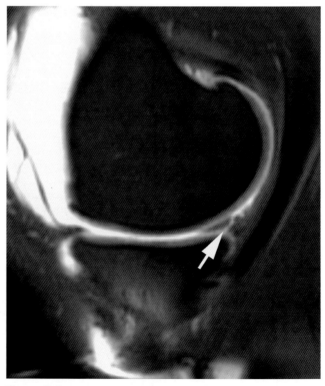

Figure 6-4 ■ MR arthrography of the knee. Sagittal image depicts a recurrent tear of the posterior horn of the medial meniscus *(arrow)* in this patient with prior partial medial meniscectomy.

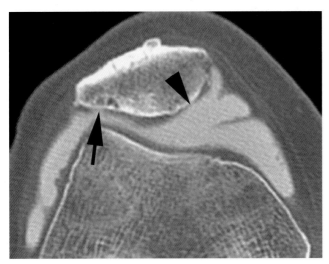

Figure 6-5 ▪ CT arthrogram of the knee. Axial image depicts focal full-thickness defects in the articular hyaline cartilage of the lateral facet of the patella *(arrow)* with underlying subchondral cystic changes and severe diffuse thinning and wear of the articular hyaline cartilage of the medial facet of the patella *(arrowhead)*.

knee joint. Therapeutic injections of the knee are commonly performed for pain relief and for viscosupplementation. A variety of agents have been introduced to alter the composition and viscosity of synovial fluid to benefit patients suffering from osteoarthritis of the knee.[17-19] Percutaneous image-guided aspiration of knee joint effusions is also useful for evaluation for infection and for obtaining synovial fluid to evaluate crystal deposition disease and other systemic processes.[6,20] Other image-guided interventions described in this chapter include proximal tibiofibular injections and popliteal cyst aspirations.

ANATOMIC CONSIDERATIONS

The knee joint is the largest and one of the most complicated joints in the body with motion limited primarily to a single plane.[21] The knee joint consists of two condylar joints between the medial and lateral condyles of the distal femur and the corresponding medial and lateral condyles of the proximal tibia. The knee joint also includes a gliding joint between the trochlear surface of the distal femur and the patella. Although often considered part of the knee joint, the proximal tibiofibular articulation is actually not part of the true knee joint.[22] The articular surfaces of the distal femur, proximal tibia, and patella are covered by hyaline cartilage (Fig. 6-6).[22]

To optimize stability with extension and to allow greater motion and rotation with flexion, the femoral condyles anteriorly are oval in shape, and posteriorly they are more rounded.[22] The medial femoral condyle supports the greatest axial load and is therefore greater in size.[22] The proximal tibial surface is expanded to form the medial and lateral tibial plateaus.[22] Between the tibial condyles is the intracondylar region, which provides the attachment sites for the cruciate ligaments, which restrict translation of the knee joint.[22,23]

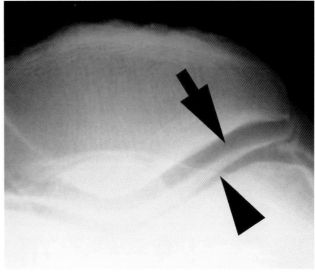

A

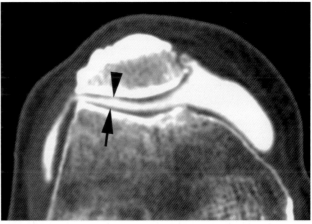

B

Figure 6-6 ▪ Articular hyaline cartilage. *A,* Conventional knee arthrogram depicting the articular hyaline cartilage of the lateral facet of the patella *(arrow)* and the lateral trochlea *(arrowhead)*. *B,* Axial image from a CT arthrogram of the knee depicting diffuse wear of the articular hyaline cartilage of both the patella *(arrowhead)* and trochlea *(arrow)*.

The articular surfaces of the femur and tibia are separated by the menisci, which are composed of fibrocartilage (Fig 6-7).[23] The menisci facilitate the articulation between the distal femur and proximal tibia and serve to absorb both axial loads and angular forces imparted upon the knee.[21] The menisci are C-shaped with a thick periphery with gradual tapering to a pointed inner margin or free edge (see Fig 6-7).[21,23] When seen in cross section, the menisci have a triangular configuration (Fig. 6-8).[22]

The cruciate ligaments are two strong knee ligaments that cross each other and provide anterior and posterior stability.[23] They are designated the anterior (ACL) and posterior (PCL) cruciate ligaments, depending on their tibial attachment (Fig. 6-9).[23] Although both ligaments are centrally located within the joint, both are excluded from the articular cavity by an enveloping synovial membrane.[22] The primary function of the ACL is to limit anterior translation

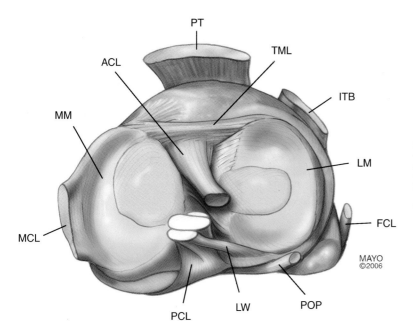

Figure 6-7 ▪ Knee joint anatomy. MM = medial meniscus; ACL = anterior cruciate ligament; PT = patellar tendon; TML = transverse meniscal ligament; ITB = iliotibial band; LM = lateral meniscus; FCL = fibulocollateral ligament; POP = popliteus tendon; LW = ligament of Wrisberg; PCL = posterior cruciate ligament; MCL = medial collateral ligament.

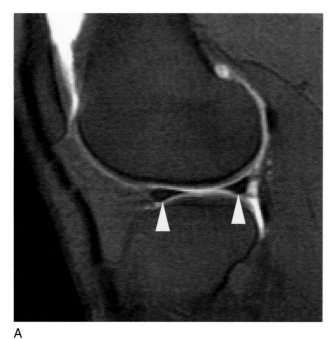

A

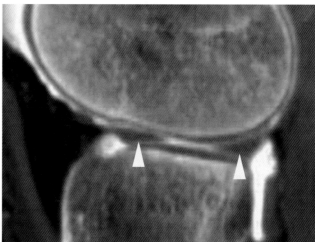

B

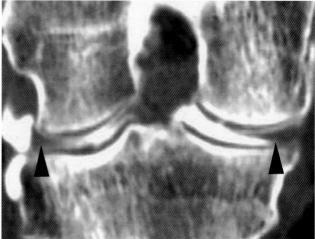

C

Figure 6-8 ▪ Normal appearance of the meniscus. *A,* Sagittal image from an MR arthrogram of the knee depicting the normal low-signal-intensity triangular configuration of the intact anterior and posterior horns of the lateral meniscus *(arrowheads). B,* Sagittal reformatted image from a CT arthrogram of the knee depicting the triangular morphology of the intact anterior and posterior horns of the lateral meniscus *(arrowheads). C,* Coronal reformatted image from a CT arthrogram of the knee depicting the normal triangular configuration of the intact body of the medial and lateral menisci *(arrowheads).*

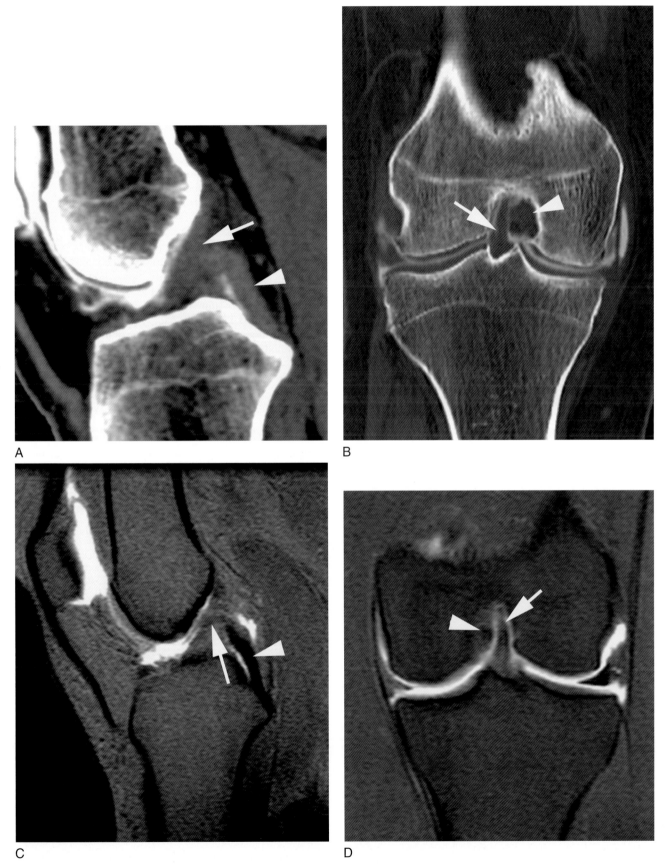

Figure 6-9 ■ Anterior and posterior cruciate ligaments. *A,* Sagittal image from a CT arthrogram of the knee depicts the intact anterior cruciate ligament (ACL) *(arrow)* and intact posterior cruciate ligament (PCL) *(arrowhead). B,* Coronal reformatted image from a CT arthrogram depicts the ACL *(arrow)* and PCL *(arrowhead)* in cross section. *C,* Sagittal image from an MR arthrogram of the knee depicting the intact ACL *(arrow)* and PCL *(arrowhead). D,* Coronal image from an MR arthrogram of the knee depicting the intact ACL *(arrow)* and PCL *(arrowhead)* in cross section.

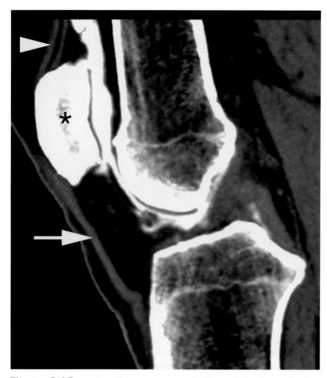

Figure 6-10 ■ Anterior extensor mechanism of the knee. Sagittal reformatted image from a CT arthrogram of the knee depicting the quadriceps tendon *(arrowhead)*, the patella *(asterisk)*, and the patellar ligament *(arrow)*.

of the tibia, and the primary function of the PCL is to limit posterior translation of the tibia.[22,23]

The periarticular ligaments and fibrous capsule of the knee provide important support and stability to the knee joint.[22] Anteriorly the knee is stabilized by the quadriceps tendon, the patella, the patellar ligament, and retinacula (Fig. 6-10).[22] Laterally the main support is provided by the lateral collateral ligament complex.[22] The lateral collateral ligament complex is composed of the fibular collateral ligament, the long head of the biceps tendon, and the iliotibial band (Fig. 6-11).[23] Additional posterolateral stabilizing structures include the popliteus muscle and tendon, the arcuate ligament, and the fabellofibular ligament.[22,23] The predominant stabilizing structure medially is the medial collateral ligament, which blends and is attached to the joint capsule (Fig. 6-12).[22]

The inner capsule of the knee joint is lined by a synovial membrane that is subdivided into several compartments that communicate.[22] Anterosuperiorly the synovial membrane forms a large recess termed the suprapatellar bursa.[22] Inferiorly the synovium is separated from the patellar ligament by the infrapatellar fat pad.[22,23] The synovium extends posteriorly along the articular surfaces of the femur and tibia both medially and laterally.[22] Centrally there are reflections of the synovium that encompass the cruciate ligaments, which are intracapsular, extrasynovial structures.[23] These reflections effectively divide the knee into medial and lateral compartments.[22] Posteromedially there is typically a small

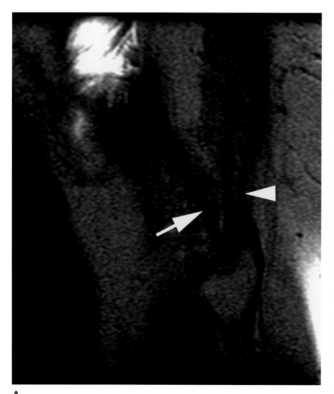

A

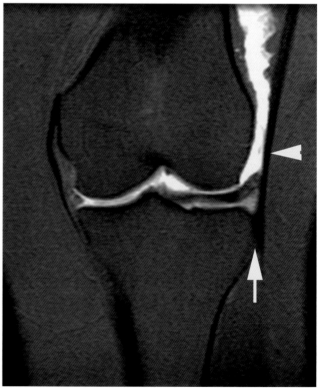

B

Figure 6-11 ■ Lateral collateral ligament complex. *A,* Sagittal image depicting the fibular collateral ligament *(arrow)* and the long head of the biceps tendon *(arrowhead)*. *B,* Coronal image depicting the iliotibial band *(arrowhead)* inserting upon Gerdy's tubercle *(arrow)*.

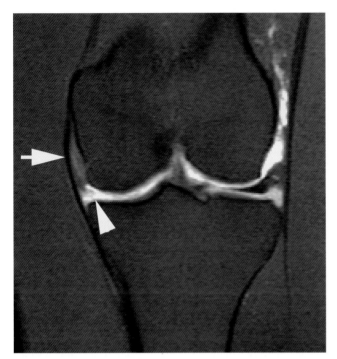

Figure 6-12 ■ Medial collateral ligament. Coronal image from an MR arthrogram depicts the intact medial collateral ligament *(arrow)*. Note the previous medial meniscectomy *(arrowhead)*.

recess termed the semimembranosus bursa, which frequently communicates with the joint.[23] Occasionally, joint fluid extends through a weakness in the joint capsule between the distal semimembranosus tendon and the proximal medial head of the gastrocnemius tendon to form an accessory bursa referred to as a popliteal cyst (Fig. 6-13).[22,23] Several addi-

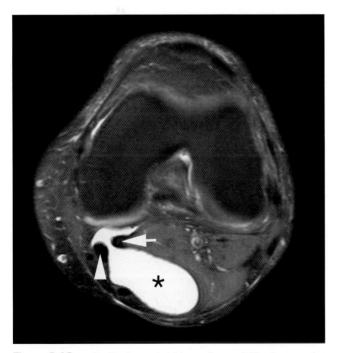

Figure 6-13 ■ Popliteal cyst. Axial image from an MR arthrogram that depicts a large popliteal cyst *(asterisk)* extending through a weakness in the joint capsule between the distal semimembranosus tendon *(arrowhead)* and the proximal medial head of the gastrocnemius tendon *(arrow)*.

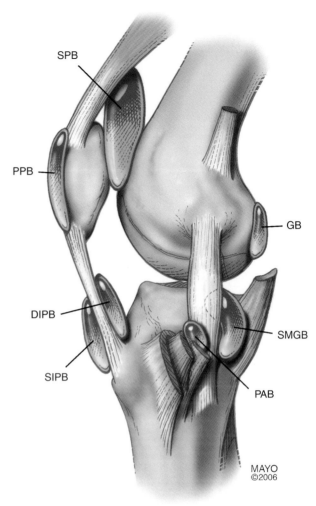

Figure 6-14 ■ Knee bursae. SPB = suprapatellar bursa; PPB = prepatellar bursa; DIPB = deep infrapatellar bursa; SIPB = superficial infrapatellar bursa; GB = gastrocnemius bursa; SMGB = semimembranosus-gastrocnemius bursa; PAB = pes anserine bursa.

tional bursae can be seen about the knee such as the prepatellar bursa and pes anserine bursa; however, these typically do not communicate with the knee joint (Fig. 6-14).[23]

PATIENT SELECTION

There are several indications for diagnostic and therapeutic injection of the knee joint. Although conventional single- and double-contrast arthrography of the knee has been largely replaced by conventional MR imaging, there are a number of other indications for image-guided interventions in the knee.[1] Therapeutic knee injections are widely used to alleviate joint pain and to differentiate intra-articular knee pain from pain related to surrounding structures.[6] Visco-supplementation is also a promising therapy that has shown efficacy in the treatment of certain knee disorders.[18,19] In addition to injections, knee aspiration can be performed to obtain knee joint fluid to evaluate for crystal deposition disease and to assess for hip joint infection.[1,20] Therapeutic injection of the proximal tibiofibular joint can also be useful for patients with symptoms specifically related to this

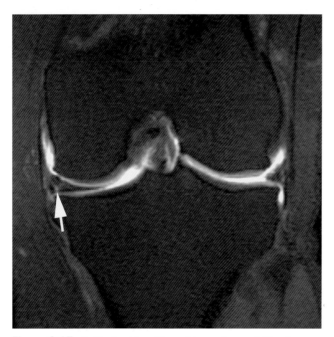

Figure 6-15 ■ Meniscal tear. Coronal image from an MR arthrogram depicts a complex tear of the body of the medial meniscus *(arrow)*.

joint.[20,24,25] Image-guided popliteal cyst aspirations and injections can be effective for short-term relief of symptoms related to these lesions.[20]

Today, most diagnostic knee arthrograms are performed with post-arthrography CT or MR.[1] This allows multiplanar image acquisition and a more precise depiction of intra-articular pathology (Fig. 6-15).[21] CT knee arthrography can be used to accurately diagnose internal derangement of the knee in patients who have contraindications to MR imaging (Fig. 6-16).[7,8] CT or MR knee arthrography is also occasionally used for the evaluation of synovial proliferative processes, osteochondral defects, and intra-articular loose bodies (Fig. 6-17).[13,15,21]

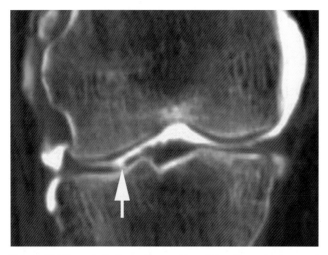

Figure 6-16 ■ Articular hyaline cartilage defect. Coronal reformatted image from a CT arthrogram of the knee depicts a large full-thickness defect involving the proximal tibial articular hyaline cartilage of the medial compartment.

Therapeutic Knee Injection/Aspiration

Therapeutic knee injections are commonly performed for knee pain.[3,23] Injections typically contain anesthetic agents such as bupivacaine or lidocaine, often in combination with long-acting corticosteroids. Substantial relief can often be obtained with therapeutic knee injections. The duration of pain relief is variable; however, occasionally lasting relief can be achieved.

In addition to anesthetic agents and corticosteroid injections, therapeutic knee injections can be used to deliver viscosupplements such as Synvisc, Orthovisc, or Hyalgan. These agents contain hyaluronan, which is found normally in the knee joint and functions to lower the viscosity of knee joint synovial fluid.[19] Typically, at least three injections are performed at varying intervals. The overall efficacy of viscosupplements in preliminary reports appears promising, although this practice remains controversial.[18,19]

MR Arthrography

MR arthrography has proved to be the best way to evaluate the postoperative meniscus.[9,10,26] Intrameniscal fibrovascular tissue, granulation tissue, and scarring, resulting from prior meniscal surgical manipulation, can result in abnormal signal within the meniscus that can extend to the articular surface.[9,12] Using conventional MR imaging alone, it may be difficult to differentiate postoperative changes in the meniscus from a recurrent tear.[9,10,12] MR arthrography allows one to differentiate these conditions by demonstrating imbibition of contrast material into the defect with recurrent tears of the meniscus (Fig. 6-18). Postoperative fibrovascular tissue prevents contrast material from entering the substance of the meniscus (Fig. 6-19).[9,21] MR arthrography may also be useful in the evaluation of articular cartilage defects, osteochondral defects, loose bodies, or synovial proliferative processes, although conventional MR imaging is often sufficient to evaluate these entities adequately (Fig. 6-20).[13,15,21]

CT Arthrography

CT arthrography can be substituted for MR imaging in patients with contraindications to MR or in patients who cannot tolerate the examination.[7] CT arthrography, like MR imaging, can precisely delineate the meniscus and evaluate for meniscal pathology (Fig. 6-21).[8] Like MR arthrography, CT arthrography can be used to evaluate the postoperative meniscus for recurrent meniscal tear.[7] CT arthrography can also be used to evaluate the articular cartilage of the femoral condyles, proximal tibia, and patella (Fig. 6-22).[7,14,16] Synovial proliferative disorders, loose bodies, and osteochondral defects can also be further characterized with CT arthrography (Fig. 6-23).[7,13]

Proximal Tibiofibular Joint Injection

Proximal tibiofibular injections can be helpful for both diagnostic and therapeutic purposes.[20,24] Therapeutic injections can be performed for pain relief associated with osteoarthritis

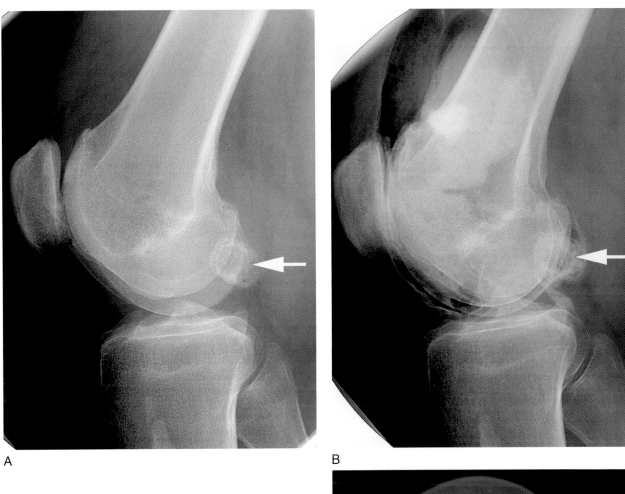

A

B

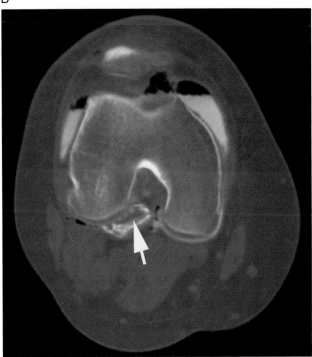

C

Figure 6-17 ■ Intra-articular loose body. *A*, Lateral radiograph depicts a large focus of ossification *(arrow)* posterior to the knee joint. *B*, Lateral radiograph following double-contrast arthrography of the knee depicting the ossification to be intra-articular in location compatible with a large loose body *(arrow)*. *C*, Axial image from a double-contrast CT arthrogram depicting an intra-articular location of the large loose body *(arrow)*, which was later surgically removed.

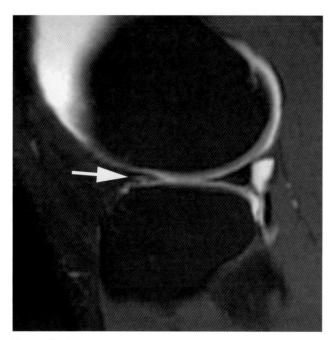

Figure 6-18 ■ Meniscal tear. Sagittal image from an MR arthrogram of the knee depicts contrast extending into the substance of the anterior horn of the lateral meniscus compatible with meniscal tear *(arrow)*.

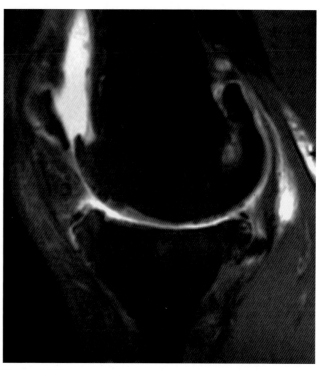

Figure 6-20 ■ Osteoarthritis of the knee. Sagittal image from an MR arthrogram reveals marked chondromalacia and osteophyte formation about the knee joint compatible with chronic osteoarthritis.

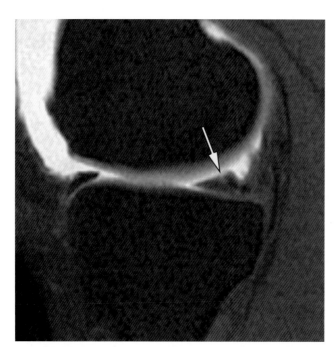

Figure 6-19 ■ Postoperative fibrovascular scar. Sagittal image from an MR arthrogram in a patient with prior medial meniscal repair depicting ill-defined increased signal within the meniscus related to fibrovascular scar *(arrow)*. No contrast material is seen entering the substance of the meniscus to suggest recurrent tear.

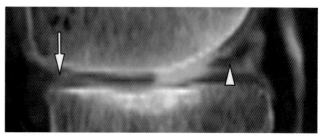

Figure 6-21 ■ Meniscal tear. Sagittal reformatted image through the medial compartment from a CT arthrogram of the knee reveals complex tearing of both the anterior horn *(arrow)* and posterior horn *(arrowhead)* of the medial meniscus.

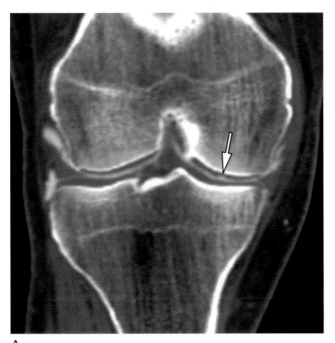

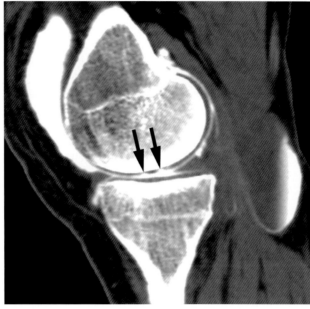

A   B

Figure 6-22 ▪ Articular hyaline cartilage defects. Coronal (*A*) and sagittal (*B*) reformatted images from a CT arthrogram of the knee show focal defects in the articular hyaline cartilage of the medial femoral condyle *(arrows)*.

and post-traumatic disorders of the joint (Fig. 6-24).[20] Diagnostic injections of the proximal tibiofibular joint can also be helpful to identify the etiology of lateral knee pain.[20,24] Relief following the injection confirms that the tibiofibular joint is the source of the pain, whereas continued symptoms following injection suggest another etiology, such as lateral compartment knee joint pathology.[20]

Popliteal Cyst or Miscellaneous Bursal Aspiration/Injection

A popliteal cyst or other bursa, such as the pes anserine bursa, can be aspirated easily utilizing image guidance. Real-time ultrasound guidance is preferable because sonography allows one to confirm the presence of the fluid-filled

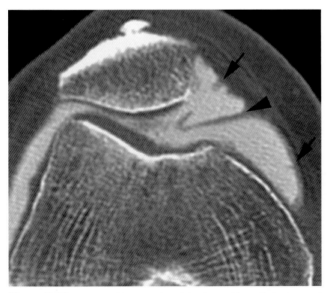

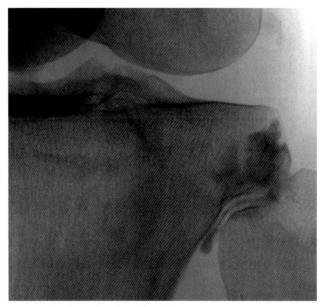

Figure 6-23 ▪ Synovitis. Synovial thickening and irregularity *(arrows)* involving the knee joint compatible with synovitis as seen on an axial image from a CT arthrogram of the knee. Note the slightly thickened medial plica *(arrowhead)*.

Figure 6-24 ▪ Proximal tibiofibular joint injection. Oblique view depicts contrast extending throughout the proximal tibiofibular joint following a diagnostic and therapeutic proximal tibiofibular joint injection.

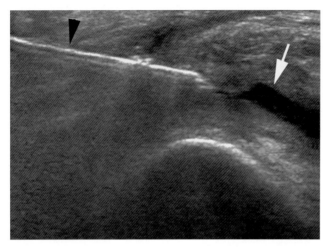

Figure 6-25 ■ Popliteal cyst aspiration. Sonographic image obtained during the performance of an ultrasound-guided popliteal cyst aspiration. The echogenic needle *(arrowhead)* has been directed into the anechoic fluid containing popliteal cyst *(arrow).*

cyst and also provides precise localization of the needle position during insertion (Fig. 6-25). Popliteal cyst aspiration or other bursal aspirations can be performed for therapeutic purposes to relieve tension and discomfort associated with large popliteal cysts or inflamed bursae.[20] Aspiration can also be performed for diagnostic purposes to identify the constituents of the fluid and evaluate for infection.[20] Injection of anesthetic agents and steroids following aspiration can also be performed for therapeutic purposes. Unfortunately, pain relief following aspiration tends to be short in duration because popliteal cysts tend to recur quickly as a result of the persistent communication between the cyst and the knee joint.[22,23]

CONTRAINDICATIONS[27]

- Coagulopathy (caution in patients with International Normalized Ratio [INR] >1.5 or platelets < 50,000/mm^3)
- Pregnancy (because of teratogenic effects of radiation)
- Systemic infection or skin infection over the puncture site
- Severe allergy to any component of the injectate
- The patient has received the maximum amount of steroid including systemic steroids allowed for a given time period unless the injection is to be performed without steroid

PROCEDURE

Equipment/Supplies

Procedural

- Spinal needle, 22-gauge, 3.5-inch (Quincke-type point, Becton Dickinson, Franklin Lakes, NJ) or 25-gauge, 1.5-inch needle
- Luer-Lock (10 or 20 mL) syringe containing injection mixture

- Sterile tubing to connect injection solution to spinal needle
- Control 12-mL syringe with 25-gauge, 1.5-inch needle containing 8 mL 1% lidocaine for local anesthesia and 2 mL 8.4% sodium bicarbonate injectable (1 mEq/mL) to alleviate burning pain associated with anesthetic
- Sterile 4 × 4 gauze pads
- Povidone-iodine (Betadine) and alcohol for preparation
- Sterile towels or fenestrated drape for draping
- Needle, 18 gauge, 1.5 inch, to draw up lidocaine and medication
- Sterile gloves
- Adhesive bandage

Medications (Injection Mixtures)

Volume

The knee joint total volume is variable. A typical volume is approximately 20 to 30 mL; however, this can range from 20 to 40 mL.[6,28] A 20-mL syringe can be utilized for most knee injections. For diagnostic knee injections prior to CT or MR arthrography, 20 mL is typically injected into the knee to result in adequate distention for imaging. For therapeutic injections, less volume is necessary and 15 to 20 mL is adequate. The proximal tibiofibular joint in comparison is very small in volume; typically only 1 to 2 mL. For tibiofibular injections a 10-mL syringe is adequate.

Therapeutic Knee Joint Injection

20-mL syringe
15- to 20-mL total injected joint volume
10 mL iodinated contrast (Reno-60, Omnipaque 300)
8 to 10 mL anesthetic agent (bupivacaine hydrochloride 0.5%, lidocaine hydrochloride 1% MPF*)
Optional: 2 mL steroid (methylprednisolone sodium succinate (Solu-Medrol 40 mg/mL, Depo-Medrol 40 mg/mL), triamcinolone (Kenalog-40), betamethasone sodium phosphate and betamethasone acetate (Celestone Soluspan 6 mg/mL)

CT Knee Arthrography

20-mL syringe
20 mL total injected joint volume
10 mL iodinated contrast
8 to 10 mL anesthetic agent
Optional: 2 mL steroid

MR Knee Arthrography

20-mL syringe
20 mL total injected joint volume
10 mL iodinated contrast
9 to 10 mL anesthetic agent
0.1 to 0.2 mL gadodiamide MR contrast (Omniscan, Magnevist)

---

*Local anesthetics should be from single-use vials and be free of paraben (MPF) and phenol to prevent flocculation of the steroid.[29]

Proximal Tibiofibular Joint Injection

10-mL syringe
1 to 2 mL total injected bursal volume
5 mL iodinated contrast
4 to 5 mL anesthetic agent
Optional: 0 to 1 mL steroid

Popliteal Cyst or Miscellaneous Bursal Injection

10-mL syringe
2 to 5 mL total injected bursal volume (variable)
9 to 10 mL anesthetic agent, 0 to 1 mL steroid

Methodology

Therapeutic Knee Joint Injection

CT Knee Arthrography

MR Knee Arthrography

Prior to knee joint interventions, routine radiographic images of the knee should be obtained and reviewed. The procedure should be explained to the patient and informed consent should be obtained.[3] The patient is placed on the fluoroscopy table in the supine position. The solution to be injected into the articulation is then drawn into a 20-mL syringe. Examples of injection mixtures are listed in the solutions section of the chapter. Flexible tubing should then be placed on the syringe and the solution should be advanced through the tubing to the tip. Any air bubbles should be expelled from the syringe and tubing. A metallic object such as a hemostat is useful with fluoroscopy to mark

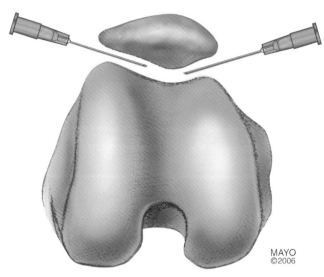

Figure 6-27 ▪ Medial and lateral approaches. For the medial or lateral approach, the space between the articular surface of the patella and the opposing femoral condyle is palpated and the target site is beneath the upper or middle portion of the patella. Most prefer a lateral approach as the soft tissues of the lateral aspect of the knee are thin and the needle does not have to traverse any muscles or other important structures.

the precise location of the injection (Fig. 6-26). The puncture site is marked on the patient with an indelible marker. There are several approaches and associated target sites for knee joint injections. A medial, lateral, or anterior approach can be used (Figs. 6-27 and 6-28).[20,30] With the medial or lateral approach, the space between the articular surface of the patella and the opposing femoral condyle is palpated. The target site for the medial or lateral approach is beneath the upper or middle portion of the patella (see Fig 6-27).[20]

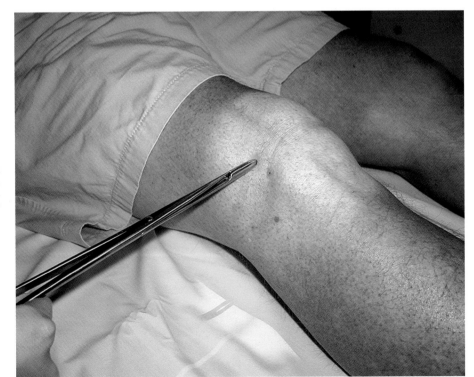

Figure 6-26 ▪ A metallic object such as a set of Kelly clamps can be utilized to identify the location of the puncture site for the injection under fluoroscopy.

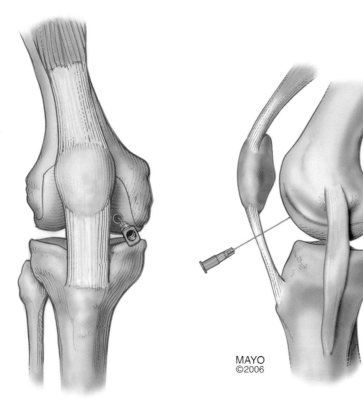

Figure 6-28 ■ Anterior approach. The target site is the anterior aspect of the medial femoral condyle just beneath the patella and medial to the patellar tendon. The needle should be advanced with a slight cephalad angulation.

MAYO
©2006

Most prefer a lateral approach as the soft tissues of the lateral aspect of the knee are thin and the needle does not have to traverse any muscles or other important structures. With a medial approach, the needle must traverse fibers of the vastus medialis; however, this is typically of little consequence. With the anterior approach, the target site is the anterior aspect of the medial femoral condyle just beneath the patella and medial to the patellar tendon (see Fig 6-28).[30] The needle should be advanced with a slight cephalad angulation.[30]

The field overlying the target site should then be prepared and draped using sterile technique. Local anesthesia of the skin and underlying subcutaneous tissue is obtained with 1% lidocaine with 8.4% sodium bicarbonate buffer (Fig. 6-29). A 22-gauge, 3.5-inch spinal needle or 25-gauge, 1.5-cm

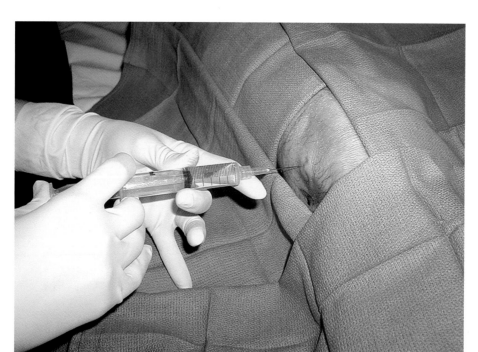

Figure 6-29 ■ Local anesthesia of the skin and underlying subcutaneous tissue is obtained with 1% lidocaine with 8.4% sodium bicarbonate buffer.

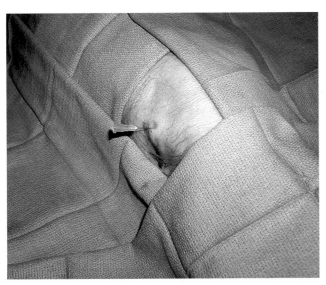

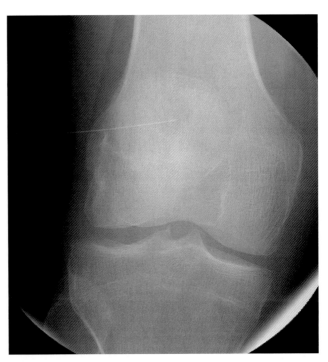

Figure 6-30 ▪ A 25-gauge, 1.5-cm needle is advanced through the overlying soft tissues until contact is made with the underlying bone. Fluoroscopy is then utilized to check the needle position.

Figure 6-31 ▪ Fluoroscopic image depicting the 25-gauge, 1.5-cm needle within the patellofemoral articulation of the knee joint.

needle can then be advanced through the overlying soft tissues until contact is made with bone (Fig. 6-30). It is not uncommon for the patient to experience discomfort when the needle enters the joint or makes contact with the periosteum of the bone. Fluoroscopy is used to verify the needle position (Fig. 6-31). Alterations in needle position can then be made to guide the needle to its intended target.

When the needle has been properly positioned, the stylet of the spinal needle is withdrawn. The syringe and tubing containing the solution to be injected into the knee joint are then connected to the indwelling needle (Fig. 6-32). A small test injection is performed to ensure appropriate intra-articular placement of the needle (Fig. 6-33). If resistance to the injection is met, the bevel of the needle may be embedded in the car-

Figure 6-32 ▪ The syringe and tubing containing the solution to be injected into the knee joint are connected to the indwelling needle.

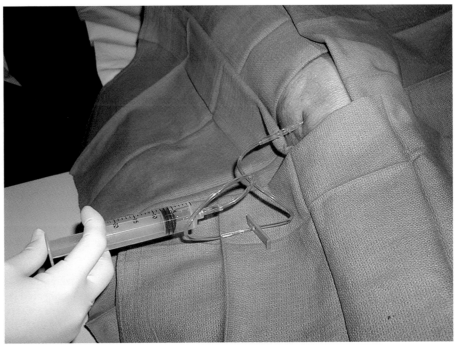

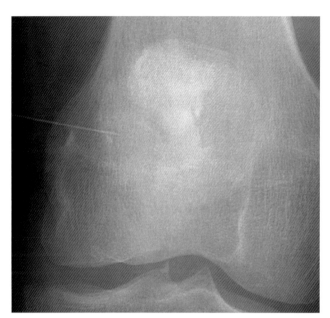

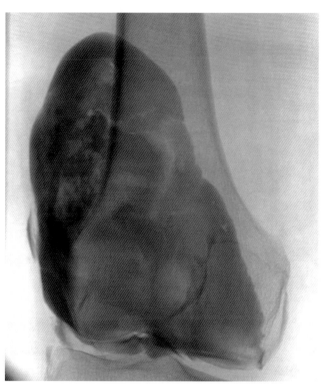

Figure 6-33 ■ A small test injection should be performed to ensure appropriate intra-articular placement of the needle. If contrast material collects at the needle tip as seen here, the needle is extra-articular and needs to be repositioned.

Figure 6-35 ■ Fluoroscopic image following a 20-mL injection of the knee joint with distention of the joint and a large amount of the injection solution pooling within the suprapatellar bursa.

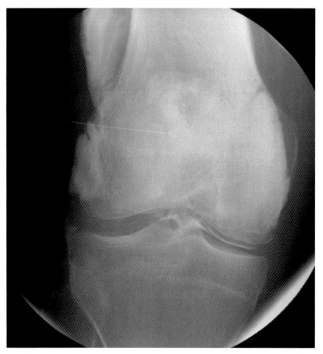

tilage. Slight withdrawal of the needle may be helpful to free the tip from the cartilage. If contrast material collects at the needle tip, the needle is extra-articular and needs to be repositioned (Fig. 6-33). If contrast flows freely away from the needle tip, the injection can be administered (Fig. 6-34). The entire injection should be performed under continuous fluoroscopic monitoring to ensure continued intra-articular placement of the needle throughout the injection and avoid inadvertent extra-articular injection. The volume of the injection depends upon the indication for the injection. For therapeutic knee injections, 15 to 20 mL is adequate volume. For CT or MR arthrography, 20 mL should be utilized to distend the knee joint (Fig. 6-35). If further distention is necessary, additional saline can be injected into the joint. The injection should not exceed 40 mL.[6,28] Following the injection, the needle is withdrawn. For CT and MR arthrography, movement of the joint should be kept to a minimum to avoid extravasation from the joint prior to imaging. The patient should be transferred to the CT or MR scanner with an MR-compatible wheelchair.

Figure 6-34 ■ Fluoroscopic image following repositioning of the needle demonstrates contrast flowing freely away from the needle tip and filling the knee joint.

Knee Joint Aspiration

Knee joint aspiration is very similar to knee joint injections. However, when the needle is in place, a 60-mL syringe and tubing are connected to the needle and aspiration of the joint is performed (Fig. 6-36). If no fluid is withdrawn, the needle is repositioned. If still no fluid can be aspirated, nonbacteriostatic saline is injected into the joint and reaspirated.

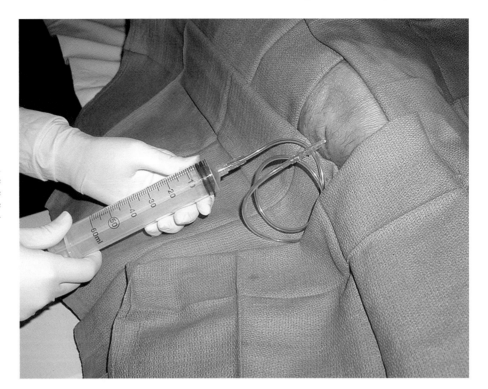

Figure 6-36 ■ Knee joint aspiration. The needle has been advanced into the knee joint under fluoroscopic guidance and a 60-mL syringe and tubing have been connected to the needle for aspiration of knee joint fluid.

Nonbacteriostatic saline is drawn up into a separate 20-mL syringe and tubing, and 10 mL is injected into the joint through the indwelling needle. The syringe tubing is then exchanged for the 60-mL syringe and tubing and the non-bacteriostatic saline is reaspirated.

The aspirated fluid or nonbacteriostatic saline wash is then sent for aerobic and anaerobic culture. If enough fluid is present, Gram stain and additional analysis of the fluid can be performed depending upon the specific clinical situation.

Proximal Tibiofibular Joint Injection

Prior radiographs or cross-sectional imaging should be obtained and reviewed prior to injection of the proximal tibiofibular joint. The patient should be placed on the fluoroscopy table in the supine position. A metallic object such as a hemostat placed on the skin surface is useful to mark the precise location of the injection site. The patient's skin should be marked with an indelible marker. An antero-lateral approach is utilized for injection of the proximal tibiofibular articulation.[20] This can be facilitated by placing the knee in slight internal rotation and flexion, which aligns the joint parallel to the fluoroscope. The field should then be prepared and draped in a sterile fashion.

Local anesthesia of the skin and underlying subcutaneous tissue is obtained with 1% lidocaine with 8.4% sodium bicarbonate buffer. A 1.5-inch, 25-gauge needle, used to anesthetize the skin, can be left at the puncture site and disconnected from the syringe. This can then be utilized to gauge the position of the planned puncture site relative to the target site. If the planned puncture site is concordant with the target site, the needle can be advanced into the proximal tibiofibular joint. Fluoroscopy is then used to

check the needle position, and alterations in needle position can be made if necessary.

The articulation between the proximal tibia and fibula is usually very narrow. When the needle has been properly positioned, the syringe and tubing containing the solution to be injected are connected to the indwelling 25-gauge needle. A small test injection should be performed to ensure intra-articular placement of the needle. The joint is typically very small, and therefore resistance to injection is typically encountered after only a small volume of fluid is injected. Imaging must be used to confirm proper position. If contrast material collects at the needle tip, the needle is extra-articular and must be repositioned. If contrast flows away from the needle tip in a linear fashion along the joint line, the remainder of the injection mixture is injected (Fig. 6-37). The proximal tibiofibular joint has a low volume, typically allowing only 1 to 2 mL to be injected. The entire injection should be performed under continuous fluoroscopic monitoring. Following the injection, the needle is withdrawn.

Popliteal Cyst or Miscellaneous Bursal Aspiration/Injection

Prior to aspiration or injection, or both, of a popliteal cyst or bursa about the knee, imaging studies should be obtained and reviewed. The position of vital structures is noted to avoid their incidental puncture. After a safe trajectory is determined, the patient is placed on the table in a position that facilitates the procedure. Preliminary sonographic evaluation is performed to identify the popliteal cyst or distended bursa. Ultrasonography shows the cyst or bursa as an anechoic or hypoechoic rounded or elongated structure (Fig. 6-38). Any adjacent vessels are identified to avoid

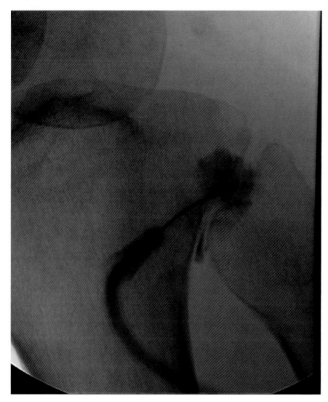

Figure 6-37 ■ Proximal tibiofibular joint injection. A 22-gauge spinal needle has been advanced into the proximal tibiofibular joint and 2 mL of the injection solution has been administered into the joint.

puncture. The skin and ultrasound probe are prepared in a sterile manner and local anesthesia is obtained with 1% lidocaine with sodium bicarbonate buffer. Under sonographic guidance, the 20- or 22-gauge spinal needle is advanced into the cyst or bursa (Fig. 6-39). A 60-mL syringe and sterile tubing are then connected to the indwelling needle and aspiration is performed (Fig. 6-40). For a cyst or bursa contain-

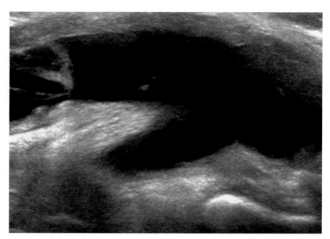

Figure 6-38 ■ Ultrasound image depicting a popliteal cyst as an anechoic elongated structure posterior to the knee joint.

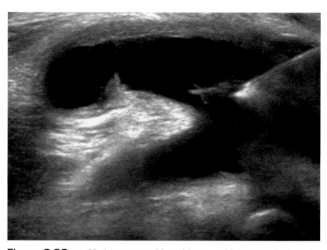

Figure 6-39 ■ Under sonographic guidance, a 22-gauge spinal needle has been advanced into the popliteal cyst.

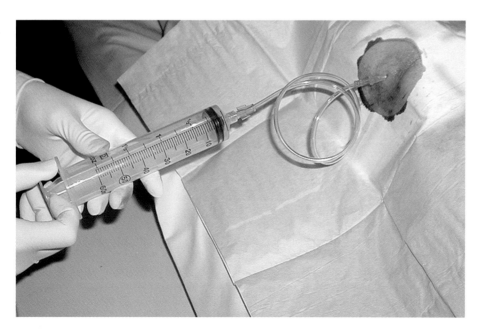

Figure 6-40 ■ Popliteal cyst aspiration. A 60-mL syringe and sterile tubing have been connected to the indwelling needle, and aspiration of the cyst is performed.

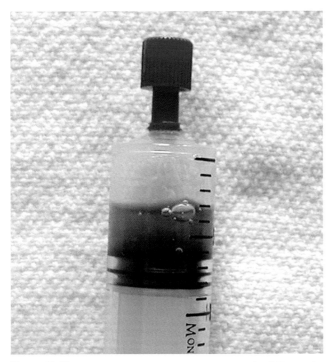

Figure 6-41 ▪ Fluid aspirated from the popliteal cyst should be sent for appropriate laboratory analysis if clinically indicated.

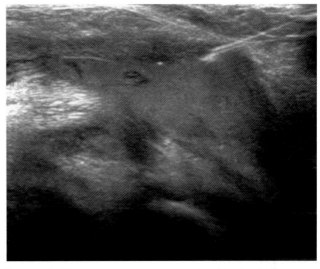

Figure 6-42 ▪ Popliteal cyst injection. The injection is seen sonographically as echogenic swirling fluid entering the cyst or bursa.

ing viscous fluid, a 20-gauge needle is better suited for the aspiration. The aspirated fluid is then sent for appropriate laboratory analysis (Fig. 6-41). The syringe containing the injection is then connected to the needle with sterile tubing. The injection is made using sonographic guidance. The injection is often seen as echogenic swirling fluid entering the cyst or bursa (Fig. 6-42). The volume depends on the structure being injected. For a popliteal cyst, an injection volume of 2 to 5 mL is typically sufficient.

POTENTIAL COMPLICATIONS[27]

- Bleeding
- Infection (cellulitis, septic arthritis, or osteomyelitis)
- Drug-related allergic reactions
- Transient synovitis
- Transitory lower extremity weakness
- Transitory lower extremity paresthesia
- Femoral or popliteal artery or vein injury

POST-PROCEDURE CARE/FOLLOW-UP[27]

Immediate

1. The patient should be observed for 15 minutes after the injection.
2. Blood pressure, pulse, heart rate, and respiratory rate are monitored as necessary.

Discharge

1. An adhesive bandage is placed on the puncture site. The bandage should remain dry for at least 24 hours, at which point it can be removed.
2. The patient is instructed to continue taking his or her prescription medication, although pain medication may be tapered as indicated.
3. A discharge sheet should be given to the patient outlining the following:
   a. The procedure performed
   b. Procedure-related symptoms that typically resolve in 7 to 10 days
   c. Treatment for mild post-procedure symptoms
      - Rest the knee for 1 to 2 days
      - Avoid movements that worsen the pain
      - Use cold compresses to the area that hurts
   d. Signs and symptoms of infection
      - Fever
      - Chills
      - Swelling or drainage from the puncture site(s)
      - New knee pain that is different from the usual pain
   e. Signs and symptoms of possible more serious problems
      - Decreased range of motion of the knee
      - Increasing pain
      - Motor dysfunction of the lower extremity
   f. Physician name and contact number if the patient has any concerns or if any problems were to arise as a result of the procedure
   g. Advice to schedule a follow-up appointment with the referring physician in 7 to 10 days

SAMPLE DICTATIONS

Knee CT Arthrogram

After the procedure was explained to the patient and informed consent was obtained, the patient was placed on the table in the supine position. The skin overlying the knee articulation was prepared and draped in the usual sterile fashion. Local anesthesia was obtained with 1% lidocaine with bicarbonate buffer. Under fluoroscopic guidance, a 25-gauge, 1.5-inch needle was advanced into the knee joint utilizing a medial approach and a 15-mL solution containing iodinated contrast material and 0.5% bupivacaine was administered into the knee articulation. The needle was withdrawn. The patient was sent to CT for additional imaging of the knee after arthrography.

Proximal Tibiofibular Joint Injection

After the procedure was explained to the patient and informed consent was obtained, the patient was placed on the table in the supine position. The knee was slightly internally rotated and flexed. The skin overlying the proximal tibiofibular articulation was prepared and draped in sterile fashion. Local anesthesia was obtained with 1% lidocaine with bicarbonate buffer. Under fluoroscopic guidance, a 25-gauge, 1.5-inch needle was advanced into the proximal tibiofibular joint and a 2-mL solution containing iodinated contrast material and 0.5% bupivacaine was administered into the joint. The needle was withdrawn. The patient reported moderate relief of symptoms immediately following the injection.

Ultrasound-Guided Popliteal Cyst Aspiration

After the procedure was explained to the patient and informed consent was obtained, the patient was placed on the table in the prone position. Preliminary real-time gray scale sonographic images demonstrated a distended popliteal cyst. The skin overlying the cyst was sterilely prepared and draped in the usual fashion. Local anesthesia was obtained with 1% lidocaine with bicarbonate buffer. Under real-time sonographic guidance, a 22-gauge spinal needle was advanced into the popliteal cyst and 15 mL of straw-colored fluid was aspirated. A 5-mL solution containing 0.5% bupivacaine and Kenalog at 40 mg/mL was administered into the cyst. The needle was withdrawn. Post-injection sonography demonstrated near-complete collapse of the popliteal cyst. The patient reported complete relief of symptoms following the procedure.

CASE REPORTS

CASE 1

Clinical Presentation

A 67-year-old female patient presented with medial right knee pain. The pain reportedly developed 1 year earlier and continued to increase in severity. The pain was exacerbated by weight bearing, walking, and twisting and relieved with rest. The patient denied any trauma or known injury. Physical examination demonstrated medial joint line tenderness with normal range of motion. No erythema, edema, or obvious knee joint effusion was noted. The orthopedic surgeon suspected medial meniscal pathology.

Imaging and Therapy

The patient had a pacemaker, and therefore MR imaging was contraindicated. Upon further consultation with the referring orthopedic surgeon, it was decided to proceed with a CT arthrogram of the knee instead. The patient was placed on the fluoroscopy table and the knee was prepared and draped in the usual sterile manner. A 25-gauge, 1.5-inch needle was advanced into the right knee joint under fluoroscopic guidance by a medial approach. A volume of 20 mL of a solution containing 10 mL of iodinated contrast medium and 10 mL of bupivacaine was administered into the knee joint. The patient was subsequently taken to CT, and a high-resolution, thin-section CT scan of the right knee was obtained in the axial plane. Sagittal and coronal reformatted images were also performed.

Results

The patient immediately reported pain relief following the injection. CT arthrography revealed the medial meniscus to be intact. However, a large full-thickness chondral flap tear involving the articular hyaline cartilage was seen involving the weight-bearing surface of the medial femoral condyle (Fig. 6-43). Two weeks later, the patient underwent arthroscopic debridement of the chondral flap tear with abrasion arthroplasty. The patient did well following the surgery with complete resolution of knee symptoms.

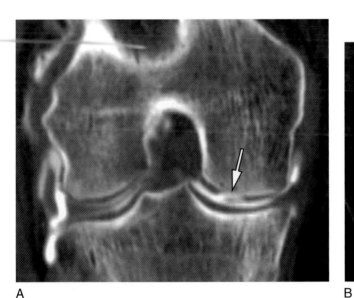
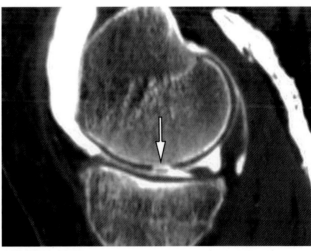

A   B

Figure 6-43 ■ Chondral flap tear of the medial femoral condyle. Coronal (*A*) and sagittal (*B*) reformatted images from a CT arthrogram of the knee depict a large chondral flap tear involving the articular hyaline cartilage of the medial femoral condyle (*arrows*).

CASE 2

Clinical Presentation

A 34-year-old patient, after ACL reconstruction and medial meniscal debridement, presented following a fall with recurrent pain and swelling about the left knee joint. The patient reported instability of the knee joint following the fall with a large "popping" noise heard during the injury. Evaluation of the knee by the orthopedic surgeon revealed a large left knee joint effusion. The knee demonstrated instability with positive Lachman and pivot shift tests. A recurrent ACL tear and possibly a recurrent meniscal tear were suspected.

Imaging and Therapy

MR arthrography of the left knee was performed. The patient was placed on the fluoroscopy table and the knee was prepared and draped in the usual sterile manner. A 25-gauge, 1.5-inch needle was advanced into the right knee joint under fluoroscopic guidance by a medial approach. Approximately 20 mL of a solution containing 10 mL of iodinated contrast medium, 10 mL of bupivacaine, and 0.1 mL of gadolinium was administered into the left knee joint. The patient was subsequently taken to MR and placed in the knee coil. T1-weighted images in all three planes as well as sagittal proton density and T2-weighted images with fat saturation were obtained.

Results

MR arthrography depicted a complete tear of the distal ACL graft near the tibial tunnel (Fig. 6-44). Bone contusion was seen in the posterolateral tibial plateau and lateral femoral condyle related to the ACL disruption. The PCL remained intact. Evidence of previous medial meniscal debridement with amputation of the free margin of the body and posterior horn of the meniscus was seen, although no recurrent meniscal tear was identified. The patient subsequently underwent repeated ACL reconstruction utilizing a hamstring autograft with good results following rehabilitation.

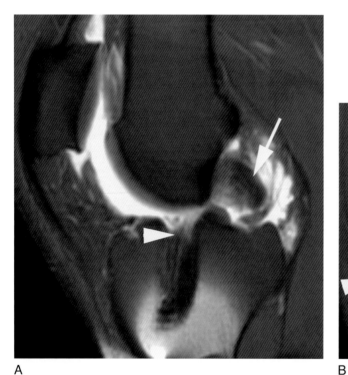

A

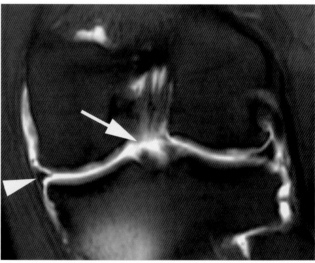

B

Figure 6-44 ■ Recurrent tear of the anterior cruciate ligament. *A,* Sagittal image from an MR arthrogram of the knee shows complete disruption of the ACL graft near the tibial tunnel; both the proximal *(arrow)* and distal *(arrowhead)* ACL graft fragments are seen. *B,* Coronal MR image following arthrography reveals the tear in the ACL distally near the tibial tunnel *(arrow).* The body of the medial meniscus is amputated, related to previous meniscal debridement *(arrowhead);* however, no recurrent meniscal tear was seen.

CURRENT PROCEDURAL TERMINOLOGY (CPT) CODES[31]

CPT codes change often and sometimes are valid only for certain states or regions. It is best to consult with coding experts to make sure that coding for one's procedures is legitimate and complete. Below is a sample of codes that are being used for knee injection procedures at this writing.

20610 Arthrocentesis, aspiration and/or injection; major joint or bursa (e.g., shoulder, hip, knee joint, subacromial bursa)

(If imaging guidance is performed, see 76942, 77002, 77012, 77021)

27370 Injection procedure for knee arthrography

(For radiologic supervision and interpretation, use 73580. Do not report 77002 in addition to 73580)

27599 Unlisted procedure, femur or knee

73560 Radiologic examination, knee; one or two views

73562 three views

73564 complete, four or more views

73565 both knees, standing, anteroposterior

73580 Radiologic examination, knee, arthrography, radiologic supervision and interpretation

(Do not report 73580 in conjunction with 77002)

73700 Computed tomography, lower extremity; without contrast material

73701 with contrast material(s)

73702 without contrast material, followed by contrast material(s) and further sections

(To report 3D rendering, see 76376, 76377)

76376 3D rendering with interpretation and reporting of computed tomography, magnetic resonance imaging, ultrasound, or other tomographic modality; not requiring image postprocessing on an independent workstation

(Use 76376 in conjunction with code(s) for base imaging procedure(s))

(Do not report 76376 in conjunction with 70496, 70498, 70544–70549, 71275, 71555, 72159, 72191, 72198, 73206, 73225, 73706, 73725, 74175, 74185, 75635, 76377, 78000–78999, 0066T, 0067T, 0144T–0151T)

76377 requiring image postprocessing on an independent workstation

(Use 76377 in conjunction with code(s) for base imaging procedure(s))

Do not report 76377 in conjunction with 70496, 70498, 70544–70549, 71275, 71555, 72159, 72191, 72198, 73206, 73225, 73706, 73725, 74175, 74185, 75635, 76376, 78000–78999, 0066T, 0067T, 0144T–0151T)

76942 Ultrasonic guidance for needle placement (e.g., biopsy, aspiration, injection, localization device), imaging supervision and interpretation

(Do not report 76942 in conjunction with 43232, 43237, 43242, 45341, 45342, or 76975)

77002 Fluoroscopic guidance for needle placement (e.g., biopsy, aspiration, injection, localization device)

(See appropriate surgical code for procedure and anatomic location)

(77002 includes all radiographic arthrography with the exception of supervision and interpretation for CT and MR arthrography)

(Do not report 77002 in addition to 70332, 73040, 73085, 73115, 73525, 73580, 73615)

77012 Computed tomography guidance for needle placement (e.g., biopsy, aspiration, injection, localization device), radiologic supervision and interpretation

77021 Magnetic resonance guidance for needle placement (e.g., for biopsy, needle aspiration, injection, or placement of localization device) radiologic supervision and interpretation

References

1. Coumas JM, Palmer WE. Knee arthrography. Evolution and current status. Radiol Clin North Am 1998; 36:703–728.
2. Werndorff KR, Robinson I. Uber Intraarticulare und Interstielle Sauerstaff-Insufflation Zu Radiologischen, Diagnostichen Und Theraputischen Zwaken. Kongr Verh Dtsch Ges Orthop 1905.
3. Freiberger RH, Kaye JJ. Arthrography. Norwalk, CT: Appleton Century Crofts, 1979, pp 1–3, 5–135.
4. Ekstrom JE. Arthrography: Where does it fit in? Clin Sports Med 1990; 9:561–566.
5. Steinbach LS, Helms C, Sims RE, et al. High resolution computed tomography of knee menisci. Skel Radiol 1987; 16:11–16.
6. Hodge JC. Musculoskeletal Imaging: Diagnostic and Therapeutic Procedures. Montreal: Karger Landes Systems, 1997, pp 73–89.
7. Vande Berg BC, Lecouvet FE, Poilvache P, et al. Spiral CT arthrography of the knee: Technique and value in the assessment of internal derangement of the knee. Eur Radiol 2002; 12:1800–1810.
8. Vande Berg BC, Lecouvet FE, Poilvache P, et al. Dual-detector spiral CT arthrography of the knee: Accuracy for detection of mensical abnormalities and unstable meniscal tears. Radiology 2000; 216:851–857.
9. Applegate GR, Flannigan BD, Tolin BS, et al. MR diagnosis of recurrent tears in the knee: Value of intraarticular contrast material. AJR Am J Roentgenol 1993; 161:821–825.
10. Magee T, Shapiro M, Rodriguez J, Williams D. MR arthrography of postoperative knee: For which patients is it useful? Radiology 2003; 229:159–163.
11. De Smet AA. MR imaging and MR arthrography for diagnosis of recurrent tears in the postoperative meniscus. Semin Musculoskeletal Radiol 2005; 9:116-124.
12. McCauley TR. MR imaging evaluation of the postoperative knee. Radiology 2005; 234:53–61.
13. Brossmann J, Preidler KW, Daenon B, et al. Imaging of osseous and cartilaginous intraarticular bodies in the knee: Comparison of MR imaging and MR arthrography with CT and CT arthrography in cadavers. Radiology 1996; 200:509–517.
14. Gagliardi JA, Chung EM, Chandnani VP, et al. Detection and staging of chondromalacia patellae: Relative efficacies of conventional MR imaging, MR arthrography, and CT arthrography. AJR Am J Roentgenol 1994; 163:629–636.
15. Kramer J, Stigbauer R, Engel A, et al. MR contrast (MRA) in osteochondrosis dissecans. J Comput Assist Tomogr 1992; 16:254–260.
16. Rand T, Brossman J, Pedowitz R, et al. Analysis of patellar cartilage: Comparison of conventional MR imaging and MR and CT arthrography in cadavers. Acta Radiol 2000; 41:492–497.
17. Aggarwal A, Sempowski IP. Hyaluronic acid injections for knee osteoarthritis. Systematic review of the literature. Can Fam Physician 2004; 50:249–256.

18. Kahan A, Lleu PL, Salin L. Prospective randomized study comparing the medicoeconomic benefits of Hylan GF-20 vs. conventional treatment in knee osteoarthritis. Joint Bone Spine 2003; 70:276-281.

19. Kotevoglu N, Iyibozkurt PC, Hiz O, et al. A prospective randomised controlled clinical trial comparing the efficacy of different molecular weight hyaluronan solutions in the treatment of knee osteoarthritis. Rheumatol Int 2006; 26:325–330.

20. Berquist TH. Diagnostic and therapeutic injections as an aid to musculoskeletal diagnosis. Semin Interv Radiol 1993; 10:326-344.

21. Kramer J, Recht MP. MR arthrography of the lower extremity. Radiol Clin North Am 2002; 40:1121–1132.

22. Berquist TH. MRI of the Musculoskeletal System, 5th ed. Philadelphia: Lippincott Williams & Wilkins, 2006, pp 303–429.

23. Resnick D. Diagnosis of Bone and Joint Disorders, 4th ed. Philadelphia: WB Saunders, 2002, pp 259–290, 3167–3285.

24. Bozkurt M, Yilmaz E, Atlihan D, et al. The proximal tibiofibular joint. An anatomic study. Clin Orthop Relat Res 2003; 406:136-140.

25. Sugita T, Matumura Y, Umehara J, Sakurai M. Proximal tibiofibular joint: A radiographic and computed tomographic study. Tohoku J Exp Med 1995; 176:35–44.

26. Palmer WE. MR arthrography: Is it worthwhile? Top Magn Reson Imaging 1996; 8:24–43.

27. Fenton DS, Czervionke LF. Image-Guided Spine Intervention. Philadelphia: WB Saunders, 2003.

28. Sahin G, Demirtas M. An overview of MR arthrography with emphasis on the current technique and application hints and tips. Eur J Radiol 2006; 58:416-430.

29. Physicians' Desk Reference, 60th ed. Montvale, NJ: Medical Economics Company, 2006.

30. Zurlo JV, Towers JD, Golla S. Anterior approach for knee arthrography. Skeletal Radiol 2001; 30:354–356.

31. CPT 2007, CPT Intellectual Property Services. Chicago: American Medical Association, 2007.

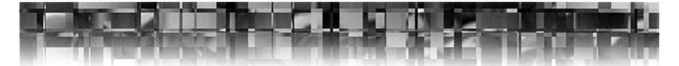

A Knee Surgeon's Perspective

Knee Injections

Cedric J. Ortiguera, MD

Injections are an integral part of the diagnosis and treatment of knee disorders. Therapeutic injections of the knee joint are performed on a daily basis utilizing corticosteroids or visco-supplementation. Although most knee surgeons are comfortable with knee injection techniques, studies have shown that even experienced knee surgeons successfully enter the knee joint without image guidance only 60% to 70% of the time. The addition of image guidance for these daily procedures can only improve our accuracy.

With the outstanding quality of today's diagnostic MR imaging, it is unusual to utilize arthrography in my practice. If a patient is contraindicated for MR imaging, CT arthrography can be useful to delineate internal derangement of the knee. In the postsurgical patient, MR arthrography can be useful in determining recurrent meniscal tearing versus postmeniscectomy changes. Standard arthrography is now rarely utilized. However, it may play a role in the evaluation of suspected mechanical failure or loosening of joint arthroplasty implants.

A number of other structures about the knee may be incidental radiologic findings or a true cause of pain. To help differentiate this, localized injections are often helpful. Many of these areas can be injected without guidance. Others, such as certain ganglia about the knee, septated popliteal cysts, and a proximal tibio fibular joint, are often best reached through image guidance. Relief as a result of the localized injections (either short or long term) may help differentiate localized pathology from referred pain from the back or hip.

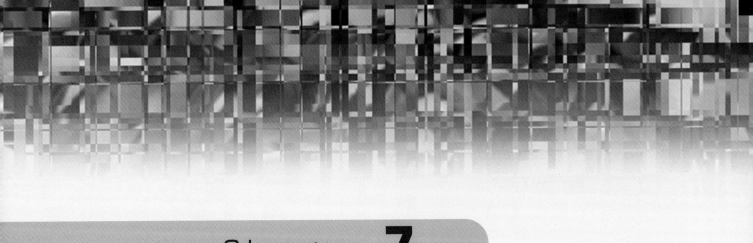

Chapter 7

Ankle and Foot Injections

- Jeffrey J. Peterson, MD

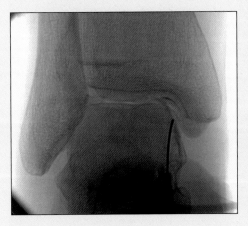

BACKGROUND

Prior to the introduction of modern cross-sectional imaging techniques, ankle arthrography and tenography were commonly used to evaluate the integrity of the tendinous and ligamentous structures of the foot and ankle.[1-3] Ankle arthrography was also commonly utilized to evaluate the integrity of the articular cartilage of the ankle joint and to characterize osteochondral defects.[4,5] With the introduction of cross-sectional imaging techniques, especially magnetic resonance (MR) imaging in the late 1980s, indications for ankle arthrography and tenography significantly diminished.[2,6] Conventional MR imaging of the foot and ankle precisely depicts the tendons and ligaments about the foot and ankle with a noninvasive technique and no ionizing radiation.[1,2]

Today, most foot and ankle joint injections are performed for either therapeutic or diagnostic purposes using MR or CT arthrography.[2,6] Therapeutic injections are useful to treat chronic foot and ankle pain and to localize the site of symptoms in cases of vague hindfoot and ankle pain or discomfort.[7-9] Tendon sheaths as well as trigger points such as the plantar fascial attachment can also be injected with anesthetic agents and corticosteroids for relief of pain and localization purposes.[10-12] Occasionally, therapeutic injections can be useful in cases of adhesive capsulitis involving the ankle joint with distention of the capsule and rupture of intra-articular adhesions.[2,13] Ankle

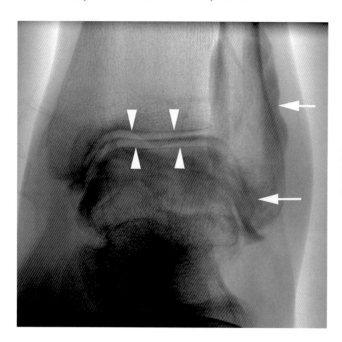

Figure 7-1 ■ AP image from following arthrography of the ankle depicting the articular hyaline cartilage of the talar dome and plafond to be intact *(arrowheads)*. Extravasation from the lateral aspect of the ankle joint indicates lateral ligamentous disruption *(arrows)*.

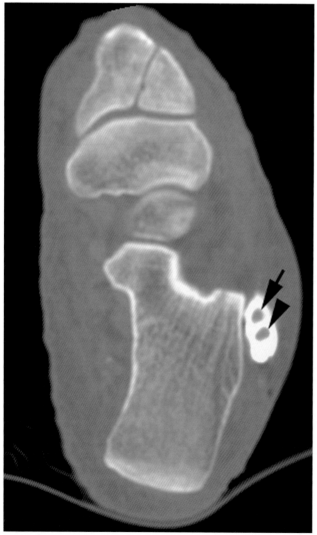

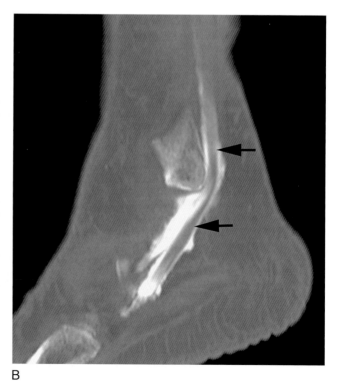

Figure 7-2 ■ CT tenography. Axial image *(A)* from a CT tenogram of the peroneal tendons precisely depicts the peroneus longus *(arrowhead)* and peroneus brevis *(arrow)* tendons outlined by contrast within the peroneal tendon sheath. Reformatted images *(B)* can be obtained in any plane to better depict tendons, in this case the peroneus longus tendon *(arrows)*, in long axis.

A

B

joint aspirations can also be performed to obtain synovial fluid for evaluation of possible infection, arthropathy, or crystal deposition disease.[2]

CT arthrography or tenography is indicated for evaluation of the ankle joint, of tendons about the ankle joint in patients who have contraindications to MR, or in patients who cannot tolerate MR for other reasons such as claustrophobia.[14,15] CT ankle arthrography can precisely define the articular cartilage of the ankle and can demonstrate sites of ligamentous disruption as foci of extravasation of contrast material (Fig. 7-1).[14,15] CT tenography can be used to assess the integrity of several of the tendons that pass near the ankle (Fig. 7-2). MR and CT arthrography of the ankle can also be useful in evaluation of the hyaline cartilage of the tibial plafond and talar dome as well as for the evaluation of osteocartilaginous lesions involving these areas (Fig. 7-3).[4,5,16] MR or CT arthrography can be useful for evaluation of suspected loose bodies within the ankle joint, synovial proliferative processes involving the ankle, and various soft tissue and osseous impingement syndromes that can be seen about the ankle.[2,13,16]

Fluoroscopically guided injections of the soft tissues of the foot and ankle and of the small joints of the foot continue to be useful in identifying the location of the source of symptoms and relief of pain (Fig. 7-4).[7–9] Localization of symptoms within the foot and ankle is often a difficult clinical task owing to the complex and compact anatomy of the articulations and surrounding structures of the foot and ankle.[8–10] Therapeutic injections, tenography, and arthrography continue to play an important clinical role in the evaluation of ankle and foot pain.

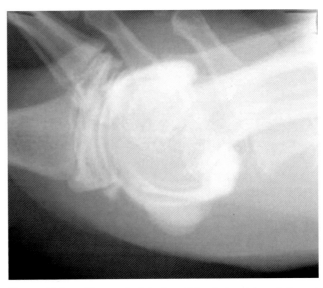

Figure 7-4 ▪ Therapeutic injection of the first metatarsophalangeal articulation in a young patient with chronic medial forefoot pain.

ANATOMIC CONSIDERATIONS

The ankle joint is a synovium-lined hinge joint.[1,17] The osseous structures that make up the ankle joint are the distal tibia, fibula, and talus.[18] The tibia forms the roof, termed the tibial plafond, of the ankle articulation and also the medial

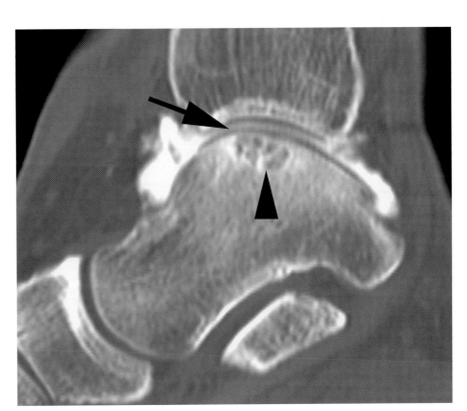

Figure 7-3 ▪ Sagittal reformatted image from a CT arthrogram of the ankle depicting cystic changes in the talar dome *(arrowhead)* with relative preservation of the overlying articular hyaline cartilage *(arrow)*.

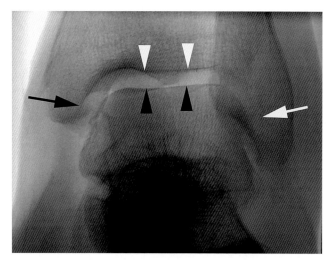

Figure 7-5 ■ Anatomy of the ankle joint. The talar dome *(black arrowheads)* is seen inferiorly. The tibial plafond *(white arrowheads)* forms the roof of the ankle articulation. The medial margin of the ankle joint is formed by the medial malleolus *(black arrow).* The lateral margin of the ankle joint is formed by the distal fibula *(white arrow).*

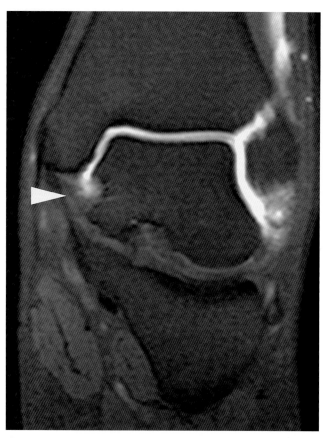

Figure 7-7 ■ Deltoid ligament. Coronal image from an MR arthrogram depicts the deltoid ligament *(arrowhead).* The apex of the triangular ligament is directed superiorly, attaching to the medial malleolus. The ligament fans out distally, attaching to the navicular, the talus, and the sustentaculum tali of the calcaneus.

margin with the medial malleolus (Fig. 7-5).[21] The lateral margin of the ankle joint is formed by the distal fibula and is called the lateral malleolus, which extends more inferiorly than the medial malleolus (see Fig. 7-5).[17] The distal tibia and fibula articulate distally and are stabilized by the intraosseous membrane, the anterior and posterior tibiofibular ligaments, and the transverse tibiofibular ligament.[17] The articular surfaces of the ankle joint are lined with hyaline cartilage except for the far posterior aspect of the tibia, which lacks

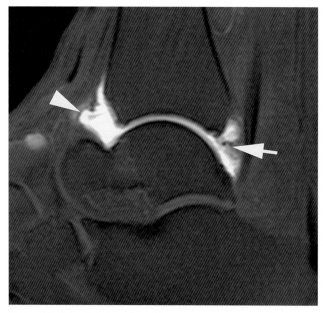

Figure 7-6 ■ Anterior and posterior recesses of the ankle joint. The ankle joint capsule is weak anteriorly and posteriorly, resulting in prominent anterior *(arrowhead)* and posterior *(arrow)* recesses.

overlying hyaline cartilage.[18] The joint capsule circumferentially extends around the joint and is weak anteriorly and posteriorly, where prominent recesses are located (Fig. 7-6).[2,17] The joint capsule medially and laterally, however, is quite strong.[17] The shape of the osseous articulations in conjunction with strong surrounding ligaments creates a strong, stable joint.[17,18]

The deltoid ligament is a strong triangular ligament that provides great medial stability to the ankle joint.[18,19] The apex of the triangular ligament is directed superiorly, attaching to the medial malleolus.[18] The ligament then fans out distally, attaching to the navicular bone, the talus, and the sustentaculum tali of the calcaneus (Fig. 7-7).[18]

The lateral stabilizing ligaments of the ankle are composed of three individual ligaments, the anterior talofibular ligament, the calcaneofibular ligament, and the posterior talofibular ligament.[1,18–20] The anterior talofibular ligament is the weakest and most susceptible to injury.[18] It extends anteriorly in an oblique course from the fibula to insert on the talus just anterior to the lateral talar facet (Fig. 7-8).[1,18–20] The longest of the three ligaments is the calcaneofibular ligament.[18] The calcaneofibular ligament extends in a nearly vertical plane from the tip of the fibula to the lateral surface of the calcaneus (Fig. 7-9).[17–19] The calcaneofibular liga-

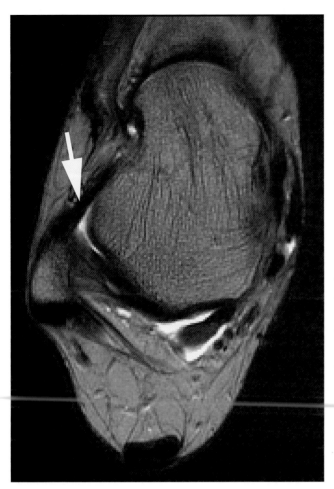

Figure 7-8 ▪ Anterior talofibular ligament. Axial image depicts the anterior talofibular ligament extending anteriorly along an oblique course from the fibula to insert on the talus just anterior to the lateral talar facet.

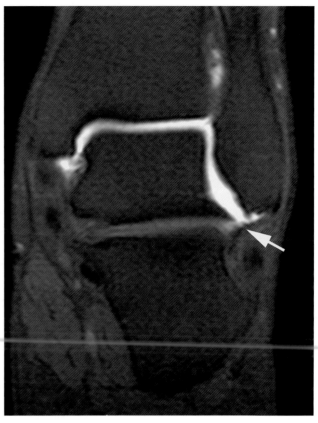

Figure 7-9 ▪ Calcaneofibular ligament. Coronal image from an MR arthrogram of the ankle depicts the calcaneofibular ligament *(arrow)* extending from the tip of the fibula to the lateral aspect of the calcaneus.

ment passes deep to the peroneal tendons, which course superficially around the distal fibula.[1,17,18] The posterior talofibular ligament is the strongest of the three ligaments.[18] The posterior talofibular ligament extends in a nearly horizontal plane, originating from the posteromedial aspect of the distal fibula, coursing posteromedially to insert in the posterior talar tubercle (Fig. 7-10).[18,19]

There are four major groups of tendons that traverse the ankle joint and comprise a total of nine tendons (Fig. 7-11).[11,12,18] The flexor tendons are found medially, with the largest tendon of the group, the tibialis posterior tendon, located anteriorly (Fig. 7-12; see Fig 7-11).[11,12,18] The tibialis posterior tendon extends posterior to the distal tibia in a small concavity.[17,18,21] The tendon then curves anteriorly and inferiorly over the medial malleolus to insert in a complex fashion upon the navicular bone, cuneiform bones, and the bases of the second, third, and fourth metatarsal bones.[21] The posterior tibialis tendon plays a critical role in maintaining integrity of the longitudinal arch of the foot and preventing abnormal valgus angulation of the hindfoot and pronation of the forefoot.[17,21] Located just posterior to the tibialis posterior tendon is the flexor digitorum longus tendon, which divides into four slips in the plantar aspect of the

foot to insert on the second through fourth phalanges (see Fig. 7-12).[17,18] Just posterior to the flexor digitorum longus tendon, at the level of the ankle, is the flexor hallucis longus tendon, which passes beneath the sustentaculum tali to insert on the base of the distal phalanx of the great toe (Fig. 7-13; see Fig. 7-12).[17,18] Not uncommonly, the flexor hallucis longus tendon sheath communicates with the posterior aspect of the ankle joint (Fig. 7-14).[17,18,22] The tendon sheaths of the tibialis posterior, the flexor digitorum longus, and the flexor hallucis longus may also communicate.[17,18,22]

Anteriorly, the extensor tendon group is composed of the large tibialis anterior, the extensor hallucis longus, and the extensor digitorum longus (Fig. 7-15; see Fig. 7-11).[11,12,17,18] The tibialis anterior tendon is the most medial and largest of the extensor tendons extending to insert upon the medial cuneiform and first metatarsal.[18] At the level of the ankle joint, just lateral to the tibialis anterior tendon, is the extensor hallucis longus tendon and more laterally are the extensor digitorum longus and peroneus tertius tendons.[17,18]

Located along the posterolateral margin of the ankle, the peroneus longus and peroneus brevis tendons pass posterior to the distal fibula (Fig. 7-16; see Fig 7-11).[11,12,17,18] These

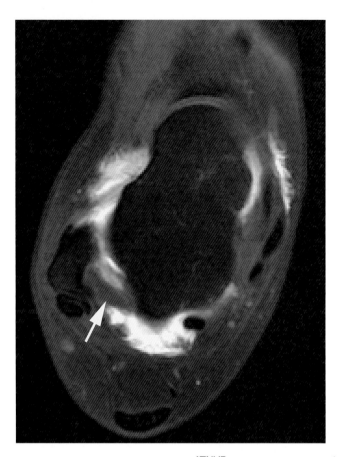

Figure 7-10 ■ Posterior talofibular ligament. Axial image from an MR arthrogram of the ankle depicts the posterior talofibular ligament *(arrow)* extending from the posteromedial aspect of the distal fibula to the posterior talar tubercle.

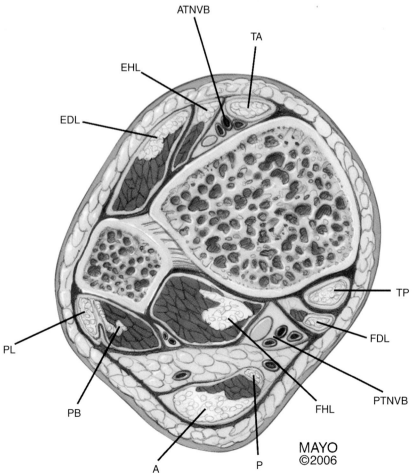

Figure 7-11 ■ Ankle anatomy. TP = tibialis posterior tendon; PTNVB = posterior tibial neurovascular bundle; FDL = flexor digitorum longus tendon; FHL = flexor hallucis longus tendon; P = plantaris tendon; A = Achilles tendon; PB = peroneus brevis tendon; PL = peroneus longus tendon; EDL = extensor digitorum longus tendon; EHL = extensor hallucis longus tendon; ATNVB = anterior tibial neurovascular bundle; TA = tibialis anterior tendon.

MAYO
©2006

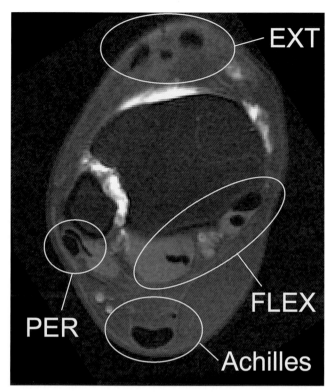

Figure 7-12 ■ Four major groups of tendons traverse the ankle joint and comprise a total of nine tendons. The flexor tendons are seen medially (FLEX), including the tibialis posterior, the flexor digitorum longus, and the flexor hallucis longus. The extensor tendons are seen anteriorly (EXT), including the tibialis anterior, the extensor hallucis longus, and the extensor digitorum longus. The peroneal tendons are seen laterally (PER), including the peroneus longus and peroneus brevis. The Achilles and plantaris tendons are seen posteriorly (Achilles).

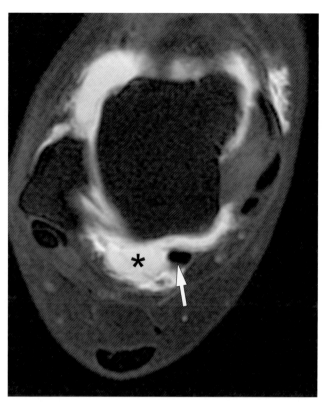

Figure 7-14 ■ Communication between the flexor hallucis longus tendon sheath *(arrow)* and posterior aspect of the ankle joint *(asterisk)*. This occurs in a high percentage of patients.

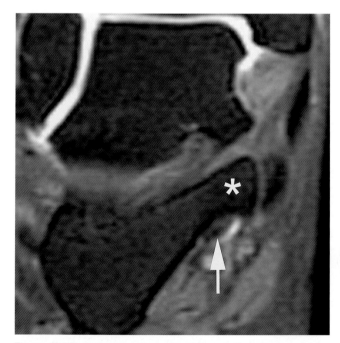

Figure 7-13 ■ Sustentaculum tali and flexor hallucis longus tendons. Coronal image from an MR arthrogram of the ankle demonstrating the flexor hallucis longus tendon *(arrow)* passing below the sustentaculum tali of the calcaneus *(asterisk)*. Note the small amount of contrast extending within the flexor hallucis longus tendon sheath, which communicates with the ankle joint.

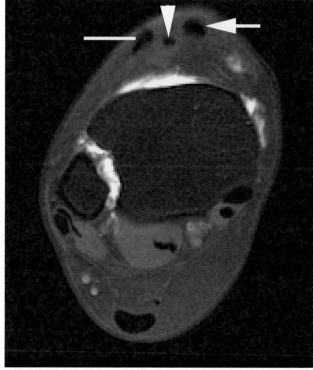

Figure 7-15 ■ Extensor tendons: tibialis anterior *(arrow)*, extensor hallucis longus *(arrowhead)*, and extensor digitorum longus *(line)*.

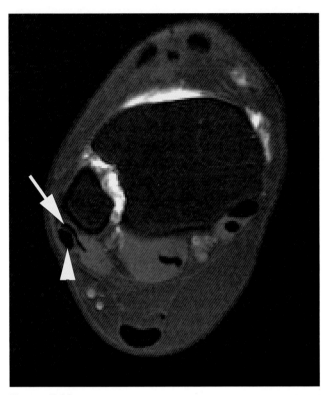

Figure 7-16 ■ Peroneal tendons: peroneus longus *(arrowhead)* and peroneus brevis *(arrow)* tendons.

tendons share a common tendon sheath and are closely applied to the posterior surface of the distal fibula.[11,12,17,18] At the level of the ankle, the peroneus longus tendon is superficial to the peroneus brevis tendon as the two tendons together curve around the distal fibula.[11,12,17,18] The peroneus brevis tendon inserts upon the base of the fifth metatarsal, and the peroneus longus tendon inserts on the base of the first metatarsal and medial cuneiform.[11,12,17,18] The peroneal tendons serve to evert and dorsiflex the foot and are important lateral stabilizers of the ankle.[18]

The longest and strongest tendon in the lower leg is the Achilles tendon.[17,18] The Achilles tendon is formed by the distal portion of the soleus and gastrocnemius musculature, and this tendon attaches to the posterior surface of the calcaneus (Fig. 7-17; see Fig 7-11).[17,18,23] The Achilles allows plantar flexion of the ankle and is approximately 10 to 15 cm in length with no associated tendon sheath.[17,18,23] Just medial to the Achilles tendon in the lower calf and ankle is the plantaris, which also inserts upon the calcaneus. The plantaris is a small muscle and tendon that provides flexion of the knee and plantar flexion of the foot.[18]

The foot is often divided into three segments, the hindfoot, the midfoot, and the forefoot (Fig. 7-18).[18] The hindfoot is composed of the talus and calcaneus; the midfoot includes the navicular, cuboid, and three cuneiforms (medial, middle, and lateral); and the forefoot is composed of the metatarsals and phalanges.[18] The primary articulation of the hindfoot is the subtalar joint, located between the talus and

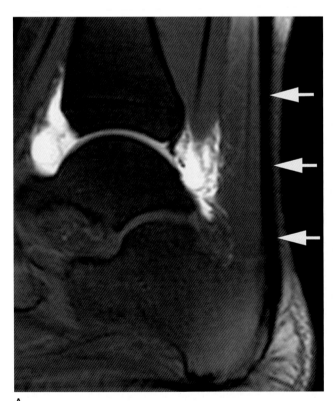

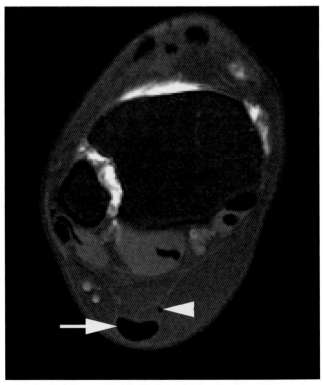

A   B

Figure 7-17 ■ Achilles tendons. Sagittal *(A)* and axial *(B)* images depicting the Achilles tendon *(arrow)* formed by the distal portion of the soleus and gastrocnemius musculature, inserting on the posterior surface of the calcaneus. The smaller plantaris tendon is seen medially *(arrowhead)*.

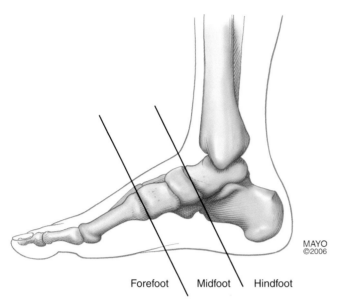

Forefoot | Midfoot | Hindfoot

MAYO
©2006

Figure 7-18 ■ The foot is often divided into three segments: the hindfoot, the midfoot, and the forefoot. The hindfoot is composed of the talus and calcaneus. The midfoot includes the navicular, cuboid, and three cuneiforms (medial, middle, and lateral). The forefoot is composed of the metatarsals and phalanges.

calcaneus.[18] The subtalar joint is subdivided into the anterior, middle, and posterior facets.[17,18] The posterior facet is the largest facet, whereas the anterior facet is the smallest and most variable in size and shape.[17,18] The sinus tarsi is a

recess that exists between the anterior and middle facets of the subtalar joint and contains fat, several ligaments, and neurovascular structures (Fig. 7-19).[18,24] The sinus tarsi is cone shaped, extending in a posteromedial to anterolateral course at approximately a 45-degree angle relative to the axis of the calcaneus.[18] There are several ligaments and retinacular elements within the sinus tarsi; the most significant are the cervical ligament and the ligament of the tarsal canal (Fig. 7-20).[18,24]

At the junction of the hindfoot and midfoot are the talonavicular and calcaneocuboid articulations.[18] There are multiple intertarsal articulations and several intervening ligaments that connect the navicular, cuboid, and cuneiform bones of the midfoot.[17,18] The tarsometatarsal articulations form the junction of the midfoot and forefoot.[18] The dorsal, plantar, and intraosseous ligaments support the tarsometatarsal articulations.[18] Distally, the five metacarpal heads are connected by the transverse metacarpal ligament.[17,181] The metatarsophalangeal articulations form between the metatarsals and the proximal phalanges and are stabilized primarily by the collateral and plantar ligaments and dorsally by the extensor tendons.[18]

The plantar aponeurosis or plantar fascia is a sophisticated combination of fibers that are composed of a network of tendinous bundles along the plantar aspect of the foot (Fig. 7-21).[18,25] The plantar fascia is a strong structure that contributes greatly to the stability of the longitudinal arch of the foot.[18,25] The plantar fascia is composed of three segments: the medial, central, and lateral segments.[18,25] The thickest portion of the plantar aponeurosis is the central

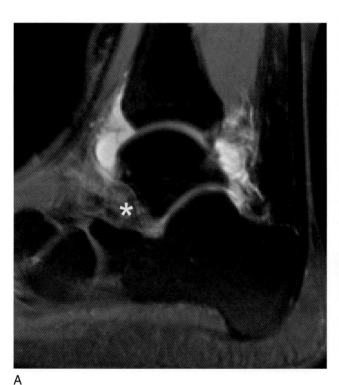

A

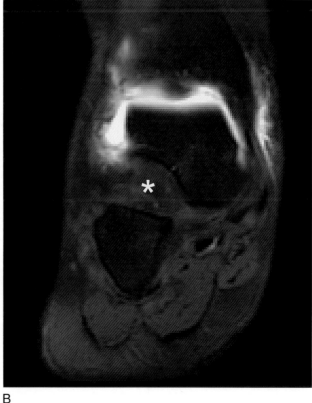

B

Figure 7-19 ■ Sinus tarsi. Sagittal (*A*) and coronal (*B*) images depict the sinus tarsi (*asterisk*) as a cone-shaped space between the anterior and middle facets of the subtalar joint, which contains fat, several ligaments, and neurovascular structures.

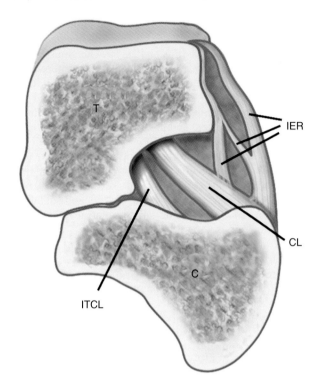

Figure 7-20 ■ Sinus tarsi. T = talus; C = calcaneus; ITCL = interosseous talocalcaneal ligament; CL = cervical ligament; IER = medial, intermediate, and lateral roots of the inferior extensor retinaculum.

segment.[17] The central segment attaches to the medial portion of the calcaneal tuberosity.[17] As the central segment passes distally it broadens, thins, and finally divides at the level of the metatarsophalangeal joints and inserts upon the phalanges.[17] The lateral band of the plantar fascia is thin and extends from the lateral process of the calcaneal tuberosity to the base of the

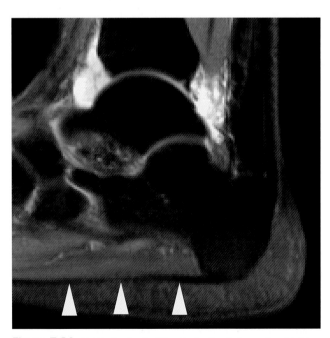

Figure 7-21 ■ Plantar fascia. The plantar fascia *(arrowheads)* represents a sophisticated combination of fibers that comprise a network of tendinous bundles along the plantar aspect of the foot.

fifth metatarsal.[17] The medial segment of the plantar fascia is also thin, extending from the medial aspect of the calcaneal tuberosity and blending distally with the central segment of the aponeurosis and the flexor retinaculum.[17]

PATIENT SELECTION

There continue to be many indications for image-guided injections of the foot and ankle. Therapeutic injections of the foot and ankle are widely utilized to alleviate joint pain and to localize the source of nonspecific pain about the foot and ankle.[7–9] CT and MR ankle arthrography can be useful to diagnose intra-articular pathology of the ankle and to define disorders of the joint and its surrounding capsule and synovium.[1,26,27] Ankle arthrography gives the most information if followed by post-arthrography CT or MR, which provides multiplanar views of the ankle joint with high spatial resolution and soft tissue contrast. Ankle joint aspiration can also be performed to obtain joint fluid for evaluation of possible crystal deposition or joint infection.[2]

Therapeutic Foot and Ankle Injections

Therapeutic injections are commonly performed for relief of foot and ankle pain (Fig. 7-22).[7–9] Injections typically contain anesthetic agents such as bupivacaine or lidocaine, often

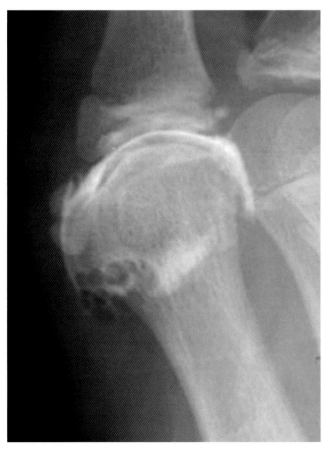

Figure 7-22 ■ Diagnostic and therapeutic metatarsophalangeal (MTP) joint injection. Patient with chronic medial forefoot pain reported significant relief following injection of the first MTP joint with bupivacaine.

used in combination with long-acting corticosteroids.[7–9] Substantial relief can often be obtained with therapeutic injections of the ankle joint and of the small joints of the foot. The duration of pain relief is variable; however, occasionally lasting relief can be achieved.

In addition to pain relief, these injections can play an important diagnostic role in the evaluation of vague or nonspecific foot and ankle pain. Intra-articular injections of anesthetic agents aid in determining the precise origin of the patient's symptoms.[7–9] Significant pain relief from an anesthetic injection localizes the joint of interest, and lack of response to a given injection suggests an alternative source of the pain.[7–9]

In addition to articular injections, injections of the soft tissues about the foot and ankle can be performed using image guidance. Painful tendons and ligaments can be injected for short-term relief of symptoms related to inflammatory processes or overuse injuries of these structures.[11,12] Therapeutic injections of the plantar fascia can also be performed for short-term relief of discomfort referable to the attachment of the plantar aponeurosis upon the plantar surface of the calcaneus.[2]

CT Ankle Arthrography

CT arthrography has proved to be an excellent means for evaluating the articular hyaline cartilage of the ankle joint.[4,5,15] Cartilaginous defects of the tibial plafond or talar dome are well demonstrated with the addition of intra-articular contrast (Fig. 7-23).[4,5,14,15] Osteochondral defects can

also be evaluated and the stability of osteochondral fragments can be assessed by the presence or absence of contrast imbibition around a fragment located within the osteochondral defect.[4,14] Post-arthrogram CT using thin slices allows isotropic reformatted images in any plane, which can help to define precisely even small cartilaginous defects. Synovial proliferative disorders and loose bodies are also well delineated with CT arthrography. CT arthrography provides an excellent alternative to patients with contraindications to MR imaging or patients who cannot tolerate MR examinations.

CT Tenography

Tenography followed by CT can clearly demonstrate the tendinous structures of the ankle. With this technique, contrast within the tendon sheath outlines the tendon, allowing visualization of the tendon configuration (Fig. 7-24).[10–12] Post-tenography CT utilizing thin slices allows one to generate isotropic reformatted images. This permits high-quality reconstructions of the tendon in any plane, which is especially useful in the ankle, as the tendons change from a vertical course in the lower leg to a more horizontal course in the foot (Fig. 7-25). The peroneal tendons can be well seen with CT tenography as they course about the distal fibula, and the flexor tendons can also be well seen along the medial aspect of the ankle. Like CT ankle arthrography, CT tenography of the ankle provides an excellent alternative to MR imaging in patients with contraindications to MR or those who cannot tolerate MR examinations.

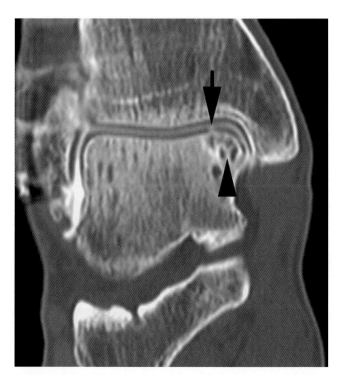

Figure 7-23 ▪ CT arthrogram of the ankle depicts an osteochondral defect involving the medial talar dome with disruption of the articular hyaline cartilage *(arrow)* and associated underlying cystic changes in the subchondral bone *(arrowhead).*

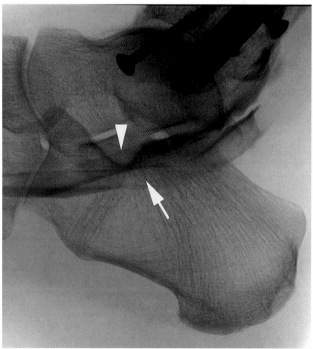

Figure 7-24 ▪ Flexor tenogram. Lateral image from a flexor tendon tenogram depicts contrast material outlining both the flexor digitorum longus *(arrowhead)* and the flexor hallucis longus *(arrow)* tendons.

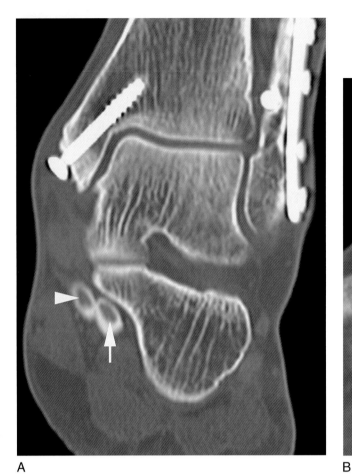

A

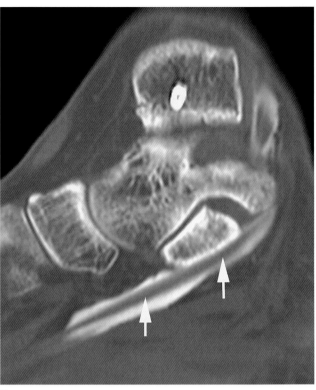

B

Figure 7-25 ■ Flexor tendon CT tenogram. Coronal (*A*) and sagittal (*B*) reformatted images from a CT tenogram of the flexor tendons depicts contrast material outlining both the flexor hallucis longus *(arrow)* and the flexor digitorum longus *(arrowhead)*.

MR Ankle Arthrography

MR arthrography can be used to precisely define the articular hyaline cartilage of the ankle joint (Fig. 7-26).[1,26,28,29] Although MR arthrography does not provide significantly more information than conventional MR of the ankle, it can occasionally be useful in patients with equivocal findings with conventional MR imaging (Fig. 7-27). In addition, as with CT arthrography of the ankle, osteochondral defects can be well evaluated and the stability of associated fragments can be established with intra-articular gadolinium injection.[3] MR arthrography can also precisely evaluate and characterize synovial disorders and synovial proliferative processes and localize loose bodies.[1,26,28,29]

CONTRAINDICATIONS[30]

* Coagulopathy (International Normalized Ratio [INR] >1.5 or platelets < 50,000/mm^3)
* Pregnancy (because of teratogenic effects of radiation)
* Systemic infection or skin infection over the puncture site
* Severe allergy to any component of the injectate
* The patient has received the maximum amount of steroid including systemic steroids allowed for a given time period unless the injection is to be performed without steroid

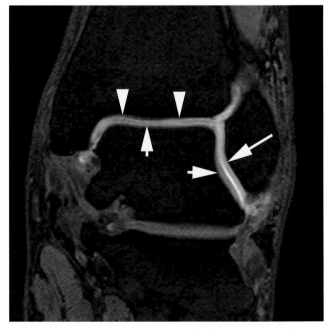

Figure 7-26 ■ Coronal image from an MR arthrogram of the ankle depicting the articular hyaline cartilage of the plafond *(arrowheads)*, talus *(short arrows)*, and distal fibula *(long arrow)*.

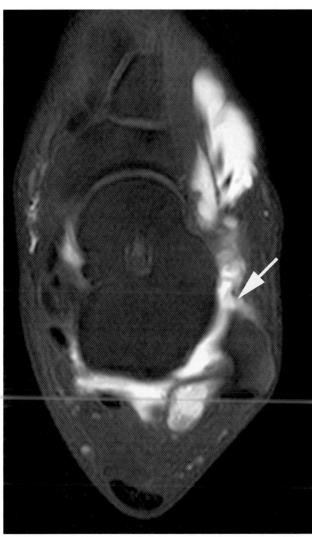

Figure 7-27 ■ Anterior talofibular ligament tear. Axial image from an MR arthrogram of the ankle demonstrating a tear of the anterior talofibular ligament *(arrow)* with extravasation of contrast material into the surrounding anterolateral soft tissues of the ankle.

PROCEDURE

Equipment/Supplies

Procedural

* Spinal needle, 22-gauge, 3.5-inch (Quincke-type point, Becton Dickinson, Franklin Lakes, NJ) or 25-gauge, 1.5-inch needle
* Luer-Lock (10- or 20-mL) syringe containing injection mixture
* Sterile tubing to connect injection solution to spinal needle
* Control 12-mL syringe with 25-gauge, 1.5-inch needle containing 8 mL 1% lidocaine for local anesthesia and 2 mL 8.4% sodium bicarbonate injectable (1 mEq/mL) to alleviate burning pain associated with anesthetic
* Sterile 4 × 4 gauze pads
* Povidone-iodine (Betadine) and alcohol for preparation
* Sterile towels or fenestrated drape for draping

* Needle, 18-gauge, 1.5-inch, to draw up lidocaine and medication
* Adhesive bandage

Imaging

* Lead apron
* Multidirectional C-arm fluoroscopy with film archiving capability

Medications (Injection Mixtures)

Volume

The typical ankle joint volume is approximately 3 to 6 mL. A 10-mL syringe is utilized for ankle injections. A 3- to 6-mL solution is typically injected regardless of the indication, whether therapeutic injection or diagnostic CT or MR arthrography. Other joints about the foot that can be injected are much smaller in volume. Commonly injected joints such as the subtalar joint, the talonavicular joint, and the calcaneonavicular joint accept an injection volume of no more than 1 to 2 mL.

Therapeutic Ankle Injection

10-mL syringe
3- to 6-mL total injected joint volume
5 mL iodinated contrast (Reno-60, Omnipaque 300)
4 to 5 mL anesthetic agent (bupivacaine hydrochloride 0.5%*, lidocaine hydrochloride 1% MPF*)
Optional: 0 to 1 mL steroid (methylprednisolone sodium succinate [Solu-Medrol 40 mg/mL, Depo-Medrol 40 mg/mL], triamcinolone [Kenalog-40], betamethasone sodium phosphate and betamethasone acetate [Celestone Soluspan 6 mg/mL])

CT Ankle Arthrography

10-mL syringe
3- to 6-mL total injected joint volume
5 mL iodinated contrast
4 to 5 mL anesthetic agent
Optional: 0 to 1 mL steroid

MR Ankle Arthrography

10-mL syringe
3- to 6-mL total injected joint volume
5 mL iodinated contrast
4 to 5 mL anesthetic agent
0.1 to 0.2 mL gadopentetate dimeglumine MR contrast (Omniscan, Magnevist)

CT Tenography

10-mL syringe
2- to 8-mL total injected joint volume

---

*Local anesthetics should be from single-use vials and be free of paraben (MPF) and phenol to prevent flocculation of the steroid.[31]

5 mL iodinated contrast
4 to 5 mL anesthetic agent
Optional: 0 to 1 mL steroid

Foot Joint Injection

10-mL syringe
1- to 2-mL total injected joint volume
5 mL iodinated contrast
4 to 5 mL anesthetic agent
Optional: 0 to 1 mL steroid

Methodology

Ankle Joint Injection

The patient is placed on the fluoroscopy table in the supine position with the foot plantar flexed (Fig. 7-28). The dorsalis pedis artery should be palpated and identified to avoid puncture (Fig. 7-29). The tibialis anterior tendon is palpated. This is the large tendon anterior to the ankle joint, which becomes prominent when the patient is asked to dorsiflex the foot against resistance. The optimal puncture site for an ankle joint injection is located just medial to the tibialis anterior tendon and approximately 1 cm below the level of the ankle joint to avoid the overhanging anterior margin of the distal tibia (Fig. 7-30). A metallic object such as a hemostat should be utilized to indicate the injection site at fluoroscopy (Fig. 7-31), and the corresponding site should be marked on the patient's skin with an indelible marker.

The field overlying the target site is sterilely prepared and draped. Local anesthesia of the skin and underlying subcutaneous tissue is obtained with 1% lidocaine with 8.4% sodium bicarbonate buffer (Fig. 7-32). A 25-gauge, 1.5-inch spinal needle can then be advanced through the soft tissues with the needle angled slightly cephalad to avoid the over-

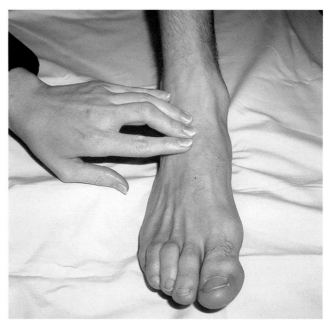

Figure 7-29 ▪ Ankle injection. The dorsalis pedis artery should be palpated and identified to avoid puncture. The puncture site for an ankle joint injection is located just medial to the tibialis anterior tendon and approximately 1 cm below the level of the ankle joint.

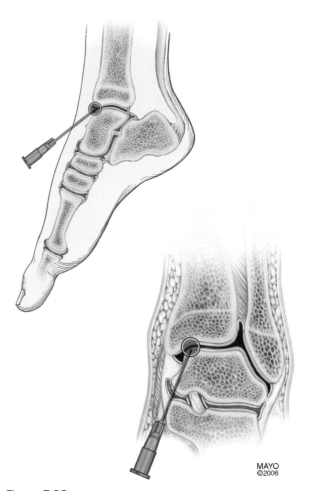

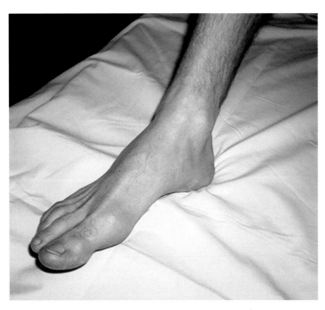

Figure 7-28 ▪ Positioning for ankle arthrography. The patient is placed on the fluoroscopy table in the supine position with the foot plantar flexed.

Figure 7-30 ▪ Ankle joint injection. The optimal puncture site for an ankle joint injection is located just medial to the tibialis anterior tendon and approximately 1 cm below the level of the ankle joint to avoid the overhanging anterior margin of the distal tibia.

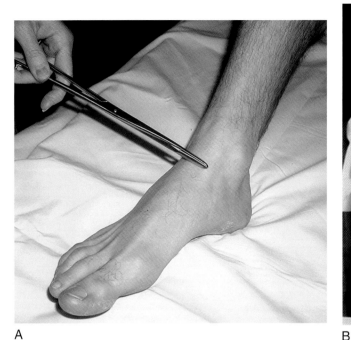

A

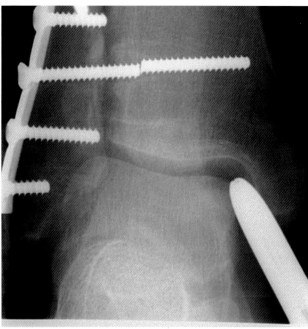

B

Figure 7-31 ■ Ankle injection. A metallic object such as a set of Kelly clamps (*A*) should be utilized to identify the precise location of the injection (*B*).

hanging anterior margin of the distal tibia (Fig. 7-33). The needle should be advanced directly into the joint. It is not uncommon for the patient to experience discomfort when the needle enters the joint or makes contact with the periosteum of the bone. Fluoroscopy is then utilized to check the needle position (Fig. 7-34). Alterations in needle position can be made to place the needle at the intended target site.

When the needle has been properly positioned, the syringe and tubing containing the solution to be injected into the

ankle joint are connected to the indwelling needle (Fig. 7-35). A small test injection should be performed to ensure appropriate intra-articular placement of the needle (Fig. 7-36). If resistance is met to the injection, the needle may be embedded in the bone or the capsule may be tented over the needle. Rotating while advancing the needle may be helpful to penetrate the capsule if it is being tented by the needle, and slight withdrawal of the needle may be helpful if the needle is embedded in the bone. If contrast material collects at the

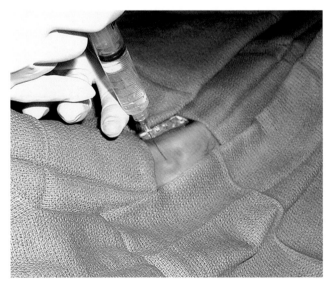

Figure 7-32 ■ Ankle injection. Local anesthesia of the skin and underlying subcutaneous tissue is obtained with 1% lidocaine with 8.4% sodium bicarbonate buffer.

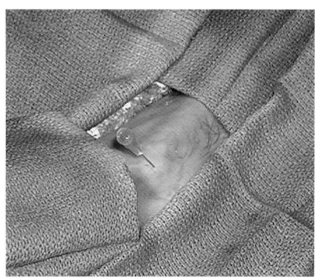

Figure 7-33 ■ Ankle injection. A 25-gauge, 1.5-inch spinal needle is advanced through the soft tissues into the ankle joint with the needle angled slightly cephalad to avoid the overhanging anterior margin of the distal tibia.

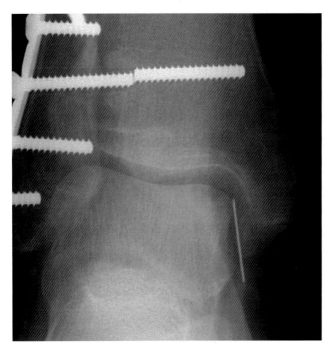

Figure 7-34 ■ Fluoroscopy is then utilized to check the needle position. A 25-gauge needle is seen with its tip within the medial aspect of the ankle joint.

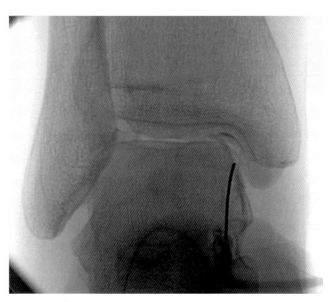

Figure 7-36 ■ A small test injection confirms intra-articular placement of the needle.

needle tip, the needle is extra-articular and needs to be repositioned. If contrast flows freely away from the needle tip, the injection mixture can be administered (Fig. 7-37). The entire injection is performed under continuous fluoroscopic monitoring to ensure continued intra-articular placement of the needle throughout the injection and avoid inadvertent extra-articular injection. The volume of the injection is typically 3 to 6 mL.

Following the injection, the needle is withdrawn. Fluoroscopic evaluation of the joint may be useful while placing

the ankle in different projectional positions. For CT and MR arthrography, movement of the joint should be kept to a minimum to avoid extravasation from the joint prior to imaging. The patient should be transferred to the CT or MR scanner in an MR-compatible wheelchair.

Foot Joint Injections

Injection of the smaller joints of the foot is similar to injections of the ankle joint; however, approaches vary depend-

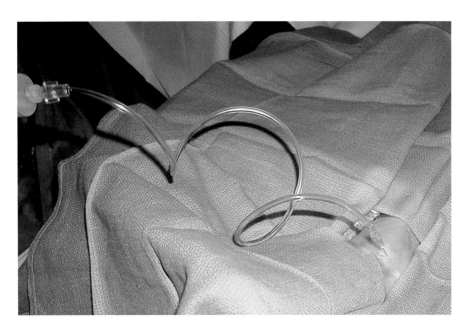

Figure 7-35 ■ Once the needle is properly positioned, the syringe and tubing containing the solution are connected to the needle.

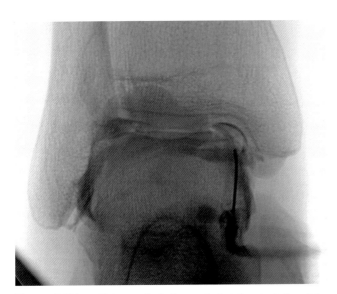

Figure 7-37 ■ If the needle in intra-articular, the remainder of the injection is performed under continuous fluoroscopic monitoring.

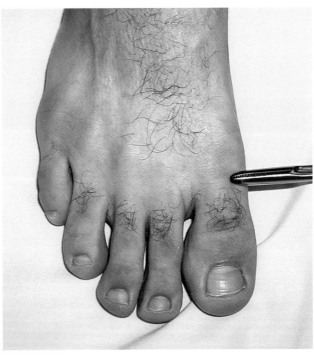

Figure 7-38 ■ The metatarsophalangeal articulations can be approached from a direct vertical approach from the dorsal aspect of the foot.

ing on the articulation to be injected. Joints that can be injected include the subtalar joint, talonavicular joint, naviculocuneiform joint, calcaneocuboid joint, and the tarsometatarsal, metatarsophalangeal, and interphalangeal articulations. The approach utilized depends on the joint to be injected. Most injections are performed with the patient in the supine or lateral position. The tarsometatarsal, metatarsophalangeal, and intertarsal articulations can be approached from a direct vertical approach from the dorsal aspect of the foot (Fig. 7-38). The talonavicular and naviculocuneiform articulations can be injected by a direct vertical or oblique dorsal medial approach (Fig. 7-39). The calcaneocuboid articulation can be injected by a lateral approach with the patient's foot placed in the opposite oblique lateral or lateral decubitus position (Fig. 7-40). A similar lateral approach can be used to inject the posterior facet of the subtalar joint. The middle facet of the subtalar joint can be approached medially with the patient in the oblique lateral or lateral decubitus position.

The solution to be injected into the articulation is then drawn into a 10-mL syringe. A metallic object such as a hemostat is used to indicate the precise location of the injec-

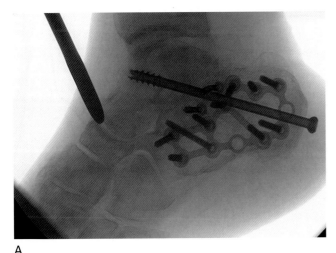

A

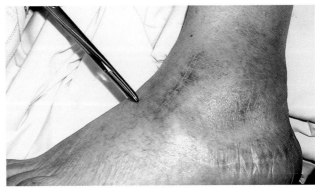

B

Figure 7-39 ■ The talonavicular articulation can be injected by a direct vertical or oblique dorsal approach with the foot oblique to the table.

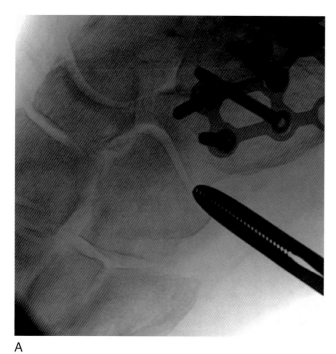

A

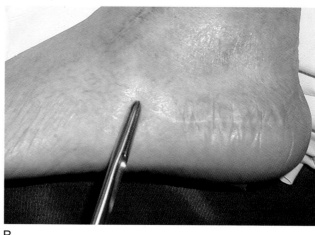

B

Figure 7-40 ■ Calcaneocuboid joint injection. The calcaneocuboid articulation can be injected by a lateral approach.

tion fluoroscopically, and the patient's skin should be marked accordingly with an indelible marker. The field is then prepared and draped in a sterile fashion. A 25-gauge needle is advanced directly into the joint. Fluoroscopy is utilized to check the needle position (Fig. 7-41). Alterations in needle position can then be made. The articulations between the small bones of the feet are usually very narrow. When the needle has been properly positioned, the syringe and

tubing containing the solution to be injected are connected to the indwelling 25-gauge needle. A small test injection should be performed to ensure appropriate intra-articular placement of the needle (Fig. 7-42). The small joints of the foot are typically very low in volume, requiring only a 1- to 2-mL injection. The entire injection should be performed under continuous fluoroscopic monitoring. Following the injection, the needle is withdrawn.

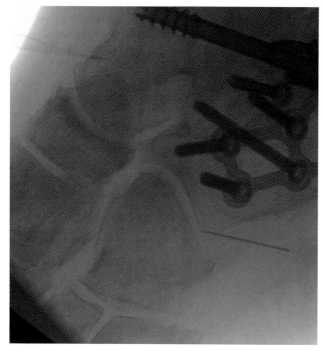

Figure 7-41 ■ Calcaneocuboid joint injection. A 25-gauge needle is advanced into the joint. Fluoroscopy is utilized to check needle position.

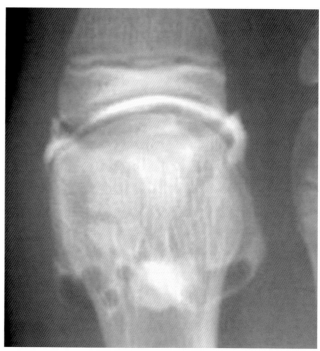

Figure 7-42 ■ First metatarsophalangeal (MTP) joint injection. AP image following injection of the first MTP joint for therapeutic purposes.

Tenography

Plantar Fascia Injection

Sinus Tarsi Injection

Several tendon sheaths around the foot and ankle are accessible to tenography. The most commonly injected tendons include the common peroneal tendon sheath and the tibialis posterior tendon sheath, but the tendon sheaths for the tibialis anterior, the flexor hallucis longus, and the flexor digitorum longus are also easily accessible. The flexor and extensor tendons distally in the foot can usually be injected with little difficulty. The plantar fascial attachment and the sinus tarsi can also be injected under image guidance in symptomatic patients.

Prior to injection, radiographs of the foot are obtained and reviewed. The patient is placed on the fluoroscopy table in the position best suited for reaching the desired tendon sheath or soft tissue structure. For tenography of the flexor tendons (tibialis posterior, flexor hallucis longus, or flexor digitorum longus) the lateral aspect of the foot and ankle is placed against the table (Fig. 7-43). For peroneal tenography (peroneus longus or peroneus brevis) the medial aspect of the ankle should rest against the table (Fig. 7-44). For tenography of the extensor tendons (tibialis anterior, extensor hallucis longus, or extensor digitorum longus) the heel is placed against the table (Fig. 7-45).

A metallic object such as a hemostat is used to indicate the precise location of the injection, and the patient's skin should be marked with an indelible marker (Fig. 7-46). The target site varies depending on the target to be injected. Two points along the course of the tendon to be injected should be identified utilizing anatomic landmarks. A line is then drawn on the skin along the expected course of the tendon (Fig. 7-47). The field is prepared and draped in the usual sterile fashion and local anesthesia is given. A 0.5- or 1.5-inch, 25-gauge needle is used to anesthetize the skin and entry site (Fig. 7-48). This same needle can be held at a 45-degree angle relative to the table and advanced along the long axis of the tendon sheath (Fig. 7-49). Typically, a firm

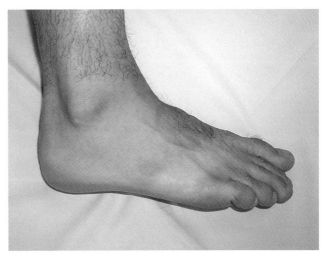

Figure 7-44 ▪ Positioning for peroneal tenography. The medial aspect of the ankle should rest against the table with the lateral aspect of the ankle exposed.

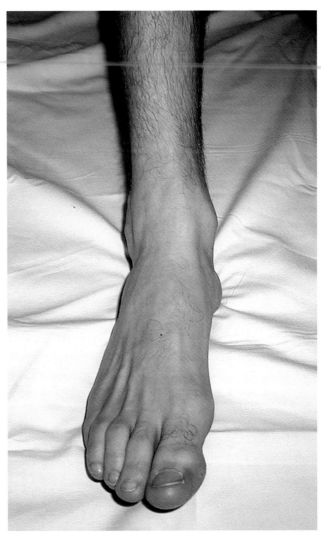

Figure 7-45 ▪ Positioning for extensor tenography. The heel and plantar aspect of the foot is placed against the table with the dorsum of the foot and ankle exposed.

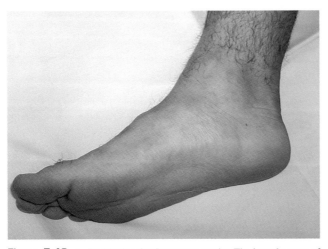

Figure 7-43 ▪ Positioning for flexor tenography. The lateral aspect of the foot and ankle is placed against the table with the medial aspect of the ankle exposed.

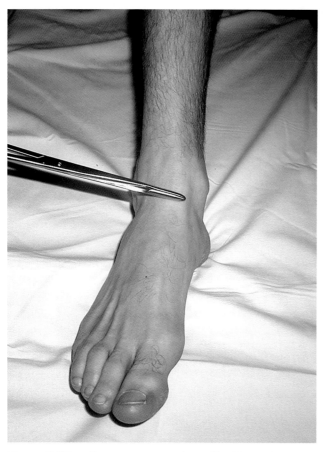

Figure 7-46 ■ Extensor tenogram. A metallic object such as a set of Kelly clamps should be utilized to identify the precise location of the puncture site.

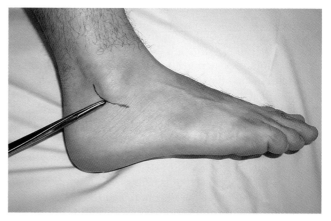

Figure 7-47 ■ A line can be drawn on the skin along the expected course of the tendon to aid in guiding the tendon sheath injection.

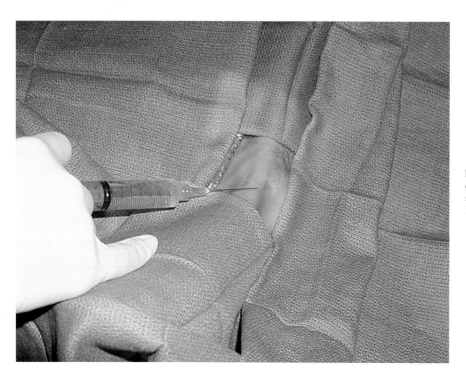

Figure 7-48 ■ Local anesthesia is obtained utilizing 1% lidocaine with 8.4% sodium bicarbonate buffer with a 0.5- or 1.5-inch, 25-gauge needle.

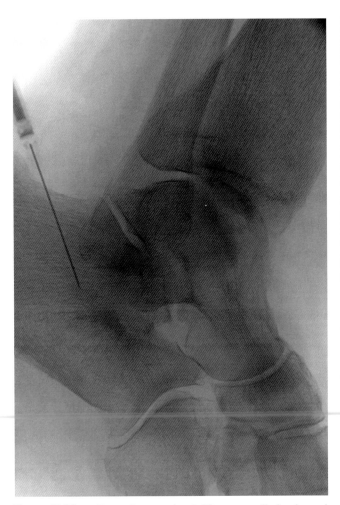

Figure 7-49 ■ Peroneal tenography. A 25-gauge needle is advanced along the long axis of the tendon to be injected.

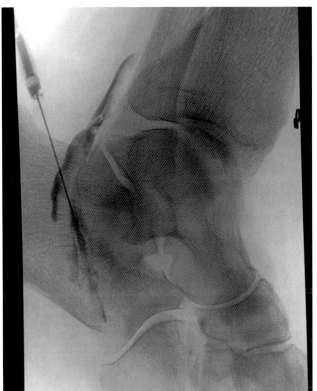

Figure 7-50 ■ A small test injection is performed to evaluate needle position. Contrast material is seen flowing away from the needle tip in a linear fashion outlining the tendon of the tendon sheath.

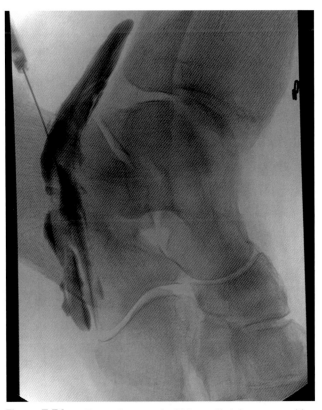

Figure 7-51 ■ Peroneal tenography. If the needle is in correct position the remainder of the injection is performed under fluoroscopic monitoring. The volume injected is variable but should be adequate to distend and visualize the entire tendon sheath.

structure can be felt as the needle makes contact with the tendon. The syringe and tubing containing the solution to be injected are connected to the indwelling needle. A small test injection should be performed to evaluate needle position. Ideally, the contrast material is seen flowing away from the needle tip in a linear fashion outlining the tendon if the tendon sheath has been penetrated (Fig. 7-50). The volume injected is variable, but typically an injection of about 2 to 8 mL should be adequate to distend and visualize the entire tendon sheath (Fig. 7-51). The entire injection is performed using continuous fluoroscopic monitoring.

The needle is withdrawn following the injection. Fluoroscopic evaluation of the tendon sheath is then performed and a spot radiographic image is obtained. Provocative maneuvers may be useful to evaluate the dynamic motion of the tendon and evaluate for subluxation or dislocation. The patient is then transferred to the CT table, where post-procedure CT is performed, obtaining thin-section high-resolution images. Obtaining isotropic multi-planar reformatted images allows one to visualize the tendon in any plane.

A similar approach is utilized for therapeutic injections of the plantar fascia and sinus tarsi. In both cases the foot is placed on the table with the medial aspect in contact with the table and the lateral aspect exposed. Site localization, sterile preparation, and local anesthesia are performed in a fashion similar to that for tenography, as described previously. For both plantar fascia injections and injections of the sinus tarsi, a 25-gauge, 1.5-inch needle is utilized. For plantar fascia injections, the needle is advanced to the plantar fascia and injection of anesthetic agent and corticosteroids is performed about the plantar fascia. For sinus tarsi injections, the needle is advanced by a lateral approach into the sinus tarsi between the talus and calcaneus and anesthetic agent and corticosteroids are injected throughout the sinus tarsi. In both cases, a specific structure is not being injected but rather the soft tissues surrounding or within the region of interest are injected with the goal of pain relief.

POTENTIAL COMPLICATIONS[30]

* Bleeding
* Infection (cellulitis, septic arthritis, or osteomyelitis)
* Drug-related allergic reactions
* Transient synovitis
* Transitory lower extremity weakness
* Transitory lower extremity paresthesia
* Arterial or venous injury

POST-PROCEDURE CARE/FOLLOW-UP[30]

Immediate

1. The patient should be observed for 15 minutes after the injection.
2. Blood pressure, pulse, heart rate, and respiratory rate are monitored as necessary.

Discharge

1. An adhesive bandage is placed on the puncture site. The bandage should remain dry for at least 24 hours, at which point it can be removed.
2. The patient is instructed to continue taking his or her prescription medication, although pain medication may be tapered as indicated.
3. A discharge sheet should be given to the patient outlining the following:
   a. The procedure performed
   b. Procedure-related symptoms that typically resolve in 7 to 10 days
      * Pain at the needle puncture site(s)
      * Mild increase in ankle or foot stiffness with a feeling of fullness in the joint
      * Deep ankle or foot pain
   c. Treatment for mild post-procedure symptoms
      * Rest the ankle or foot for 1 to 2 days
      * Avoid movements that worsen the pain
      * Use cold compresses to the area that hurts
   d. Signs and symptoms of infection
      * Fever
      * Chills
      * Swelling or drainage from the puncture site(s)

* New ankle or foot pain that is different from the usual pain
   e. Signs and symptoms of possible, more serious problems
      * Decreased range of motion of the ankle or foot
      * Increasing pain
      * Motor dysfunction of the lower extremity
   f. Physician name and contact number if the patient has any concerns or if any problems were to arise as a result of the procedure
   g. Advice to schedule a follow-up appointment with the referring physician in 7 to 10 days.

SAMPLE DICTATIONS

MR Ankle Arthrography

After the procedure was explained to the patient and informed consent was obtained, the patient was placed on the table in the supine position. The skin overlying the ankle articulation was prepared and draped in the usual sterile fashion. Local anesthesia was obtained with 1% lidocaine with bicarbonate buffer. Under fluoroscopic guidance, a 25-gauge, 1.5-inch needle was advanced into the ankle joint and a 5-mL solution containing iodinated contrast material, bupivacaine, and gadolinium was administered into the ankle articulation. The needle was withdrawn. The patient was sent to MR for additional imaging of the ankle after arthrography.

CT Peroneal Tenography

After the procedure was explained to the patient and informed consent was obtained, the patient was placed on the table with the foot in the lateral position. The course of the peroneus longus tendon was identified and the skin overlying it was sterilely prepared and draped in the usual fashion. Local anesthesia was obtained with 1% lidocaine with bicarbonate buffer. Under fluoroscopic guidance, a 25-gauge, 0.5-inch needle was advanced into the peroneal tendon sheath and a 5-mL solution containing iodinated contrast material and bupivacaine was administered into the tendon sheath. The needle was withdrawn. The patient reported moderate relief of symptoms immediately following the injection. The patient was sent to CT for additional imaging of the ankle after tenography.

Calcaneocuboid Injection

After the procedure was explained to the patient and informed consent was obtained, the patient was placed on the table with the foot in the lateral position. The skin overlying the calcaneocuboid articulation was sterilely prepared and draped in the usual fashion. Local anesthesia was administered with 1% lidocaine with bicarbonate buffer. Under fluoroscopic guidance, a 25-gauge, 0.5-inch needle was advanced into the calcaneocuboid articulation and a 2-mL solution containing iodinated contrast material, bupivacaine, and Kenalog-40 was administered into the joint. The needle was withdrawn. The patient reported prompt relief of symptoms following the injection.

CASE REPORTS

CASE 1

Clinical Presentation

A 46-year-old male patient presented with lateral ankle pain following a fall resulting in inversion of the foot. Several months of swelling and tenderness followed. Soft tissue edema subsided after 2 months, but pain persisted. The patient reported a clicking noise and feeling of instability with inversion of the foot. Pain was localized at the distal tip of the fibula. Physical examination demonstrated no instability of the ankle joint.

Imaging and Therapy

An MR arthrogram of the ankle was requested to evaluate the integrity of the lateral ankle ligaments and assess whether ankle injection relieved the patient's symptoms. The patient was placed on the fluoroscopy table with the foot in plantar flexion. The tibialis anterior tendon and dorsalis pedis artery were identified. The puncture site overlying the medial aspect of the ankle joint was identified fluoroscopically and marked. The ankle was prepared and draped in the usual sterile fashion. A 22-gauge needle was advanced into the ankle joint under fluoroscopic guidance (Fig. 7-52). A 6-mL solution containing bupivacaine, iodinated contrast material, and gadolinium was injected. The needle was removed and post-arthrography MR of the ankle was performed.

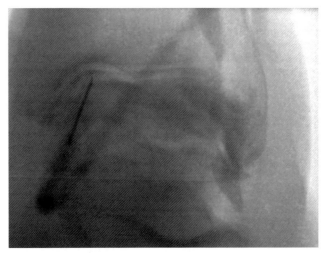

Figure 7-52 ■ Ankle arthrography. A 22-gauge needle has been advanced into the ankle joint under fluoroscopic guidance. A small test injection confirms intra-articular position of the needle tip.

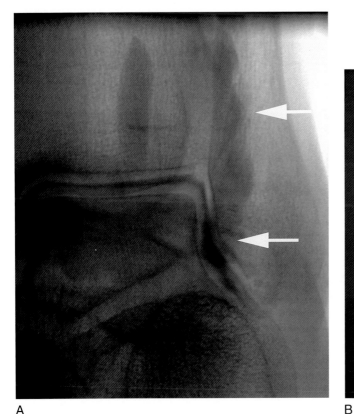

A

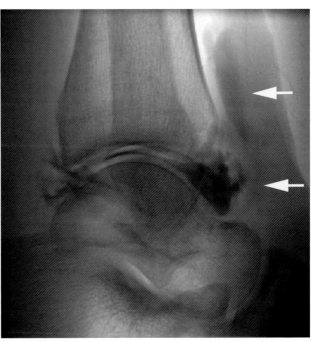

B

Figure 7-53 ■ Conventional ankle arthrography. Oblique (*A*) and lateral (*B*) images depict extravasation (*arrows*) from the lateral aspect of the ankle joint anteriorly.

Results

Conventional arthrography depicted extravasation from the lateral aspect of the ankle joint (Fig. 7-53). Fluoroscopic images in various projections depicted the extravasation to be anterior at the level of the distal fibula. Findings were compatible with rupture of the anterior talofibular ligament. This was confirmed with MR arthrography with absence of visualization of the anterior talofibular ligament compatible with rupture and associated extravasation of contrast material from this site into the anterolateral soft tissues of the ankle and foot (Fig. 7-54). The calcaneofibular and posterior talofibular ligaments remained intact. The ankle injection provided minimal short-term improvement in symptoms. Conservative therapy was chosen with physical therapy to strengthen the peroneal tendon group and increase lower extremity conditioning. The patient's symptoms significantly improved by 3 months and did not require surgical intervention.

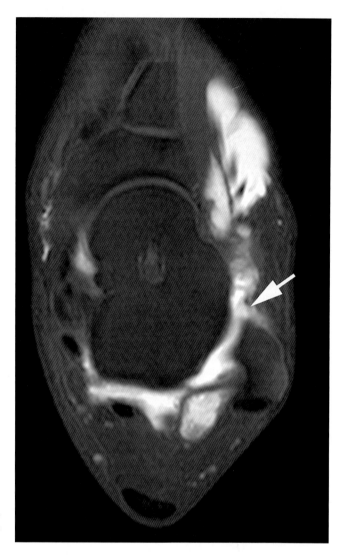

Figure 7-54 ■ Anterior talofibular ligament tear. MR arthrography depicts rupture of the anterior talofibular ligament with extravasation anteriorly and laterally into the surrounding tissues.

CASE 2

Clinical Presentation

The patient is a 70-year-old man with prior calcaneal fracture after open reduction and internal fixation with lateral side plate and screws 2 years previously. The patient now presents with pain about the left lateral ankle that has increased over the last year. Physical examination localizes the pain just posterior to the distal fibula in the region of the peroneal tendons. No peroneal subluxation is noted. The pain is worse with weight bearing and walking. The patient reports little relief from nonsteroidal anti-inflammatory medications.

Imaging and Therapy

Peroneal CT tenography was performed. Metallic hardware limited visualization of the peroneal tendons with MR imaging. The patient was placed on the fluoroscopic table with the left ankle in the lateral position with the medial ankle against the table and the lateral ankle exposed. The precise location of the left distal fibula was identified by palpation and fluoroscopy. The peroneal tendons could also be palpated coursing posterior to the lateral malleolus. The course was identified and marked on the skin. The skin was prepared and draped in the usual sterile fashion. A 25-gauge needle was advanced along the long axis of the peroneal tendons at the level of the distal tip of the fibula. A small test injection confirmed adequate position of the needle within the peroneal tendon sheath, and 6 mL of a solution containing bupivacaine and iodinated contrast material was administered into the tendon sheath (Fig. 7-55). The needle was withdrawn. Thin-section CT images were then obtained through the left ankle. Reformatted images were obtained in several planes.

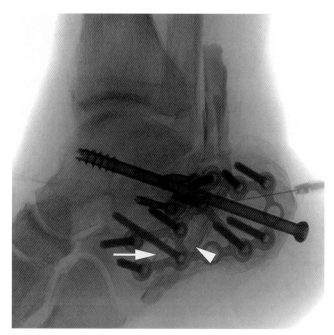

Figure 7-55 ▪ Peroneal tenography. A 25-gauge needle has been advanced into the peroneal tendon sheath and 6 mL of contrast material outlines both the peroneus longus *(arrowhead)* and brevis *(arrow)* tendons.

Results

The peroneal tendons coursed alongside the lateral plate and screws. Several of the screws protruded and directly touched the peroneal tendons, resulting in marked tendonopathy and partial tearing of the peroneus longus and brevis tendons (Fig. 7-56). This corresponded precisely to the site of pain. The patient reported approximately 24 hours of near-complete relief of symptoms following the injection. Surgical removal of the orthopedic hardware was performed in addition to debridement of the peroneal tendons. Longitudinal tears were seen in the tendons directly corresponding to contact with the protruding screws. The patient did well following the surgery with complete resolution of pain.

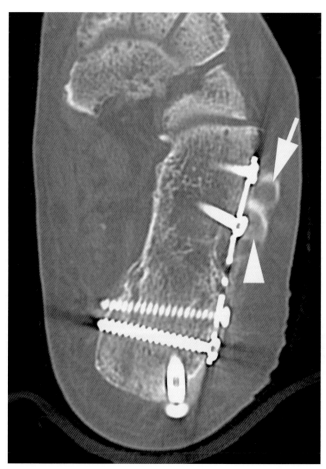

A

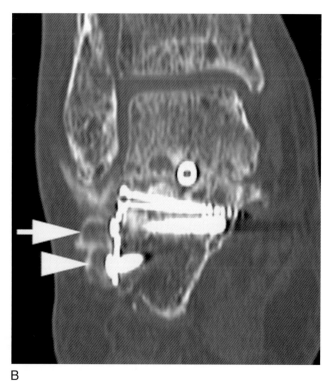

B

Figure 7-56 ▪ Tendonopathy and partial tearing of the peroneus longus and brevis tendons. Several of the screws protruded and directly touched the peroneal tendons, resulting in marked tendonopathy and partial tearing of the peroneus longus *(arrowhead)* and peroneus brevis *(arrow)* tendons.

CURRENT PROCEDURAL TERMINOLOGY (CPT) CODES[32]

CPT codes change often and sometimes are valid only for certain states or regions. It is best to consult with coding experts to make sure that coding for one's procedures is legitimate and complete. Below is a sample of codes that are being used for ankle and foot injection procedures at this writing.

20600 Arthrocentesis, aspiration and/or injection; small joint or bursa (e.g., fingers, toes)

20605 intermediate joint or bursa (e.g., temporomandibular, acromioclavicular, wrist, elbow or ankle, olecranon bursa)

(If imaging guidance is performed, see 76942, 77002, 77012, 77021)

27648 Injection procedure for ankle arthrography

(For radiologic supervision and interpretation, use 73615. Do not report 77002 in addition to 73615)

73590 Radiologic examination; tibia and fibula, two views

73600 Radiologic examination, ankle; two views

73610 complete, minimum of three views

73615 Radiologic examination, ankle, arthrography, radiologic supervision and interpretation

(Do not report 73615 in conjunction with 77002)

73620 Radiologic examination, foot; two views

73630 complete, minimum of three views

73650 Radiologic examination; calcaneus, minimum of two views

73660 toe(s), minimum of two views

73040 Radiologic examination, shoulder, arthrography, radiologic supervision and interpretation

(Do not report 76003 in addition to 73040)

73700 Computed tomography, lower extremity; without contrast material

73701 with contrast material(s)

73702 without contrast material, followed by contrast material(s) and further sections

(To report 3D rendering, see 76376, 76377)

73721 Magnetic resonance (e.g., proton) imaging, any joint of lower extremity; without contrast material(s)

73722 with contrast material(s)

73723 without contrast material(s), followed by contrast material(s) and further sequences

76376 3D rendering with interpretation and reporting of computed tomography, magnetic resonance imaging, ultrasound, or other tomographic modality; not requiring image postprocessing on an independent workstation

(Use 76376 in conjunction with code[s] for base imaging procedure[s])

(Do not report 76376 in conjunction with 70496, 70498, 70544-70549, 71275, 71555, 72159, 72191, 72198, 73206, 73225, 73706, 73725, 74175, 74185, 75635, 76377, 78000-78999, 0066T, 0067T, 0144T-0151T)

76377 requiring image postprocessing on an independent workstation

(Use 76377 in conjunction with code[s] for base imaging procedure[s])

(Do not report 76377 in conjunction with 70496, 70498, 70544-70549, 71275, 71555, 72159, 72191, 72198, 73206, 73225, 73706, 73725, 74175, 74185, 75635, 76377, 78000-78999, 0066T, 0067T, 0144T-0151T)

76942 Ultrasonic guidance for needle placement (e.g., biopsy, aspiration, injection, localization device), imaging supervision and interpretation

(Do not report 76942 in conjunction with 43232, 43237, 43242, 45341, 45342, or 76975)

77002 Fluoroscopic guidance for needle placement (e.g., biopsy, aspiration, injection, localization device)

(See appropriate surgical code for procedure and anatomic location)

(77002 includes all radiographic arthrography with the exception of supervision and interpretation for CT and MR arthrography)

(Do not report 77002 in addition to 70332, 73040, 73085, 73115, 73525, 73580, 73615)

77012 Computed tomography guidance for needle placement (e.g., biopsy, aspiration, injection, localization device), radiologic supervision and interpretation

77021 Magnetic resonance guidance for needle placement (e.g., for biopsy, needle aspiration, injection, or placement of localization device) radiologic supervision and interpretation

References

1. Helgason JW, Chandnani VP. MR arthrography of the ankle. Radiol Clin North Am 1998; 36:729–738.
2. Hodge JC. Musculoskeletal Imaging: Diagnostic and Therapeutic Procedures. Montreal: Karger Landes Systems, 1997, pp 91–108, 189–201.
3. Trnka HJ, Ivanic G, Tattnig S. Arthrography of the foot and ankle. Foot Ankle Clin 2000; 5:49–62.
4. Schmid MR, Pfirrmann CWA, Hodler J, et al. Cartilage lesions in the ankle joint: Comparison of MR arthrography and CT arthrography. Skel Radiol 2003; 32:259–265.
5. Stroud CC, Marks RM. Imaging of osteochondral lesions of the talus. Foot Ankle Clin 2000; 5:119–133.
6. Berquist TH. Diagnostic and therapeutic injections as an aid to musculoskeletal diagnosis. Semin Interv Radiol 1993; 10:326–344.
7. Hurwitz S, Lucas PE. Image guided anesthetic injection into the painful foot or ankle as a guide to orthopedic treatment. Appl Radiol 2000; 29:24–27.
8. Lucas PE, Hurwitz SR, Kaplan PA, et al. Fluoroscopically guided injections into the foot and ankle: Localization of the source of pain as a guide to treatment—Prospective study. Radiology 1997; 204:411–415.
9. Newman JS. Diagnostic and therapeutic injections of the foot and ankle. Semin Roentgenol 2004; 39:85–94.
10. Jaffee NW, Gilula LA, Wissman RD, Johnson JE. Diagnostic and therapeutic ankle tenography: Outcomes and complications. AJR Am J Roentgenol 2001; 176:365–371.
11. Schreibman KL, Gilula LA. Ankle tenography. A therapeutic imaging modality. Radiol Clin North Am 1998; 36:739–756.

12. Schreibman KL. Ankle tenography: What, how, and why. Semin Roentgenol 2004; 39:95–113.

13. Freiberger RH, Kaye JJ. Arthrography. Norwalk, CT: Appleton Century Crofts, 1979, pp 1–3, 237–260.

14. Davies AM, Cassar-Pullicino VN. Demonstration of osteochondritis dissecans of the talus by coronal computed tomographic arthrography. Br J Radiol 1989; 62:1050–1055.

15. El-Khoury GY, Alliman KJ, Lundberg HJ, et al. Cartilage thickness in cadaveric ankles: Measurement with double-contrast multi-detector row CT arthrography versus MR imaging. Radiology 2004; 233:768–773.

16. Palmer WE. MR Arthrography: Is it worthwhile? Top Magn Reson Imaging 1996; 8:24–43.

17. Resnick D. Diagnosis of Bone and Joint Disorders, 4th ed. Philadelphia: WB Saunders, 2002, pp 290–304, 3285–3343.

18. Berquist TH. MRI of the Musculoskeletal System, 5th ed. Philadelphia: Lippincott Williams & Wilkins, 2006, pp 430–556.

19. Lee SH, Jacobson J, Trudell D, Resnick D. Ligaments of the ankle: Normal anatomy with MR arthrography. J Comput Assist Tomogr 1998; 22:807–813.

20. Erickson SJ, Smith JW, Ruiz ME, et al. MR imaging of the lateral collateral ligament of the ankle. AJR Am J Roentgenol 1991; 156:131–136.

21. Schweitzer ME, Karasick D. MR imaging of disorders of the posterior tibialis tendon. AJR Am J Roentgenol 2000; 175: 627–635.

22. Na JB, Bergman AG, Oloff LM, Beaulieu CF. The flexor hallucis longus: Tenographic technique and correlation of imaging findings with surgery in 39 ankles. Radiology 2005; 236:974–982.

23. Schweitzer ME, Karasick D. MR imaging of disorders of the Achilles tendon. AJR Am J Roentgenol 2000; 175:613–625.

24. Lektrakul N, Chung CB, Lai Y, et al. Tarsal sinus: Arthrographic, MR imaging, MR arthrographic, and pathologic findings in cadavers and retrospective study data in patients with sinus tarsi syndrome. Radiology 2001; 219:802–810.

25. Theodorou DJ, Theodorou SJ, Farooki S, et al. Disorders of the plantar aponeurosis: A spectrum of MR imaging findings. AJR Am J Roentgenol 2001; 176:97–104.

26. Helgason JW, Chandnani VP. Magnetic resonance imaging arthrography of the ankle. Top Magn Reson Imaging 1998; 9:286–294.

27. Kramer J, Recht MP. MR arthrography of the lower extremity. Radiol Clin North Am 2002; 40:1121–1132.

28. Cerezal L, Abascal F, Garcia-Valtuille R, Canga A. Ankle MR arthrography: How, why, when. Radiol Clin North Am 2005; 43:693–707.

29. Grainger AJ, Elliott JM, Campbell RSD, et al. Direct MR arthrography: A review of current use. Clin Radiol 2000; 55:163–176.

30. Fenton DS, Czervionke LF. Image-Guided Spine Intervention. Philadelphia: WB Saunders, 2003.

31. Physicians' Desk Reference, 60th ed. Montvale, NJ: Medical Economics Company, 2006.

32. Derived from CPT 2007, CPT Intellectual Property Services. Chicago: American Medical Association, 2007.

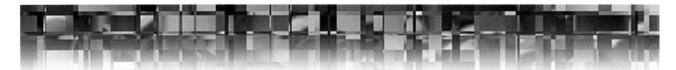

A Foot and Ankle Surgeon's Perspective

Foot and Ankle Injections

James K. DeOrio, MD

With 28 bones (including the sesamoids of the flexor hallucis brevis) and 33 joints in the foot and ankle as well as a myriad of soft tissue problems involving ligaments, tendons, and nerves, anesthetic injections serve as a significant way to differentiate among the various sources of pain. When the solution is mixed with cortisone, there can also be a therapeutic effect. I rarely inject an area, either joint or soft tissue, more than two times and never more than three. The way I see it, if the patient needs that many injections for relief of pain, it is often possible to provide more permanent relief through surgery.

The anatomic joints most frequently injected include the hallux interphalangeal, metatarsal phalangeal, tarsometatarsal, navicular-cuneiform, talonavicular, calcaneal cuboid, subtalar, and ankle joints. Of these, the subtalar joint is the one most often injected, because it is critical to assess the difference between pain coming from the ankle and pain coming from the subtalar joint. This difference can be subtle, and not infrequently patients can have their ankle joint treated with arthroscopic surgery when, in fact, the true pain is coming from the subtalar joint. The treatments for the ankle and the subtalar joint are completely different.

Soft tissue areas are also frequently injected. The most common is the intermetatarsal areas for irritation or compression of the intermetatarsal nerve (Morton's neuroma). Other soft tissue areas that can be injected include the peroneal tendons and occasionally the sural, superficial peroneal, posterior tibial, deep peroneal, or saphenous nerves to block the sources of neurogenic pain. Although injection is usually done for diagnosis, a therapeutic treatment can also be obtained by adding a steroid. I do not inject the Achilles tendon region or posterior tibial tendon with steroid mixed in the solution. These are high-stress areas and an inadvertent injection of cortisone into the tendon can result in rupture.

CT and MR are invaluable in making diagnoses around the foot and ankles. I typically use CT to assess remaining joint space and subchondral cysts or the actual size of an osteochondral lesion of the talus. By getting the CT scan parallel and perpendicular to the metatarsals when scanning the foot, it is easy to assess joint space width. MR is, of course, more useful in assessing posterior tibial tendon dysfunction, peroneal tendon tears, or areas of avascular necrosis in the metatarsal head (Freiberg infraction), sesamoid, or talus. It is also the most sensitive way to see a stress fracture and the competence of the anterior talofibular ligament and to locate the areas involved with soft tissue tumor of the synovium such as pigmented villonodular synovitis or giant cell tumor of the tendon sheath.

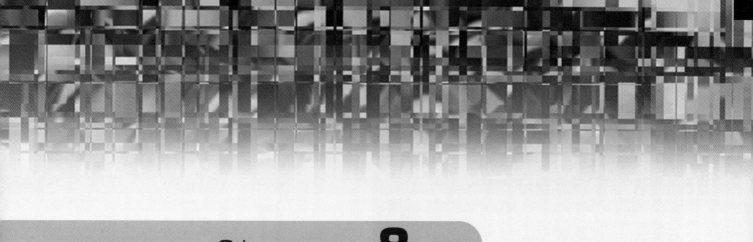

Chapter 8

Percutaneous Image-Guided Biopsy and Radiofrequency Ablation

- Jeffrey J. Peterson, MD

PERCUTANEOUS IMAGE-GUIDED BIOPSY

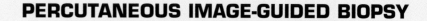

BACKGROUND

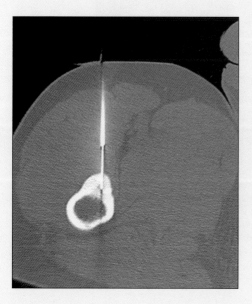

Although an experienced radiologist can often make the diagnosis of bone lesions based on imaging alone, it may be necessary to obtain tissue specimens for histologic confirmation. Osseous and soft tissue tumors often have a nonspecific imaging appearance, not infrequently requiring biopsy for diagnosis. Most soft tissue and osseous tumors require specific tissue diagnosis before definitive therapeutic interventions are undertaken.[1,2] This can be achieved by "open" surgical biopsy or by "closed" percutaneous image-guided biopsy.[3,4] In many cases, image-guided percutaneous biopsy is preferred to open biopsy, as the procedure is typically much less invasive with less trauma to the surrounding tissues.[2,4–6] Following percutaneous biopsy, therapy can often be initiated immediately and there is often less risk of tumor dissemination.[7] Radiation therapy and neoadjuvant chemotherapy can be initiated more rapidly, as wound healing is less of a concern.[7] For bone biopsy, percutaneous image-guided techniques result in less insult to the structural integrity of the osseous structure and allow a more rapid return to normal activity.[5,7] Percutaneous biopsy allows preoperative planning and results in a lower risk of complications.[2,6,7] The overall morbidity and

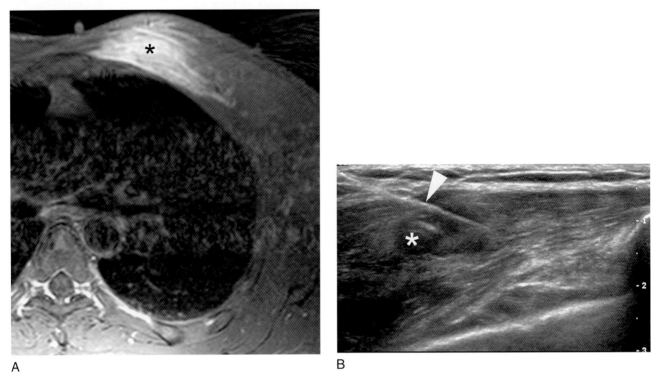

A   B

Figure 8-1 ■ Ultrasound-guided soft tissue mass biopsy; 39-year-old man with palpable mass in the left pectoral region. Axial post-contrast T1-weighted MR image with fat saturation *(A)* demonstrates a heterogeneous mass in the left pectoral region *(asterisk)*. Ultrasound-guided biopsy *(B)* of the mass *(asterisk)* was then performed with an 18-gauge Temno biopsy needle *(arrowhead)*.

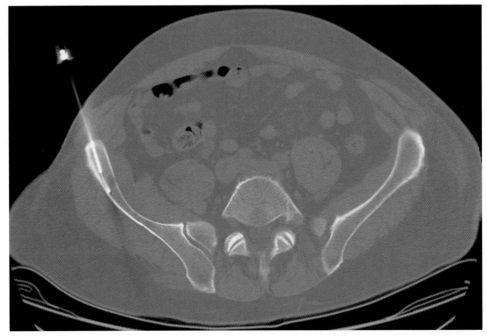

Figure 8-2 ■ Strict adherence to orthopedic oncologic consultation and compartmental anatomy is mandatory to avoid complications of the biopsy for future surgery. After consultation with the orthopedic oncologist, an approach in this case of a left iliac lytic lesion was utilized to minimize contamination of the overlying gluteal or abdominal wall musculature.

mortality with image-guided needle biopsy are less than with open biopsy, and general anesthesia is avoided.[2,7,8] Finally, cost is significantly less with image-guided needle biopsy than with open surgical techniques.[6,7,9]

Martin and Ellis first introduced needle biopsies in 1930 for diagnosing skeletal neoplasms utilizing needle aspiration.[2,10] In 1947 Ellis introduced the first trephine bone biopsy needle.[2,11] Since then, advances have continued in techniques and equipment for the performance of percutaneous biopsies.[2,4,8] Improvements have been made in the design of the needles that allow higher quality specimens to be obtained and with greater ease.[1,2,8] A large variety of biopsy needles are currently available, and needles continue to be developed and revised.[1,8] Several selected needles commonly utilized for both bone and soft tissue biopsies are presented in this chapter.

Percutaneous image-guided biopsy can be performed for both soft tissue tumors and osseous lesions (Fig. 8-1). The approach to both soft tissue and bone biopsy is similar, although the needles required are quite different.[1,8] In both cases, the shortest and most direct approach to a lesion is desirable, although care should be taken to avoid vital structures and contaminating overlying tissue that may be necessary for operative reconstruction.[7,12,13] Strict adherence to orthopedic oncologic consultation and compartmental anatomy is mandatory to avoid complications of the biopsy for future surgery (Fig. 8-2).[7,12,13] Techniques commonly utilized for soft tissue and bone biopsy are presented in this chapter, as well as a detailed delineation of the compartmental anatomy that must be understood before proceeding with image-guided biopsy.

In addition to tissue sampling for oncologic purposes, soft tissue and bone biopsies can be performed to isolate organisms in cases of infection and to sample the skeletal structures in cases of metabolic bone disease.[3,8] In suspected cases of osteomyelitis, percutaneous image-guided needle biopsy can be very useful to isolate the offending organism and optimize antibiotic therapeutic regimens (Fig. 8-3).[3,8] Biopsy can also be helpful in cases of metabolic bone disease to evaluate conditions that affect structural homeostasis such as osteoporosis, Paget's disease, or other diseases that affect mineral homeostasis such as hyperparathyroidism and osteomalacia.[3,8]

In addition to tissue sampling, techniques used for image-guided biopsy can be modified to facilitate treatment of lesions.[8] Therapeutic injections of materials can be utilized to treat lesions such as solitary bone cysts with percutaneous steroid injections or bone graft (Fig. 8-4).[8] The same techniques for percutaneous biopsy can also be applied to treat lesions using radiofrequency ablation.[14,15] There are currently several indications for percutaneous radiofrequency ablation therapy, and these therapies continue to evolve. Currently, the most common musculoskeletal indication for percutaneous radiofrequency ablation is the treatment of osteoid osteoma[16–18] (Fig. 8-5), although the technique can also be used to treat small intracortical chondromas[19] and for palliative treatment in cases of advanced osseous metastatic disease (Fig. 8-6).[20,21] Image-guided percutaneous radiofrequency ablation of osteoid osteoma is described in detail in this chapter.

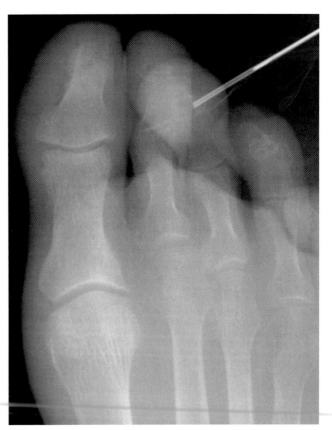

Figure 8-3 ▪ Bone biopsy of osteomyelitis. Percutaneous image-guided needle biopsy was used to isolate the offending organism to optimize antibiotic treatment in this case of septic arthritis and osteomyelitis about the third distal interphalangeal joint.

ANATOMIC CONSIDERATIONS

Knowledge of compartmental anatomy is critical when planning the approach for image-guided percutaneous biopsies.[7,12,13] Percutaneous biopsy involves the risk of seeding malignant cells along the biopsy tract.[7,12,13] For this purpose, the needle tract is typically resected en bloc with the tumor when operative treatment is indicated.[12] The approach should therefore be carefully selected in consultation with the orthopedic oncologist, as the biopsy may have devastating consequences for the patient if performed improperly.[12] In previous reports, as many as 25% of the biopsies of soft tissue sarcoma were inadequately performed, resulting in alteration of surgical treatment in 10% and limb amputation in 3%.[7] Knowledge of and strict adherence to the principles of compartmental anatomy are critical for the optimum management of many types of musculoskeletal malignancy.[7,12,13] A more thorough description of compartmental anatomy and the planning necessary for successful biopsy can be found in a 1999 manuscript by Anderson and colleagues.[12]

In the extremities, tissues are separated into distinct anatomic compartments by the bones, muscles, tendons, ligaments, fascia, and joint capsules (Fig. 8-7).[12] Tumors confined to one compartment (intracompartmental) have a

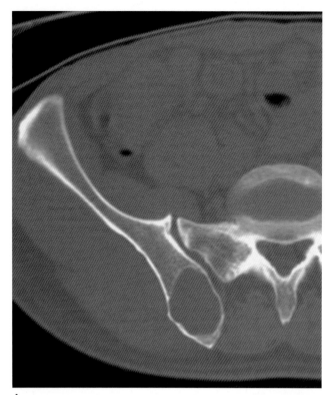

A

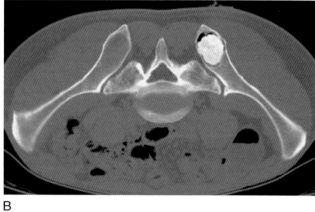

B

Figure 8-4 ■ Percutaneous bone graft placement in a simple bone cyst in the right posterior ilium. Preliminary CT image (*A*) shows a large lytic lesion with expansile remodeling involving the posterior ilium. An 11-gauge needle was advanced under CT guidance into the lesion and the cyst contents were aspirated. Injectable bone graft was then administered into the lesion (*B*). Nine-month follow-up CT demonstrates interval decrease in size of the lesion with bone ingrowth from the margins of the lesion, which is now at less risk for fracture (*C*).

C

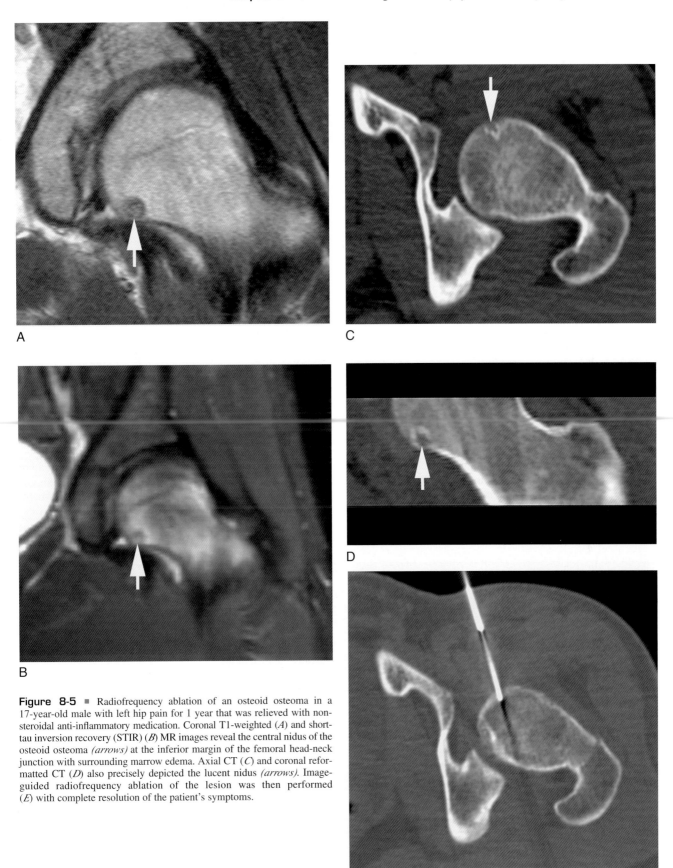

Figure 8-5 ▪ Radiofrequency ablation of an osteoid osteoma in a 17-year-old male with left hip pain for 1 year that was relieved with non-steroidal anti-inflammatory medication. Coronal T1-weighted (*A*) and short-tau inversion recovery (STIR) (*B*) MR images reveal the central nidus of the osteoid osteoma *(arrows)* at the inferior margin of the femoral head-neck junction with surrounding marrow edema. Axial CT (*C*) and coronal refor-matted CT (*D*) also precisely depicted the lucent nidus *(arrows)*. Image-guided radiofrequency ablation of the lesion was then performed (*E*) with complete resolution of the patient's symptoms.

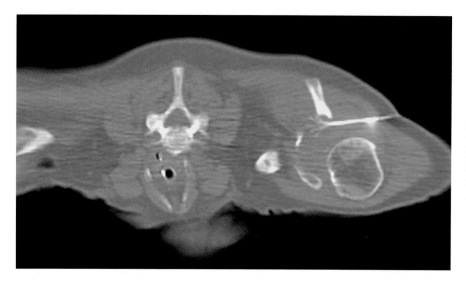

Figure 8-6 ■ Radiofrequency ablation of osseous metastatic disease in a 73-year-old male with metastatic renal cell carcinoma who presented with excruciating pain related to a scapular metastasis. Percutaneous radio-frequency ablation of the lesion was performed for palliative purposes. The electrode was repositioned several times within the lesion to ablate the majority of the lesion adequately.

lower stage than those that have spread beyond one compartment into another (extracompartmental) and generally require a less radical resection.[12] Extracompartmental spread may occur by direct tumor extension or by contamination by fracture, hemorrhage, or iatrogenic causes such as an unplanned resection or biopsy utilizing an inappropriate approach.[12]

Figure 8-7 illustrates the various compartments of the extremities. Although a comprehensive list of rules and restrictions for percutaneous image-guided biopsies is impossible, there are several points that, if followed, can decrease the chance of complications related to biopsy.[12,13]

When planning approaches for image-guided biopsy, consultation with the surgeon who plans to perform the definitive surgery is very important.[12,13] Often there are certain muscles or other soft tissues that should be avoided, as they will provide coverage through myocutaneous flaps for the operative defect.[7,12] Contaminating the tissues to be utilized for this coverage may radically change the intended operative plan or limit the surgical options.[7,12,13] It is very helpful to choose an approach that places the needle path close to the intended surgical incision so that the tract can be easily excised along with the tumor.[7,12,13] Care should always be taken to avoid crossing compartments with the

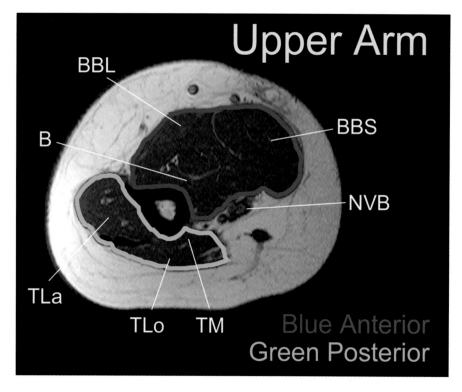

Figure 8-7 ■ A–G, Extremity anatomic compartments.
A, Upper arm. Anterior compartment: BBL = long head of biceps brachii; BBS = short head of biceps brachii; B = brachialis. Posterior compartment: TM = medial head of triceps brachii; Tlo = long head of triceps brachii; Tla = lateral head of triceps brachii; NVB = neurovascular bundle including brachial artery and vein and median and ulnar nerve.

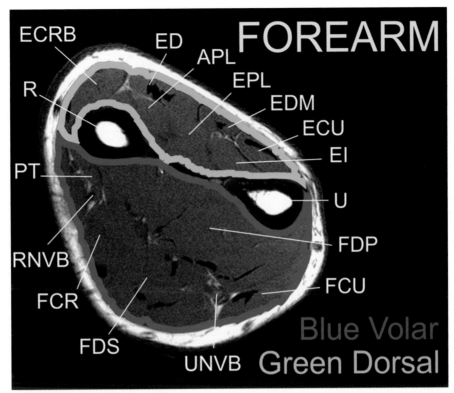

B, Forearm. Volar compartment: FDP = flexor digitorum profundus; FCU = flexor carpi ulnaris; UNVB = ulnar neurovascular bundle; FDS = flexor digitorum superficialis; FCR = flexor carpi radialis; RNVB = radial neurovascular bundle; PT = pronator teres. Dorsal compartment: ECRB = extensor carpi radialis brevis; ED = extensor digitorum; APL = abductor pollicis longus; EPL = extensor pollicis longus; EDM = extensor digitorum; ECU = extensor carpi ulnaris; EI = extensor indicis; R = radius; U = ulna.

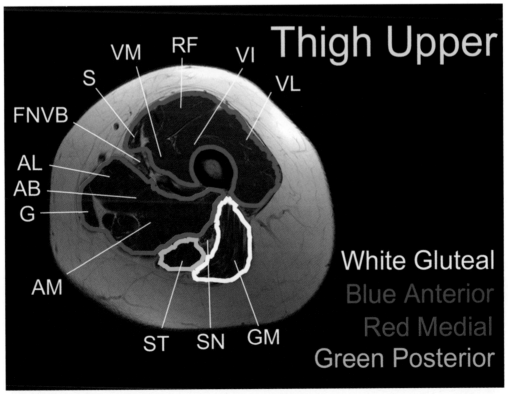

C, Upper thigh. Anterior compartment: S = sartorius; VM = vastus medialis; RF = rectus femoris; VI = vastus intermedius; VL = vastus lateralis. Medial compartment: AL = adductor longus; AB = adductor brevis; AM = adductor magnus; G = gracilis. Posterior compartment: ST = semitendinosus; GM = gluteus maximus; SN = sciatic nerve; FNVB = femoral neurovascular bundle.

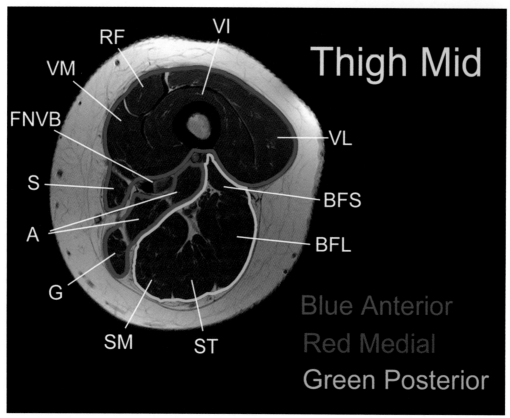

Figure 8-7 ■ (con't) *D*, Middle thigh. Anterior compartment: S = sartorius; VM = vastus medialis; RF = rectus femoris; VI = vastus intermedius; VL = vastus lateralis. Medial compartment: A = adductor magnus and longus; G = gracilis. Posterior compartment: SM = semimembranosus; ST = semitendinosus; BFS = short head of biceps femoris; BFL = long head of biceps femoris; FNVB = femoral neurovascular bundle.

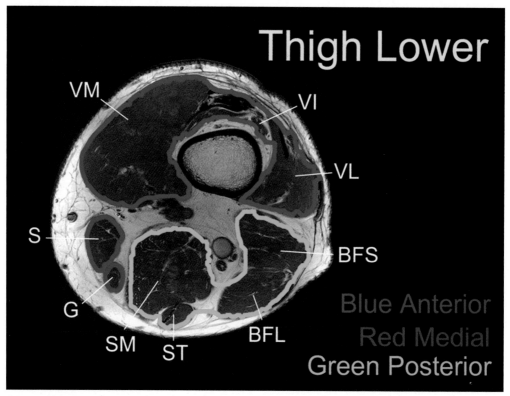

E, Lower thigh. Anterior compartment: S = sartorius; VM = vastus medialis; VI = vastus intermedius; VL = vastus lateralis. Medial compartment: G = gracilis. Posterior compartment: SM = semimembranosus; ST = semitendinosus; BFS = short head of biceps femoris; BFL = long head of biceps femoris.

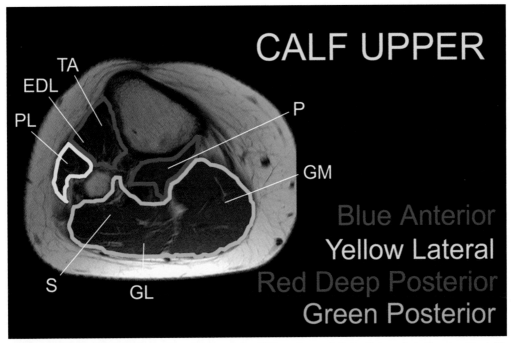

F, Upper calf. Anterior compartment: TA = tibialis anterior; EDL = extensor digitorum longus. Lateral compartment: PL = peroneus longus. Deep posterior compartment: P = popliteus. Posterior compartment: GM = medial head of gastrocnemius; GL = lateral head of gastrocnemius; S = soleus.

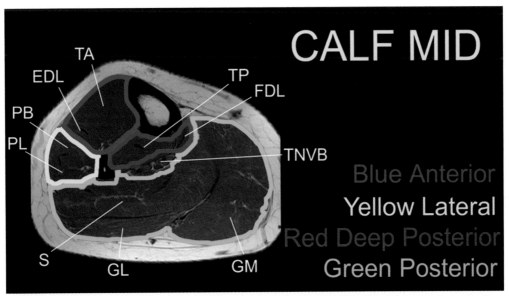

G, Mid calf. Anterior compartment: TA = tibialis anterior; EDL = extensor digitorum longus. Lateral compartment: PB = peroneus brevis; PL = peroneus longus. Deep posterior compartment: TP = tibialis posterior; FDL = flexor digitorum longus. Posterior compartment: GM = medial head of gastrocnemius; GL = lateral head of gastrocnemius; S = soleus; TNVB = tibial neurovascular bundle.

needle path, which could contaminate much of the soft tissues of the extremity and possibly even result in limb amputation.[12,13] Each tumor has a unique set of factors that guide the selection of approach, and critical evaluation of the preoperative imaging with the orthopedic oncologist is critical to optimize therapeutic outcomes.[12,13]

PATIENT SELECTION

Indications for percutaneous image-guided osseous and soft tissue biopsy include tissue sampling for diagnosing neoplasm, culture of osseous and soft tissue infection, and bone sampling for metabolic bone disease.[3,8] Prior to biopsy, appropriate thorough evaluation with noninvasive imaging such as radiographs, CT, MR, or nuclear medicine investigations should be performed. Often the need for biopsy can be obviated with appropriate high-quality imaging studies. Large-caliber core biopsy needles are typically needed for metabolic bone disease with a needle caliber diameter greater than 3 mm.[8] For this reason, most biopsies for metabolic bone disease are performed utilizing open surgical technique or large-bore needles.[8] Fine-needle aspiration and core biopsy techniques utilizing 18- or 20-gauge needles are typically adequate for diagnosis for soft tissue mass biopsy.[8] Such small needles unfortunately are often insufficient for osseous biopsies, which typically require 16-gauge or larger needles for adequate samples.[8]

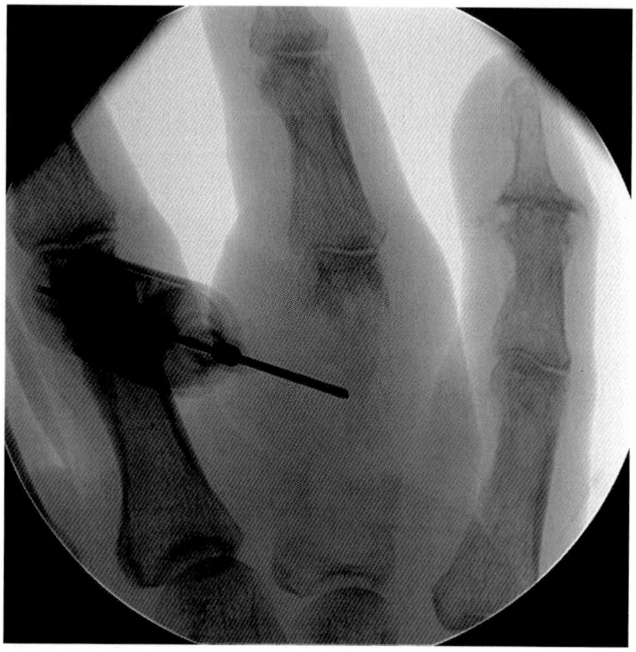

Figure 8-8 ■ Fluoroscopic bone biopsy. Fluoroscopic guidance was utilized for biopsy of this lytic lesion involving the fourth proximal phalanx. The lesion is well seen under fluoroscopy and the biopsy path is very short, making fluoroscopy a quick and inexpensive option for percutaneous biopsy.

Image Guidance

Choices for image guidance include fluoroscopy, CT, sonography, and MR imaging.[1,8]

Fluoroscopic Guidance

Fluoroscopic guidance for biopsies is faster, easier, and less costly than other methods, namely ultrasonography or CT (Fig. 8-8).[1,8] The main disadvantage with fluoroscopic guidance is that often the lesion cannot be adequately visualized under fluoroscopy, which necessitates use of cross-sectional image guidance.[1,8] This is more of a concern with soft tissue masses than with osseous structures. Another disadvantage of fluoroscopically guided biopsy is that there is suboptimal visualization of anatomic structures along the biopsy path, even if the lesion itself is visible.[1,8] Preliminary imaging studies should be assessed closely to evaluate the adequacy of visualization of the lesion and for the presence of vital structures such as a neurovascular bundle along the expected biopsy trajectory.[3,8] A thorough knowledge of the anatomy is necessary to plan fluoroscopically guided biopsies and to establish the safest and most appropriate needle trajectory.[12] If the lesion is large enough, is well seen with fluoroscopy, and no vital structures lie within the expected biopsy tract, fluoroscopic guidance can be used for biopsy.[1,3,8] Very rarely are fluoroscopically guided techniques indicated for biopsy of a soft tissue mass. A small percentage of osseous lesions are best approached with fluoroscopic guidance.

Ultrasound Guidance

Ultrasound guidance has several advantages over other imaging techniques. Ultrasonography can typically define most soft tissue masses and provide the guidance for precise needle placement (Fig. 8-9).[22,23] A major requirement of ultrasonography is the use of real-time imaging, which allows fast and precise manipulations of the biopsy needle.[1,22,23] In addition, ultrasonography does not expose the patient to ionizing radiation.[1,22,23] Ultrasonography nicely demonstrates the biopsy path, allowing a safe approach to the lesion.[1,22,23] Sonography also allows Doppler imaging, which demonstrates surrounding vascular structures and avoids puncture or vascular injury (Fig. 8-10).[1,22,23] Ultrasonography can readily demonstrate necrotic areas within lesions to guide needle placement to areas with more viable tumor, thus avoiding a sampling error.[1,22,23] For these reasons, ultrasound guidance is the preferred imaging modality for image-guided soft tissue mass biopsies.[22,23] Unfortunately, the ultrasound beam cannot penetrate osseous structures and therefore is not useful for osseous biopsies unless the osseous lesion is associated with a soft tissue component.[22,23]

CT Guidance

CT guidance has considerable advantages over fluoroscopic guidance. CT guidance allows accurate depth perception and enables visualization of the tip of the needle, which may

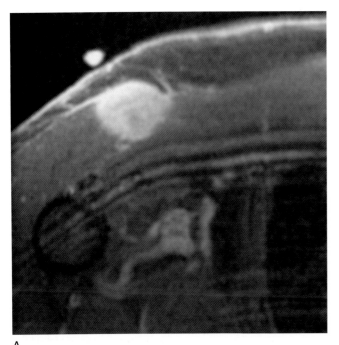

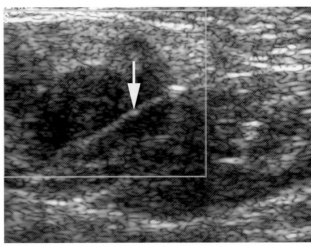

A   B

Figure 8-9 ■ Ultrasound-guided soft tissue mass biopsy. An older man with acute myelogenous luekemia presented with a palpable mass in the right pectoral region. Axial post-contrast T1-weighted MR image with fat saturation (*A*) depicts a rounded enhancing mass in the right deltopectoral interval corresponding to the palpable abnormality. Ultrasound-guided percutaneous biopsy (*B*) was performed with an 18-gauge Temno biopsy needle *(arrow).*

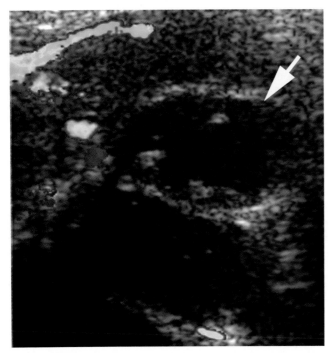

Figure 8-10 ■ Doppler imaging demonstrated the surrounding vascular structures about this soft tissue mass *(arrow)*, allowing an approach to be used that avoided vascular injury.

be difficult with fluoroscopic guidance.[1,2,24] CT also allows superior visualization of the soft tissues overlying the lesion, which provides more precise visualization of structures along the path to the bone lesion (Fig. 8-11).[1,2,24] In contrast to fluoroscopy, CT guidance allows visualization of vital structures adjacent to the biopsy site.[1,2,24] This is especially critical when important structures such as arteries or nerves overlie the lesion and need to be avoided.[8] Soft tissue components of bone lesions, which may be easier to biopsy, are well seen with CT in contrast to fluoroscopy (Fig. 8-12).[23,24] CT guidance allows specific regions inside a target lesion to be selected and thus ensures that necrotic regions are avoided and that viable tumor is sampled (Fig. 8-13).[2,8,24]

CT fluoroscopy has become widely available and can be very helpful when performing CT-guided bone biopsies.[8] CT fluoroscopy combines the superior soft tissue resolution of CT and the real-time imaging capability of fluoroscopy and sonography.[1,8] This reduces examination time, which results in less discomfort for the patient.[8]

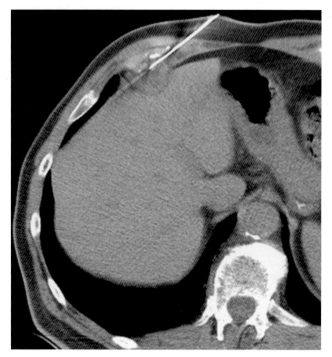

Figure 8-11 ■ CT-guided soft tissue mass biopsy. CT also allows superior visualization of the tissues overlying the lesion along the tract used to reach the lesion. This allows a more precise path to approach this lesion without traversing the adjacent lung tissue.

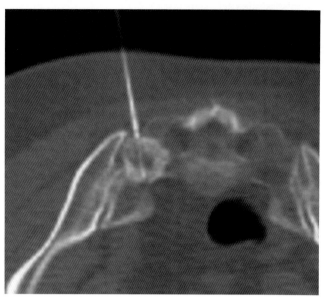

Figure 8-13 ■ CT-guided bone biopsy. CT guidance allows specific regions inside a target lesion to be selected, thus ensuring that necrotic regions are avoided and that viable tumor is sampled. In this case, the periphery of this sacral osseous lesion is biopsied and the necrotic center is avoided.

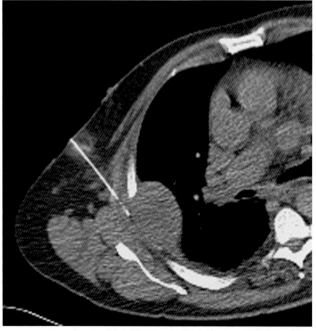

Figure 8-12 ■ CT-guided biopsy of the soft tissue component of an osseous neoplasm. CT allows specific targeting of components of the lesion, allowing, in this case, targeting of the soft tissue component of this bone lesion, which typically results in better quality tissue samples obtained with greater ease.

MR Guidance

MR-guided procedures have become more common with the proliferation of open configuration MRI units.[25] Several investigators have demonstrated that MR-guided percutaneous bone biopsy is both safe and accurate.[25,26] Advantages of MR include unlimited slice orientation, easy localization of neurovascular structures, and lack of ionizing radiation.[25,26] All equipment utilized during the procedure, including the needles, must be MR compatible.[25,26] MR-guided biopsies may not be safe in some patients with pacemakers, defibrillators, cochlear implants, or certain cerebral aneurysm clips.[25,26] The needles result in susceptibility artifact on imaging, and the artifact may obscure lesions smaller than 1 to 2 cm.[25,26] In general, we have found CT to be adequate for most bone biopsies and have encountered few patients who would benefit from MR guidance as opposed to CT. We therefore have performed few MR-guided procedures and utilize other modalities for guidance in most cases.

CONTRAINDICATIONS[8]

- Coagulopathy (caution in patients with International Normalized Ratio [INR] >1.5 or platelets < 50,000/mm^3)
- Pregnancy (because of teratogenic effects of radiation, excluding sonographic biopsy)
- Systemic infection or skin infection over the puncture site

- Severe allergy to any medication needed to perform the procedure
- Tumor inaccessible to percutaneous biopsy secondary to adjacent vital structures, intervening bowel, and so forth

PROCEDURE

Equipment/Supplies

- Control 12-mL syringe with 25-gauge, 1.5-inch needle containing 8 mL 1% lidocaine for local anesthesia and 2 mL 8.4% sodium bicarbonate injectable (1 mEq/mL) to alleviate burning pain associated with anesthetic
- Sterile 4 × 4 gauze pads
- Povidone-iodine (Betadine) and alcohol for preparation
- Sterile towels or fenestrated drape for draping
- Radiopaque marker or grid for CT-guided procedures
- Scalpel
- Sterile gloves
- Adhesive bandage
- Selected needle biopsy/aspiration system(s)
- Lead apron for fluoroscopic or CT fluoroscopic procedures

Medications (Injection Mixtures)

Intravenous sedation is usually not required for most routine soft tissue biopsies and selected osseous biopsies if small-caliber needles (18 to 20 gauge or less) are utilized.[8] For biopsies utilizing larger caliber needles such as those often used for bone biopsies, intravenous sedation is required.[8] Several agents can be utilized for anesthesia and sedation including but not limited to the following:

Lidocaine 1% (Xylocaine 1%, AstraZeneca LP, Wilmington, DE) for short-acting subcutaneous and periosteal anesthesia.[8]
Bupivacaine 0.5% (Sensorcaine-MPF injection 0.5%, AstraZeneca LP, Wilmington, DE) for long-acting subcutaneous and periosteal anesthesia.[8]
Midazolam (Versed, Roche Laboratories, Nutley, NJ), 1 mg, administered intravenously is the standard dose for relief of anxiety.[8] Maximum dose is 5 mg. Caution should be exercised in older patients, who may experience respiratory depression with even small doses (0.5 to 1 mg) of midazolam.[8] If sedation is required for patients older than 65 years, start dose at 0.5 mg intravenously.[8]
Fentanyl, 50 to 100 μg administered intravenously to alleviate pain during the procedure.[8]

In addition to medications for sedation and anesthesia, atropine should be available for treatment of vasovagal reactions, which are not uncommon[8]; 0.6 to 1 mg of atropine is administered intravenously as needed.[27]

General Principles of Soft Tissue and Osseous Biopsy

Pre-Procedure[8]

Percutaneous image-guided soft tissue mass or osseous biopsy can be performed as an outpatient or inpatient procedure.[8] Pre-procedure laboratory studies that should be obtained include prothrombin time, partial thromboplastin time, complete blood count, platelet count, and INR.[8] If the patient has a potential risk for renal failure and is to receive intravenous contrast material, serum creatinine, blood urea nitrogen, or calculation of glomerular filtration rate should be obtained before the procedure.[8] Patients are instructed to be accompanied by a responsible adult who can provide transportation home.[8] This person should be able to report any procedure-related difficulties should these occur after the patient has left the department.[8] A history of any allergies should also be noted before the procedure.[8]

Patient Preparation[8]

For all soft tissue mass and osseous biopsies, the procedure and potential risks should be thoroughly explained to the patient.[8] Informed consent should then be obtained. The decision about the type of image guidance must be made. The patient is placed on the table in a position that facilitates the biopsy.[8] Positions that are uncomfortable for the patient should be avoided (Fig. 8-14). If intravenous sedation is to be given, monitoring of the patient's vital signs is necessary.[8]

A large area surrounding the needle puncture site is scrubbed three successive times with povidone-iodine using sterile technique.[8] Then the entry site is draped with sterile

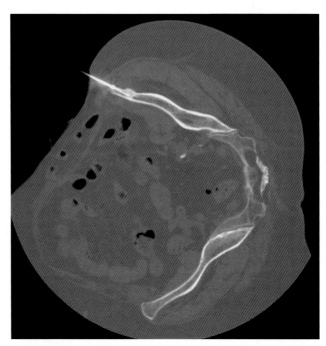

Figure 8-14 ■ CT-guided bone biopsy. The patient should be placed on the table in a position that facilitates the biopsy. Positions that are uncomfortable for the patient should be avoided.

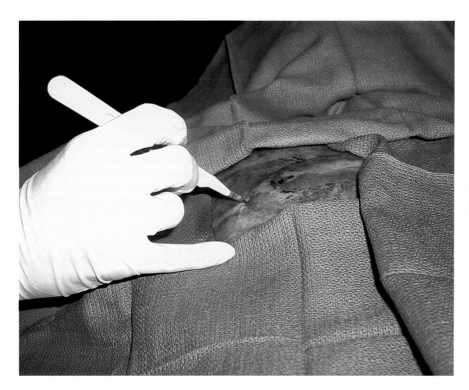

Figure 8-15 ■ Dermatotomy. A dermatotomy is performed with the scalpel to facilitate placement of the larger caliber biopsy needle through the skin.

towels or a fenestrated sterile drape. Local anesthesia of the skin and subcutaneous tissues is then achieved with lidocaine 1% buffered with 8.4% sodium bicarbonate. This is performed with a 25-gauge, 1.5-inch needle. If necessary, local anesthesia of the deeper tissues is obtained with a 22-gauge, 3.5-inch spinal needle (or longer if necessary).[8] A dermatotomy is then performed with the scalpel to facilitate placement of the larger caliber biopsy needle through the skin (Fig. 8-15). The actual technique and needle system used are specific to the given patient and anatomic location of the lesion. After all procedures, the skin at the puncture site is cleansed with hydrogen peroxide to remove the povidone-iodine, and an adhesive bandage is applied to the puncture site.[8]

Image Guidance Techniques

Fluoroscopic Guidance

When possible, fluoroscopic guidance for percutaneous biopsy provides a simple and quick way to obtain tissue samples.[1,2,8] Using fluoroscopic guidance, the puncture site should be selected before preparing the sterile field and the patient should be placed on the table in a position that most facilitates placement of the needle without causing undo discomfort to the patient.[8] Positioning to allow a near-vertical approach with the needle as parallel to the fluoroscopic beam as possible is preferred. Thorough knowledge of the anatomy is necessary to choose a needle path that is safe and efficient.[3,8] A radiopaque marker such as a metallic clamp is placed on the skin surface to identify the precise location of the needle puncture.[8] Sterile skin preparation is then performed. Under intermittent fluoroscopy, the needle can be guided precisely into the lesion and specimens obtained (Fig. 8-16).

CT Guidance

CT guidance provides the best means for biopsy of most osseous lesions and some soft tissue masses when ultrasonography is not appropriate. Prior to sterile preparation of the skin, the precise puncture site should be determined utilizing a nonsterile radiopaque grid or radiopaque marker (Fig. 8-17).[8] Initial AP and lateral CT scout views demonstrate the grid or marker in relation to the nearby anatomic landmarks. If the grid or marker is in good position, no

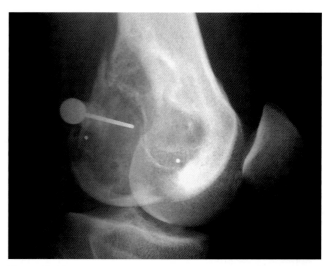

Figure 8-16 ■ Percutaneous fluoroscopic bone biopsy. This large lytic lesion involving the distal femur was easily accessible to biopsy under fluoroscopic guidance. The lesion was large enough to be well seen under fluoroscopy, and knowledge of the overlying anatomy allowed avoidance of vital overlying structures.

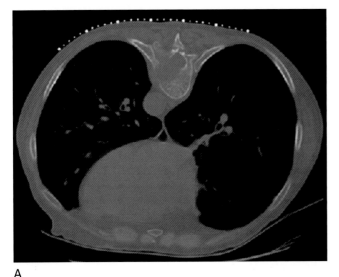

A

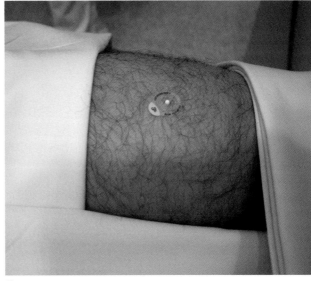

C

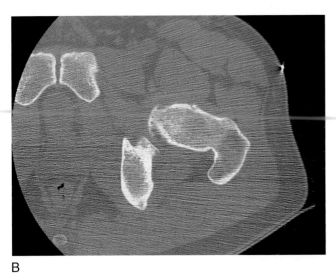

B

Figure 8-17 ▪ Radiopaque grid and marker. Prior to sterile preparation of the skin, the precise puncture site can be determined utilizing either a radiopaque grid (*A*) or radiopaque marker (*B* and *C*).

adjustment is needed in position.[8] If the grid or marker does not overlie the target, the grid position is adjusted and additional scout views are obtained.[8]

A field of view large enough to allow visualization of not only the pathology but also the skin surface and entire grid or marker should be utilized.[8] CT images of 1 to 3 mm are obtained through the area of interest to localize the lesion.[8] The images are carefully analyzed to determine the optimal needle trajectory.[8] A CT image is then selected that depicts both the pathologic target and the desired needle trajectory.[8] The image location number of this image is noted. Utilizing the measurement software on the CT scanner, a line is drawn on this CT image along the desired needle trajectory to measure the distance from the skin entry site to the target location.[8] The CT gantry is then moved to the image location number previously noted.[8] The CT laser localizer light that projects on the skin surface is used to mark the skin surface with an indelible marker at the expected skin puncture site (Fig. 8-18). The grid or marker is then removed and the skin is prepared and draped in a sterile fashion.[8]

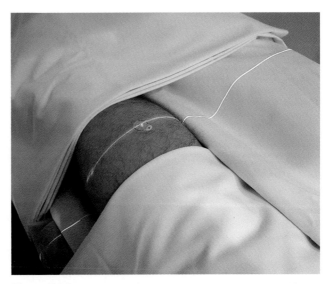

Figure 8-18 ▪ The CT laser localizer light that projects on the skin surface is utilized to mark the expected skin puncture site at the radiopaque marker.

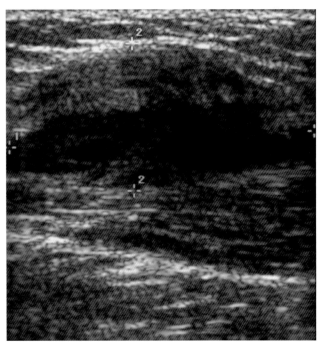

Figure 8-19 ■ Preliminary ultrasound imaging. Preliminary real-time sonographic imaging is performed through the lesion to identify the location and size of the lesion and to plan the appropriate approach for the biopsy needle.

Ultrasound Guidance

Sonography provides an efficient way to biopsy many soft tissue masses. With ultrasonography, the needle entry site is determined before the skin preparation. The patient is placed on the table in a position that optimizes exposure to the region of interest. Preliminary real-time imaging should be performed through the lesion and the expected needle approach (Fig. 8-19). Duplex Doppler imaging should also be performed to demonstrate adjacent vascular structures that should be avoided. The needle puncture site should then be marked and the skin should be prepared and sterilely draped in the usual manner. The ultrasound probe should then be cleansed and sterilized with either ethyl alcohol or Betadine, or a sterile ultrasound probe cover can be placed over the probe. Local anesthesia is then obtained with 1% lidocaine with sodium bicarbonate buffer. The 25-gauge needle used for local anesthesia can be visualized sonographically to check needle trajectory and ensure adequate local anesthesia along the entire tract used to reach the lesion (Fig. 8-20). Real-time sonographic guidance is available for guidance of the needle biopsy.

Basic Needle Biopsy Techniques

Coaxial Needle Technique[8]

Coaxial needle techniques are preferred for biopsy of deep skeletal and soft tissue masses. This technique minimizes damage to surrounding normal tissue by using a single needle placement to obtain multiple tissue samples.[1,8] This is achieved with a needle system that uses a combined large- and small-caliber needle set (Fig. 8-21).[1,8] The large-caliber, shorter needle with an inner stylet is first guided to the margin or into the lesion or structure to be sampled (Fig. 8-22).[1,8] The smaller gauge, longer biopsy needle is then advanced through the indwelling larger gauge needle in a coaxial fashion (Fig. 8-23).[1,8] Multiple tissue samples can be obtained

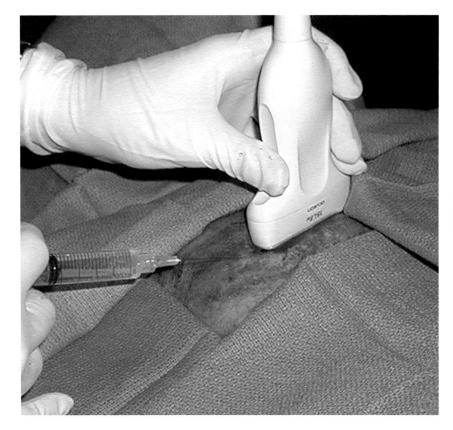

Figure 8-20 ■ Local anesthesia. Local anesthesia is obtained with 1% lidocaine with sodium bicarbonate buffer. The anesthesia needle can then be imaged to check needle trajectory and ensure adequate local anesthesia along the entire tract utilized to reach the lesion.

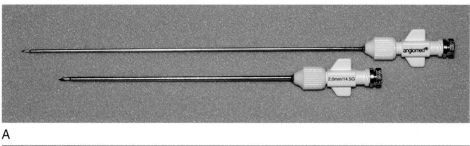

A

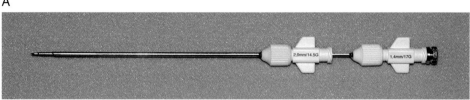

B

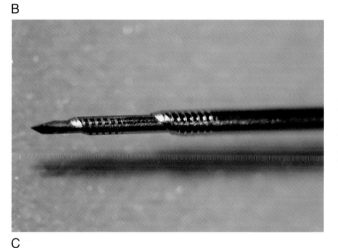

Figure 8-21 ■ Coaxial biopsy needles: 14.5- and 17-gauge Ostycut needles (*A*) can be utilized by a coaxial technique (*B*) to minimize damage to surrounding normal tissue by using a single needle placement to obtain multiple tissue samples. The large-caliber, shorter needle is first guided to the margin or into the lesion or structure to be sampled, and the smaller gauge, longer biopsy needle is then advanced through the indwelling larger gauge needle in a coaxial fashion (*C*) to obtain the specimen.

C

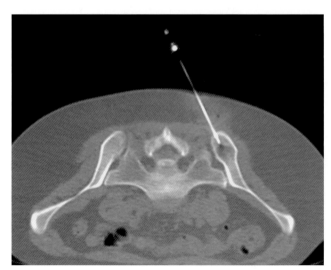

Figure 8-22 ■ Coaxial biopsy technique. The large-caliber, shorter needle with an inner stylet is guided to the margin or into the lesion or structure to be sampled. In this case, the needle tip is at the margin of a lytic lesion in the posterior ilium.

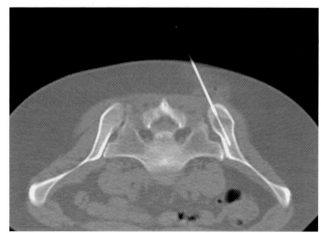

Figure 8-23 ■ Coaxial biopsy technique. The smaller gauge, longer biopsy needle is advanced through the indwelling larger gauge needle in a coaxial fashion to obtain the specimen. This can be repeated to obtain multiple specimens through a single needle placement.

without having to redirect the needle and relocalize the lesion between passes.[1,8] A large core sample is then finally obtained with the larger caliber needle by advancing the needle into the lesion, and the needle is withdrawn.

Biopsy needles utilized for a given lesion may be selected from one or multiple biopsy needle systems or needle sets.[8] Regardless of the needle systems utilized, it is important to verify before the procedure that the selected inner coaxial needle will fit through the outer cannula and that the inner needle is sufficiently long to project out from the end of the outer cannula into the target lesion.[8]

Single-Needle Technique[8]

A single-pass needle technique can be used for biopsies that are superficial (Fig. 8-24).[1,8] A needle of any caliber with an inner stylet can be used to biopsy osseous or soft tissue masses. In general, smaller gauge needles produce less damage to surrounding structures and should be used when possible.[1,8] The disadvantage of this technique is that only one biopsy sample can be obtained unless repeated passes are performed, which require repeated localization of the needle in the lesion.[1,8] This technique is ideal for superficial soft tissue lesions in which the tumor can be repeatedly sampled with little risk of damage to deeper, more vital structures.[1,8] This technique should be avoided in difficult or deep biopsies, which require precise placement of the needle to avoid damage to surrounding structures.[1,8]

Selection of Needle Biopsy System

Numerous biopsy needles are commercially available, and it is not our intention to mention each. We describe specific needle biopsy systems that we commonly utilize in our practice. These descriptions provide specific examples and help illustrate the general instructional message of this chapter.[8] Please note that we do not advocate or recommend a specific vendor or needle biopsy system and do not present any needle system as having an advantage over another.[8] We receive no financial support from any of these vendors and are not shareholders in any of the companies that manufacture these needle biopsy systems.[8]

Physicians performing image-guided biopsies, based on their training and personal experience, should strive to become proficient at utilizing no more than two or three needle biopsy systems.[8] This ensures familiarization with these specific needle systems and mastery of these techniques. If one is unfamiliar with a certain type of needle system, one should seek specific training in the proper use and handling of the needle for optimum specimen collection and for patients' safety.[8] The specific type of needle biopsy system is carefully selected based on the type of lesion to be sampled, the location of the mass, and the familiarity of the operator with the needle biopsy system.[8]

In general, larger caliber biopsy needles provide better specimens but are associated with increased risk and morbidity. The diameter of the needle chosen should balance

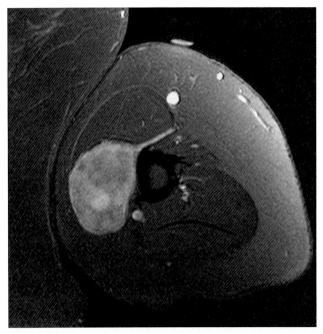

A

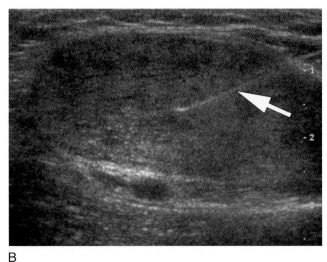

B

Figure 8-24 ▪ Single-pass biopsy technique. Middle-aged female patient with a palpable mass in the left upper arm. Axial fat-suppressed T1-weighted image of the upper arm following intravenous contrast administration (*A*) depicts an enhancing soft tissue mass corresponding to the palpable abnormality. An ultrasound-guided percutaneous biopsy (*B*) was performed with a Temno biopsy needle (*arrow*). Because the lesion was superficial with no overlying obstacles to avoid in the subcutaneous fat, a single-pass technique was used. This was repeated twice to obtain a total of three core specimens.

these factors for the individual case to be performed. The chosen needle biopsy system should in all cases be utilized in accordance with the manufacturer's technical recommendations and guidelines.[8] Frequent, if not continuous, image guidance is necessary to ensure precise placement of the needle and avoid deviation from the intended pathway.[8] Proper technique is mandatory to avoid inadvertent injury to surrounding tissues, including blood vessels and nerves.[8]

Examples of Soft Tissue Biopsy Needle Systems

Temno Adjustable Throw Biopsy Device

Available from Bauer Medical (Clearwater, FL), Temno is a registered trademark of Allegiance Healthcare (Fig. 8-25)

  18-gauge, 6-, 11-, 15-, and 20-cm length (orange)
  20-gauge, 6-, 11-, 15-, and 20-cm length (green)
  22-gauge, 6-, 11-, 15-, and 20-cm length (clear)
  Nonremovable notched inner stylet
  Spring-loaded mechanism, semiautomated gun mechanism
  Optional coaxial introducer cannulas available separately or combined in a package with the appropriate biopsy needle

METHOD

The Temno biopsy needle can be utilized with a single-pass technique or in a coaxial fashion with coaxial cannulas that are available in packages with the appropriate-sized biopsy

needles. Coaxial needles are one gauge lower and 5 cm shorter than the corresponding biopsy needle (Fig. 8-26). For example, a package is available with an 18-gauge, 11-cm Temno biopsy needle with a 17-gauge, 6-cm coaxial needle. This 5-cm difference is matched to allow only the 2-cm specimen collection segment of the inner stylet of the biopsy needle to extend beyond the distal tip of the coaxial needle (Fig. 8-27). Multiple core biopsy specimens can be obtained in this fashion through the indwelling coaxial needle.

The Temno biopsy needle can also be utilized coaxially through other larger caliber biopsy needles such as the Bonopty or Ostycut needles, although the exact lengths are not matched (Fig. 8-28). It is necessary to verify before proceeding with the biopsy that the selected Temno biopsy needle will fit through the outer coaxial needle to be utilized and that the Temno biopsy needle is sufficiently long for the specimen collection segment of the inner stylet of the biopsy needle to project out from the end of the outer coaxial needle.

Before using this needle, the operator must be keenly aware of the tissues in and near the intended target tissue being sampled that could be within the throw length of the needle to avoid injury to important normal structures such as blood vessels or neural tissue. If a coaxial technique is to be utilized, the first step is to place the larger gauge coaxial needle to the margin of the lesion under image guidance (Fig. 8-29).

The spring-loaded Temno biopsy needle is cocked by withdrawing the plunger, which pulls the inner stylet and cannula back a short distance and compresses the spring

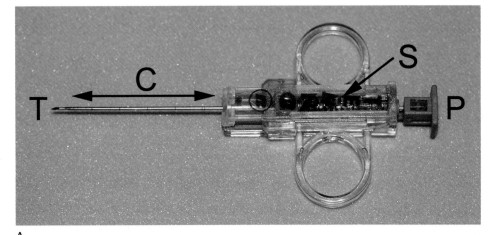

Figure 8-25 ▪ Temno biopsy needle. *A,* An 18-gauge, 6-cm Temno biopsy needle. The distal tip of the inner stylet (T) with the remainder of the inner stylet covered by the outer cannula (C). The plunger (P) is used to cock the spring mechanism (S). *B,* The distal tip of the Temno biopsy needle with needle cocked and the notch or specimen collection segment (SCS) extended beyond the outer cannula (C).

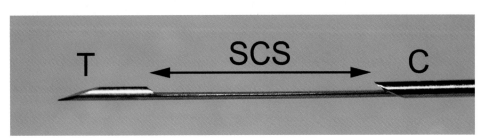

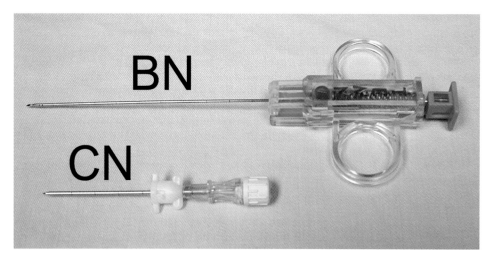

Figure 8-26 ■ Coaxial Temno biopsy needle system. This image shows the coaxial Temno biopsy needle system consisting of a 17-gauge, 6-cm outer coaxial needle (CN) and an 18-gauge, 11-cm inner Temno biopsy needle (BN). These needles are matched to allow only the 2-cm notch or specimen collection segment of the inner stylet of the biopsy needle to extend beyond the tip of the coaxial needle.

mechanism (Fig. 8-30). The biopsy needle is then advanced to the proximal margin of the lesion (Fig. 8-31). The biopsy needle is held by placing the thumb on the plunger and two fingers through the loops (Fig. 8-32). The plunger is advanced halfway to allow the specimen collection segment of the inner stylet of the biopsy needle to protrude beyond the tip of the coaxial needle and into the lesion (Fig. 8-33). To obtain the biopsy specimen, the plunger is then advanced fully, which activates the spring-loaded biopsy system

(Fig. 8-34). The outer cannula snaps forward over the inner stylet, and a small piece of tissue is captured in the specimen collection segment of the inner stylet. The needle is withdrawn from the lesion. To expose the specimen, the needle is again cocked by withdrawing the plunger, which pulls back the outer cannula, followed by partial advancement of the plunger, which exposes the specimen in the specimen collection notch of the inner stylet. The specimen is then rolled onto a sterile slide (Fig. 8-35).

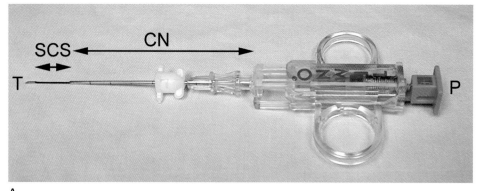

A

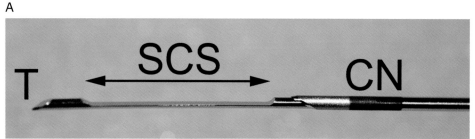

B

Figure 8-27 ■ Coaxial Temno biopsy needle system. The Temno biopsy needle has been cocked by withdrawing the plunger (P). The biopsy needle has then been advanced through the coaxial needle (CN) and the plunger has been depressed to a point at which the 2-cm specimen collection segment (SCS) protrudes beyond the tip of the coaxial needle (A). Only the distal 2 cm of the inner stylet of the biopsy needle including the specimen collection segment and tip (T) extends beyond the tip of the coaxial needle (B).

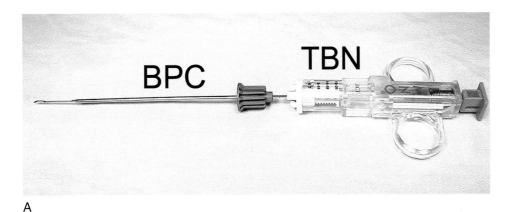

A

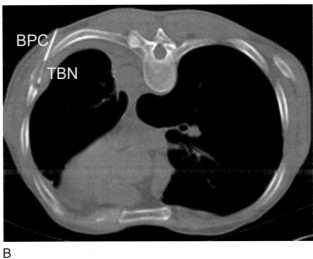

B

Figure 8-28 ■ Temno biopsy needle and Bonopty penetration cannula utilized in a coaxial fashion (*A*). An 18-gauge, 15-cm Temno biopsy needle (TBN) can be advanced through a Bonopty penetration cannula (BPC) to biopsy lytic osseous lesions. The BPC is used to breach the cortex of the lesion and the TBN is utilized to obtain specimens of the central lytic focus of the lesion (*B*).

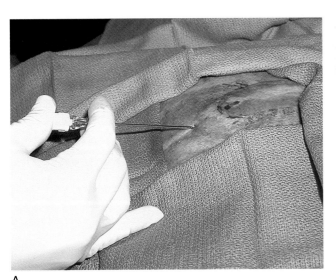

A

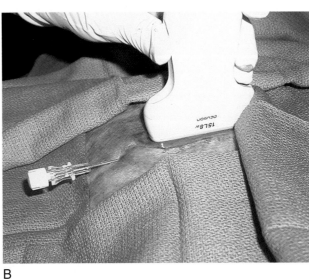

B

Figure 8-29 ■ Coaxial Temno biopsy needle. Initial needle puncture (*A*). The larger gauge coaxial needle is placed to the margin of the lesion under image guidance (*B*).

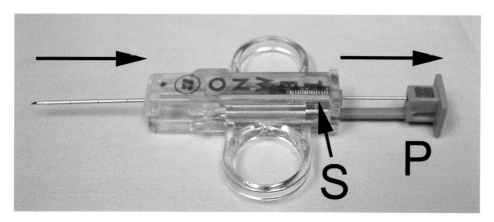

Figure 8-30 ■ Cocking the Temno biopsy needle. The needle is cocked by withdrawing the plunger (P), which pulls the inner stylet and cannula back a short distance and compresses the spring mechanism (S).

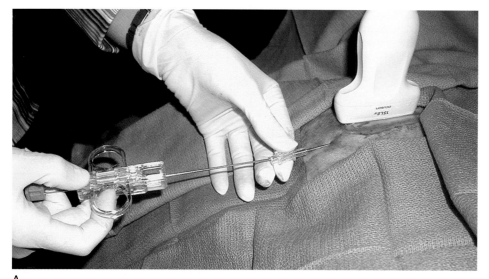

A

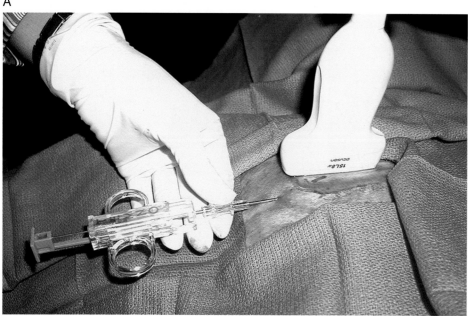

B

Figure 8-31 ■ Coaxial Temno biopsy needle. The Temno biopsy needle is advanced through the indwelling coaxial needle (*A*). The biopsy needle is hubbed within the coaxial needle, (*B*) which places the biopsy needle tip precisely at the level of the tip of the coaxial needle at the margin of the lesion.

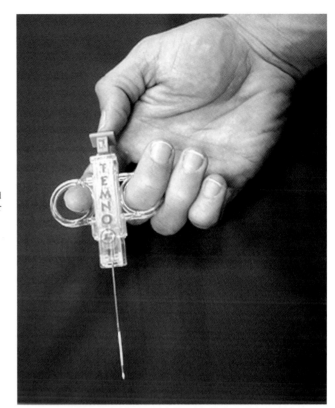

Figure 8-32 ▪ Temno biopsy needle. The Temno biopsy needle is held by placing one's thumb on the plunger and two fingers through the finger loops.

Figure 8-33 ▪ Coaxial Temno biopsy needle. The plunger (P) of the Temno biopsy needle is gently advanced to allow the specimen collection segment (SCS) of the inner stylet of the biopsy needle to project beyond the outer cannula (C).

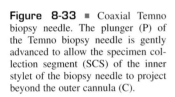

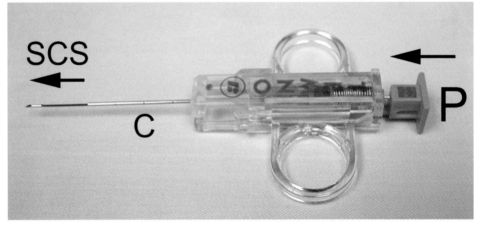

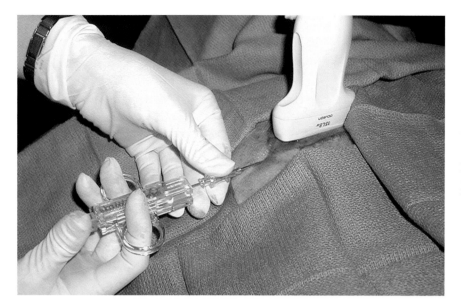

Figure 8-34 ■ Coaxial Temno biopsy needle. To obtain the biopsy specimen, the plunger (P) is advanced fully, which activates the spring-loaded biopsy system. The outer cannula snaps forward over the inner stylet and a small piece of tissue is captured in the specimen collection segment of the inner stylet.

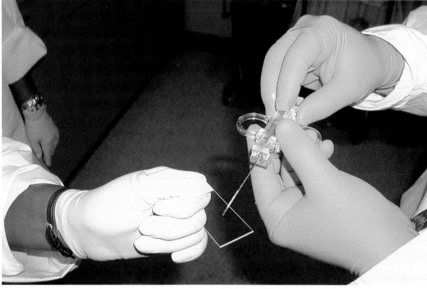

A

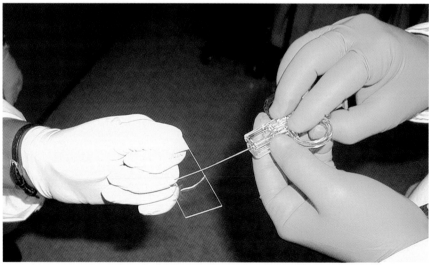

B

Figure 8-35 ■ Temno biopsy needle. To expose the specimen, the needle is again cocked by withdrawing the plunger, which pulls back the outer cannula, followed by slow advancement of the plunger, which exposes the specimen in the specimen collection notch of the inner stylet (*A*). The specimen is then rolled onto a sterile slide (*B*).

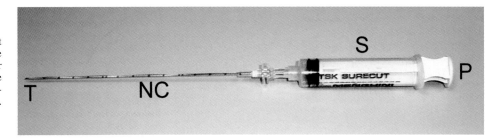

Figure 8-36 ▪ TSK SureCut modified Menghini biopsy needle (20 gauge, 15 cm). When the plunger (P) is pushed into the syringe (S), the needle tip of the inner stylet (T) protrudes from the needle cannula (NC).

TSK SureCut Modified Menghini Biopsy Needle

Available from TSK Laboratory, Japan; SureCut Biopsy needle, Boston Scientific/Medi-Tech (Fig. 8-36).

  Modified stainless steel Menghini needle with a beveled tip
  Needle calibers available: 15, 16, 17, 18, 19, 20, 21, and 22 gauge
  Needle lengths available: 4, 5, 7, 9, 10, 12, 15, and 23 cm
  Needle removable from biopsy syringe
  Syringe plunger permanently attached to inner pencil-point stylet

METHOD

When the plunger is pushed into the syringe, the needle tip of the inner stylet protrudes from the needle cannula. The needle is advanced into the target biopsy tissue (Fig. 8-37). The plunger of the biopsy syringe is withdrawn until the plastic clip stopper locks in place to provide negative pressure at the needle tip (Fig. 8-38). The needle is briskly advanced a few millimeters into the target tissue while rotating 360 degrees to collect the specimen. The needle is removed from the tissue while continuing to apply suction with the clip lock in place. Following the biopsy, the sample is deposited onto a sterile slide or into a collection tube by releasing the plastic plunger clip by gently depressing the clip and advancing the plunger. The inner stylet then pushes the sample out of the tip of the needle cannula (Fig. 8-39). This biopsy needle may be used alone for a single pass into a soft tissue mass or coaxially through a larger caliber needle (Fig. 8-40).

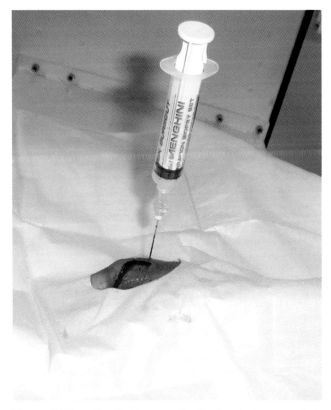

Figure 8-37 ▪ SureCut biopsy needle. The SureCut biopsy needle is advanced into the target tissue under image guidance with the plunger pushed into the syringe.

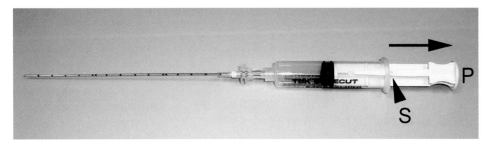

Figure 8-38 ▪ SureCut biopsy needle. The plunger (P) of the biopsy syringe (S) is withdrawn until the plastic clip stopper locks in place, which provides negative pressure at the needle tip.

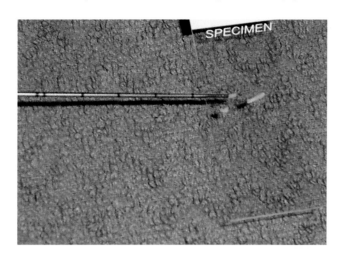

Figure 8-39 ■ SureCut biopsy needle. Following the biopsy, the plastic plunger clip is released by depressing the clip and gently advancing the plunger until the inner stylet pushes the sample out of the tip of the needle cannula.

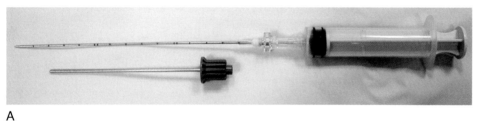

A

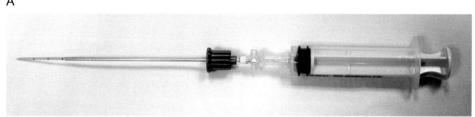

B

Figure 8-40 ■ SureCut biopsy needle and Bonopty penetration cannula (*A*). A 20-gauge, 15-cm SureCut biopsy needle can be advanced through a Bonopty penetration cannula to biopsy osseous lesions in a coaxial manner (*B*).

Examples of Bone Biopsy Needle Systems

Bonopty

Available from RADI Medical Systems (Uppsala, Sweden) (Fig. 8-41)

14-gauge, 9.5-cm length penetration cannula with diamond-pointed stylet (green)
15-gauge drill stylet, 12.2-cm length (white)
15-gauge, 16-cm length biopsy needle with diamond-pointed stylet (blue)
18-gauge blunt ejector pin (white)
15-gauge, 16-cm-length extended-length drill stylet

Depth gauges included to control precisely the depth of the biopsy needle when advanced in a coaxial fashion through the penetration cannula

METHOD

Local anesthesia is obtained at the puncture site with a 25-gauge, 1.5-inch needle followed by deeper anesthesia of the soft tissues and periosteum with a 22-gauge spinal needle. The spinal needle can then be left in place to guide the penetration cannula by a tandem needle technique or withdrawn. A small dermatotomy is made at the puncture site, and the penetration cannula and stylet are advanced through the soft tissues toward the bone surface (Fig. 8-42). If necessary, the stylet can be removed to inject additional

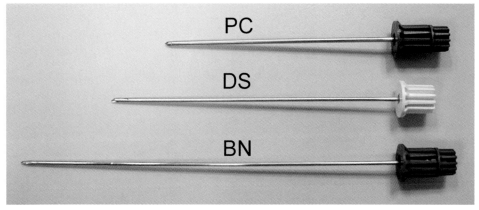

A

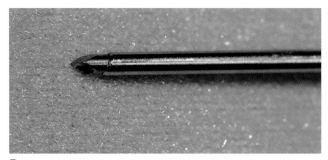

B

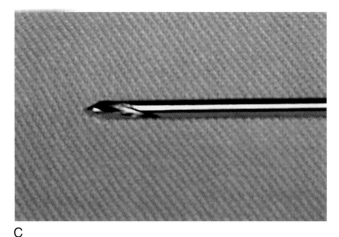

C

D

Figure 8-41 ■ Bonopty biopsy system (*A*). The Bonopty biopsy system consists of the Bonopty penetration cannula (PC), the Bonopty drill stylet (DS), and the Bonopty biopsy needle (BN). The tip of the penetration cannula (*B*) has a sharpened diamond-pointed stylet used to traverse the overlying soft tissues. The tip of the drill stylet (*C*) has two low-pitched helices and is used to penetrate the cortex of the bone. The tip of the biopsy needle (*D*) has a gentle inward reduction in diameter to aid in obtaining specimens while minimizing crush artifact.

anesthetic through the Luer-Lock opening of the penetration cannula. When the bone is reached, the diamond-pointed stylet is exchanged for the drill stylet (Fig. 8-43). The drill stylet extends approximately 8 mm beyond the penetration cannula and has two low-pitch helices that allow penetration through the cortex of the bone (Fig. 8-44). The drill stylet is rotated clockwise until the drill is anchored in the bone. Imaging is then performed to verify the position and direction of the drill and penetration cannula. It is important to have the needle well aligned along the expected path before entering the bone. At this point, correction and minor adjustments of the position and angulation are easy; however, when the drill and cannula significantly enter the bone, changes in course of the biopsy system become more difficult. The drill is then rotated further in the clockwise

direction, embedding the stylet and cannula further in the bone. When the drill has breached the inner cortex of the bone and entered the softer medullary bone, the penetration cannula can be advanced by careful clockwise rotation to a point at which its tip is a few millimeters into the bone. The drill stylet is then removed and the penetration cannula can be used as a fixed pathway for biopsy with a variety of other needles by a coaxial technique (Fig. 8-45).

If the Bonopty biopsy needle is selected for use, it can be advanced through the indwelling Bonopty penetration cannula (Fig. 8-46). The Bonopty biopsy needle protrudes 45 mm beyond the tip of the penetration cannula (Fig. 8-47). This can be shortened with the use of the depth gauge. The depth gauge can be placed onto the Luer opening on the hub of the penetration cannula (Fig. 8-48) and can be adjusted

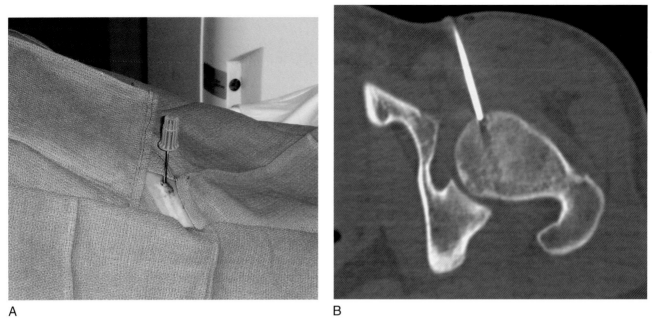

A   B

Figure 8-42 ■ Bonopty biopsy system. The Bonopty penetration cannula and stylet are advanced through the soft tissues to the bone surface (*A*). Image guidance is utilized to place the needle on the bone surface precisely above the lesion or above the tract to be used to reach the lesion (*B*).

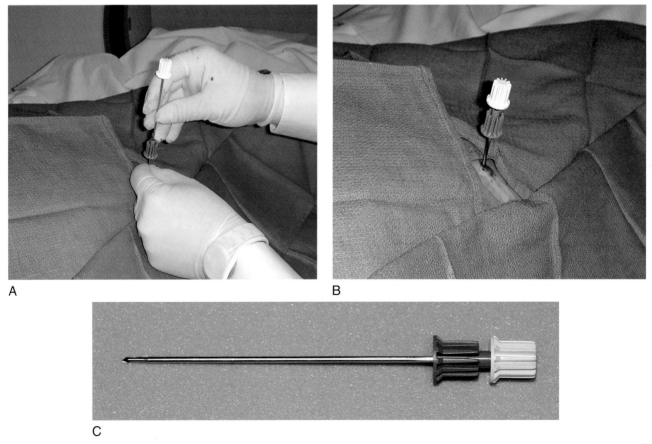

A   B

C

Figure 8-43 ■ Bonopty biopsy system. After the penetration cannula is placed on the bone surface, the diamond-pointed stylet of the penetration cannula (green handle) is exchanged for the drill stylet (white handle) (*A* and *B*). The drill stylet extends approximately 8 mm beyond the tip of the penetration cannula (*C*).

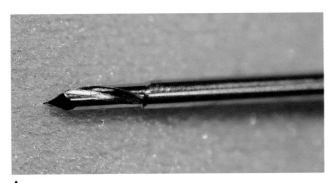

A

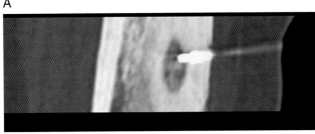

B

Figure 8-44 ■ Bonopty biopsy system. Magnified view of the tip of the drill stylet protruding beyond the tip of the penetration cannula (*A*). The drill stylet has two low-pitched helices that allow penetration through the cortex of the bone (*B*).

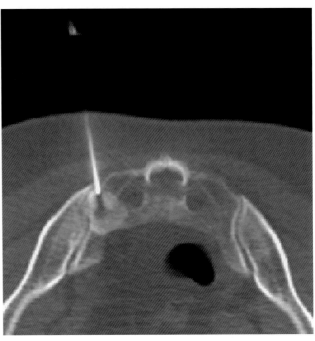

Figure 8-45 ■ Bonopty biopsy system. When the Bonopty penetration cannula is at the margin of the lesion, the drill stylet is removed and the penetration cannula can be used as a fixed pathway for biopsy with a variety of other needles by a coaxial technique.

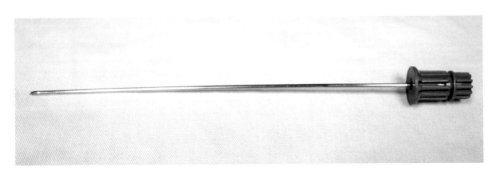

Figure 8-46 ■ Bonopty biopsy needle (blue handle).

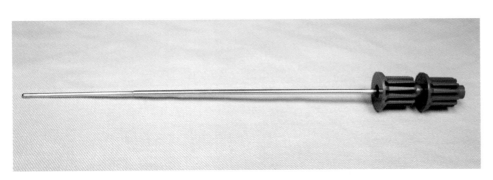

Figure 8-47 ■ Bonopty biopsy system. The Bonopty biopsy needle (blue handle) is advanced through the Bonopty penetration cannula (green handle) in a coaxial fashion. The Bonopty biopsy needle will protrude 45 mm beyond the tip of the penetration cannula.

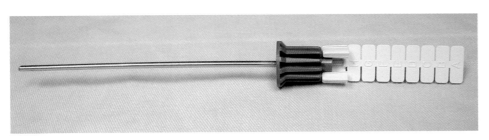

Figure 8-48 ■ Bonopty biopsy system. The depth gauge (white) can adjust the length that the Bonopty biopsy needle protrudes beyond the tip of the Bonopty penetration cannula. The depth gauge can be adjusted by breaking the component at predetermined break points located every 5 mm. The depth gauge is first placed onto the Luer-Lock opening on the hub of the penetration cannula.

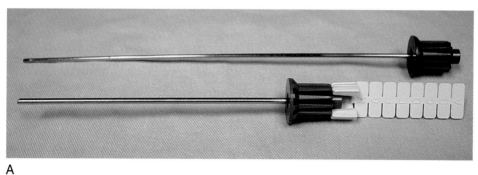

A

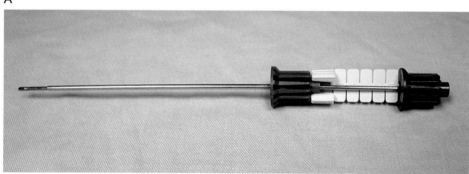

B

Figure 8-49 ■ Bonopty biopsy system. The Bonopty biopsy needle is placed next to the Bonopty penetration cannula and depth gauge (*A*). The length that the biopsy needle is to protrude from the distal tip of the cannula is determined and the depth gauge is broken off at the appropriate level. The length the Bonopty biopsy needle protrudes beyond the penetration cannula is then modified accordingly by the depth gauge when the biopsy needle is placed through the penetration cannula and depth gauge in a coaxial fashion (*B*).

by breaking the component at predetermined break points located every 5 mm (Fig. 8-49). The Bonopty biopsy needle is then placed through the penetration cannula and rotated with moderate force in the clockwise direction until the needle reaches the margin of the lesion. The stylet of the bone biopsy needle is then withdrawn and the biopsy needle is advanced into the lesion by rotating the needle clockwise (Fig. 8-50). It is often helpful to apply suction to the Luer opening of the biopsy needle with a syringe and tubing during advancement of the needle. The Bonopty biopsy needle

is then withdrawn with clockwise rotation. The ejector pin is used to remove the specimen from the needle. To avoid crush artifact from the inward reduction of diameter of the Bonopty cannula tip, the ejector pin should be placed through the distal tip of the cannula and the specimen should be ejected from the Luer opening of the cannula hub (Fig. 8-51).

For sclerotic lesions in which the Bonopty biopsy needle cannot penetrate, the drill stylet can be utilized to obtain fragments of bone from the helices of the drill. The drill

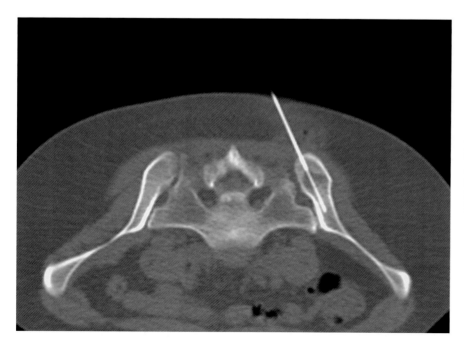

Figure 8-50 ■ Bonopty biopsy system. CT image depicting the Bonopty biopsy needle passing through the Bonopty penetration cannula in a coaxial fashion to obtain a specimen of this osseous lesion involving the posterior ilium.

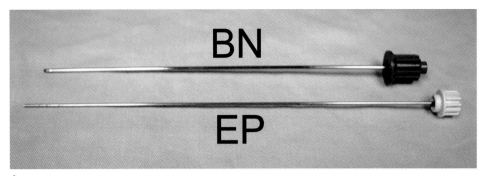
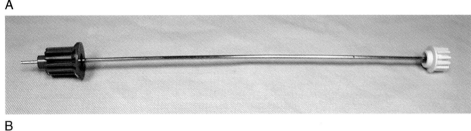

Figure 8-51 ▪ Bonopty biopsy needle and ejector pin (*A*). To avoid crush artifact from the inward reduction of diameter of the tip of the Bonopty needle (BN), the dull-tipped ejector pin (EP) should be placed through the distal tip of the biopsy needle and the specimen should be ejected from the Luer opening of the needle hub (*B*).

stylet can be inserted through the penetration cannula similarly to the Bonopty biopsy needle. The drill stylet is advanced into the lesion with clockwise rotation. It is important not to spin the drill excessively as this may hard-pack the specimen within the helix and thereby alter the architecture of the specimen and create crush artifact. The drill stylet should then be removed by simultaneously rotating it clockwise while withdrawing it. The specimen can be removed from the helices of the drill tip of the stylet (Fig. 8-52).

Angiomed Ostycut Biopsy Needle

Available from C.R. Bard (Covington, GA), Ostycut Biopsy Needle and Angiomed are both registered trademarks of C.R. Bard (Fig. 8-53).

17-gauge, 5-, 7.5-, 10-, 12.5-, and 15-cm length
16-gauge, 5-, 7.5-, 10-, 12.5-, and 15-cm length
15-gauge, 5-, 7.5-, 10-, 12.5-, and 15-cm length
14-gauge, 5-, 7.5-, 10-, 12.5-, and 15-cm length

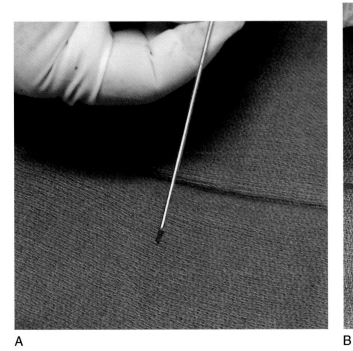
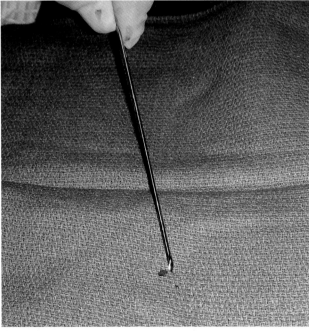

Figure 8-52 ▪ Bonopty biopsy system. For sclerotic lesions into which the Bonopty biopsy needle will not penetrate, the drill stylet can be used to obtain fragments of bone from the helices of the drill (*A*). The drill stylet is inserted through the penetration cannula with clockwise rotation. The drill stylet is then removed by withdrawal and simultaneous clockwise rotation. The specimen is removed from the helices of the drill tip of the stylet (*B*).

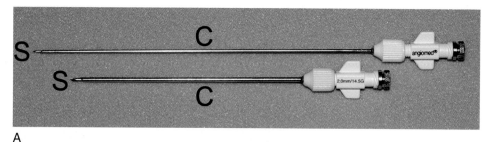

A

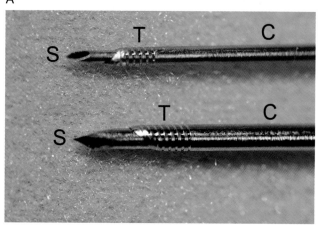

B

Figure 8-53 ▪ Ostycut biopsy needles. Ostycut needles are available in a wide variety of lengths and diameters and consist of a threaded cannula (C) and inner trocar point stylet (S) with a cutting edge (*A*).(Upper needle, 17 gauge, 15 cm. Lower needle, 14.5 gauge, 10 cm.). Magnified view of the distal tips of these needles (*B*) depicts the high pitch threading (T) at the tip of the cannula, which allows penetration into cortical bone with clockwise rotation. The inner trocar point stylet (S) is also seen protruding from the cannula.

13-gauge, 10- and 15-cm length
10-mL Luer-tipped aspiration syringe
Blunt obturator
Reusable handgrip
Two-part needle consisting of a threaded cannula and a trocar point stylet with a cutting edge capable of penetrating bone
Handgrip attaches to the needle cannula hub and can be resterilized and reused

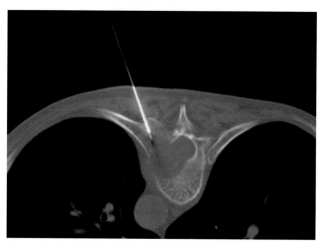

Figure 8-54 ▪ Ostycut biopsy needle. CT image of an Ostycut needle that has been advanced into the bone with firm pressure and clockwise rotation.

METHOD

The soft tissues and periosteum overlying the lesion should be anesthetized. A dermatotomy is made at the skin surface. The Ostycut biopsy needle and stylet are then advanced utilizing image guidance to the bone surface overlying the lesion. If necessary, the stylet can be removed to allow additional anesthetic injections through the Luer opening on the Ostycut needle. When the bone is reached, imaging is performed to verify the position and direction of the drill and penetration cannula. The needle is then advanced into the bone under firm pressure while rotating the needle in the clockwise direction, which embeds the stylet and needle into the bone. When the threaded portion of the needle obtains a grip in the bone, the stylet is withdrawn. The needle is then advanced further into the bone with the same firm pressure and clockwise rotation (Fig. 8-54). If desired, the Ostycut handgrip can be connected to the needle hub, facilitating the pressure and clockwise motion, simplifying the biopsy procedure. When the lesion has been reached and traversed, the handgrip is removed and the 10-mL Luer tip syringe is attached to the Luer opening of the needle hub. The plunger is withdrawn to create negative pressure (Fig. 8-55). The needle is removed while suction is applied. The syringe is removed from the needle. The biopsy specimen is removed by inserting the blunt obturator into the needle. The Ostycut needle can be used with a single-pass technique or in tandem utilizing a coaxial technique. A 15-cm, 17-gauge Ostycut needle fits precisely through a 10-cm, 14-gauge needle with the tip of the 17-gauge needle extending a very short distance beyond the tip of the 14-gauge needle (Fig. 8-56). This setup is ideal for coaxial technique bone biopsies (Fig. 8-57).

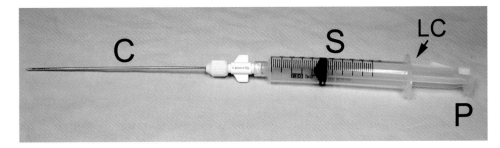

Figure 8-55 ■ Ostycut biopsy needle. When the tip of the needle cannula (C) has been placed within the lesion, the 10-mL Luer tip syringe (S) is attached to the Luer opening of the needle hub. The plunger (P) is withdrawn until the plastic locking clip (LC) locks in place, which provides negative pressure at the needle tip.

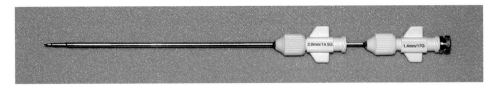

A

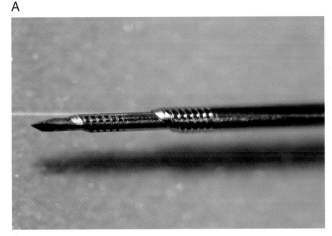

Figure 8-56 ■ Ostycut needles used in a coaxial fashion. A 15-cm, 17-gauge Ostycut needle fits precisely through a 10-cm, 14.5-gauge needle (*A*) with the tip of the 17-gauge needle extending a very short distance beyond the tip of the 14-gauge needle (*B*).

B

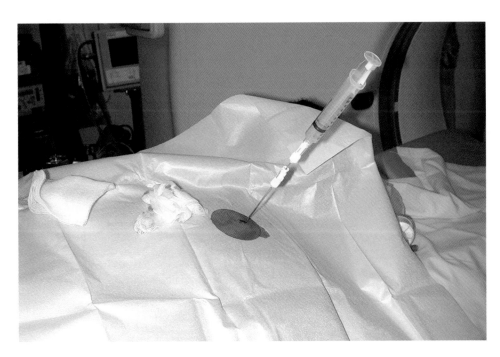

Figure 8-57 ■ Ostycut needles used in a coaxial fashion. A 15-cm, 17-gauge Ostycut needle and a 10-cm, 14.5-gauge needle utilized in a coaxial fashion with the syringe attached applying negative pressure.

POTENTIAL COMPLICATIONS[8]

In experienced hands, the complication rate of percutaneous soft tissue and bone biopsy is probably less than 1% to 3%, depending on the type and location of the tissue biopsied.
* Bleeding
* Infection (cellulitis, septic arthritis, or osteomyelitis)
* Drug-related allergic reactions
* Inadvertent nerve injury
* Arterial or venous injury
* Pneumothorax
* Vasovagal reaction
* Dissemination of tumor along the biopsy tract

POST-PROCEDURE CARE/FOLLOW-UP[8]

Immediate

1. The patient should be observed for at least 30 minutes after the biopsy.
2. Blood pressure, pulse, heart rate, and respiratory rate are monitored as necessary.

Discharge

1. The patient should be discharged into the care of a responsible person.
2. The patient is instructed not to drive or perform any other tasks that require clear thought and quick reactions for the remainder of the day, especially if sedation was given.
3. A 2- to 3-day nonrenewable prescription for a narcotic pain reliever or a muscle relaxant, or both, may be given to the patient.
4. Patients are instructed to continue to take their prescription medication, although the pain medication may be tapered as indicated.
5. An adhesive bandage may be placed on the puncture site. The bandage should remain dry for at least 24 hours, at which point it can be removed.
6. A discharge sheet should be given to the patient outlining the following:
   a. The procedure performed
   b. Procedure-related symptoms that typically resolve in 7 to 10 days
      * Pain at the needle puncture site(s)
      * Mild stiffness with a feeling of fullness in the biopsy region
      * Deep pain in the biopsy region
   c. Treatment for mild post-procedure symptoms
      * Rest the affected area for 3 to 4 days
      * Avoid movements that aggravate the pain
      * Use cold compresses to the area that hurts
   d. Signs and symptoms of infection
      * Fever
      * Chills
      * Swelling or drainage from the puncture site(s)
      * New pain that is different from the usual pain
   e. Signs and symptoms of possible more serious problems
      * Increasing pain

* Motor dysfunction of the affected region or extremity
* Bowel or bladder dysfunction

   f. Physician name and contact number if the patient has any concerns or if any problems were to arise as a result of the procedure
   g. Advice to schedule a follow-up appointment with the referring physician in 7 to 10 days

RADIOFREQUENCY ABLATION

BACKGROUND

The most common musculoskeletal application for image-guided radiofrequency ablation is the treatment of osteoid osteoma.[14–16,28] Osteoid osteoma is a benign tumor that occurs mainly in young adults.[29–31] The clinical hallmark is local pain, which is often more severe at night and typically responds promptly to aspirin and other nonsteroidal anti-inflammatory medications (Fig. 8-58).[16–18,30] Osteoid osteomas release excess prostaglandins, which produce local vasodilatation, inflammatory effects, and pain.[16] Nonsteroidal anti-inflammatory medications block the arachidonic acid pathway, thereby reducing the prostaglandin burden and ultimately decreasing pain associated with the lesions.[16] Lesions are most common in the lower extremities and often involve the cortex of the long bones.[29,30]

The pain associated with osteoid osteoma can subside with conservative medical therapy although treatment may be lengthy, requiring long exposures to often high doses of nonsteroidal anti-inflammatory medications.[18] For this reason, for many years, the common curative treatment of osteoid osteoma has been en bloc surgical excision.[18,29] Unfortunately, intraoperative localization can be difficult and surgical removal often necessitates significant bone resection.[15,18,29] In a small percentage of cases, the nidus may be missed at surgery.[14,18]

To improve upon surgical treatment, several CT-guided percutaneous techniques have been employed to achieve destruction of the nidus of the osteoid osteoma with minimal invasiveness.[18] These techniques include percutaneous trephine resection or drill resection with or without ethanol injection, cryoablation, and thermal destruction with either radiofrequency ablation or laser photocoagulation.[16,18,28] Radiofrequency ablation has proved to be the most effective technique and has gained popularity because of its high technical and clinical success rate and low complication rate.[16,30] With radiofrequency ablation of osteoid osteomas, patients may resume normal activities immediately after the procedure, which is a significant reduction in the period of convalescence compared with surgical resection.[15,17] Success rates range in the literature from 76% to 100%.[16] Radiofrequency ablation, rather than surgical excision or other options, has become the treatment of choice for osteoid osteoma.

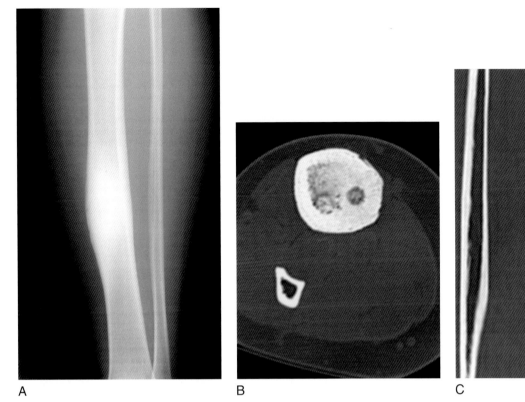

A   B   C

Figure 8-58 ■ Osteoid osteoma in a 16-year-old female with calf pain that is worse at night and improved with nonsteroidal anti-inflammatory medications. Radiograph (*A*) depicts solid continuous periosteal reaction circumferentially about the tibial diaphysis, most marked medially. Axial CT (*B*) and coronal reformatted CT (*C*) images of the tibia depict a central lucent nidus within this surrounding periosteal reaction compatible with an osteoid osteoma.

CONTRAINDICATIONS[8]

- Coagulopathy (caution in patients with INR >1.5 or platelets < 50,000/mm^3)
- Pregnancy (because of teratogenic effects of radiation)
- Systemic infection or skin infection over the puncture site
- Severe allergy to any medication needed to perform the procedure
- Tumor inaccessible to ablation secondary to adjacent vital structures such as blood vessels or nerves. The lesion should be 5 cm away from vital structures; however, at the very least it must be more than 1 cm away from adjacent vital structures.

PROCEDURE

Equipment/Supplies

- Radiofrequency ablation generator (Radionics) (Fig. 8-59)
- Radiofrequency ablation electrode (Fig. 8-60)
- Radiofrequency ablation insulation cannula (Fig. 8-61)
- Radiofrequency ablation cutaneous self-adhesive grounding pad
- Bone biopsy needle (Bonopty Penetration Cannula and Drill Stylet)
- Povidone-iodine (Betadine) scrub
- Sterile drapes, towels and gloves
- Sterile gauze
- Adhesive bandage
- CT guidance (CT fluoroscopy preferred)
- Lead apron
- Anesthesia equipment

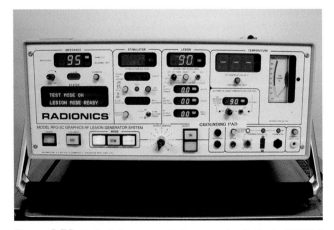

Figure 8-59 ■ Radiofrequency ablation generator. Radionics RFG-3C Graphics RF Lesion Generator System.

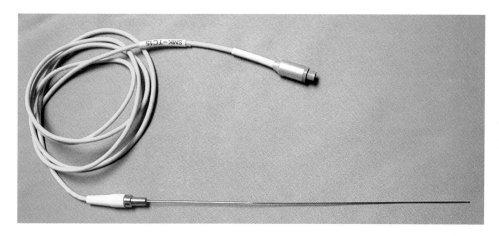

Figure 8-60 ■ Radiofrequency ablation electrode. Radionics SMK-TC 15 Thermocouple Electrode. When it is connected to the generator and activated, heating occurs along the entire length of the electrode.

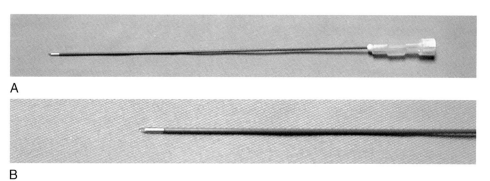

A

B

Figure 8-61 ■ Radiofrequency ablation insulating cannula. Radionics SMK-C15 Insulated Cannula. The insulating cannula (*A*) is insulated along its entire length apart from the distal noninsulated tip and protects the tissues along the tract used to reach the lesion against unwanted heating. Magnified view of the distal tip of the electrode (*B*) demonstrates the insulation along the entire length of the cannula apart from the distal tip, which allows exposure of the electrode within the lesion.

Methodology

The procedure, including the risks, benefits, and alternative treatment options, should be discussed with the patient and the patient's parents if applicable. Ideally, this should be performed in advance of the procedure in the clinic setting to allow the patient and family time to make an informed decision about treatment options. Informed consent is obtained on the day of the procedure. The procedure is performed under general or spinal anesthesia, as the procedure itself can be painful. Following the pre-anesthesia work-up, the patient is placed on the CT scanner in a safe position that facilitates access to the lesion (Fig. 8-62). The self-adhesive grounding pad is then placed on the patient. A patch of skin on the patient's thigh is shaved and the grounding pad is affixed to the skin surface (Fig. 8-63). Members of the department of anesthesia then perform general anesthesia for most lesions, although spinal anesthesia may be sufficient for lower extremity lesions.

Preliminary 1-mm-thick CT images through the lesion are then obtained. The images are carefully analyzed to determine the optimal needle trajectory. A CT image is selected that optimally demonstrates the pathologic target and the desired needle trajectory. The image location number of this image is noted. The skin puncture site can be localized using either a grid or BB pellet as described in the CT guidance section of this chapter. When the puncture site is marked, the skin is prepared and draped in a sterile fash-

ion. A dermatotomy is then performed with a scalpel to facilitate placement of the biopsy needle through the superficial soft tissues. Several options are available for the biopsy needle system used to reach the lesion. A 16- to 18-gauge needle is adequate, as larger gauge needles are not necessary. The needle should allow the chosen radiofrequency ablation electrode and insulating cannula to pass through the needle in a coaxial fashion and must be short enough to allow the cannula and electrode to extend well (more than 3 cm)

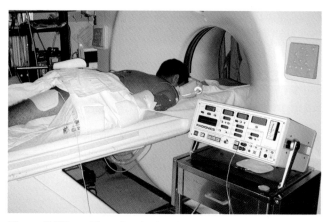

Figure 8-62 ■ The patient is placed on the CT scanner in a safe position that facilitates access to the lesion.

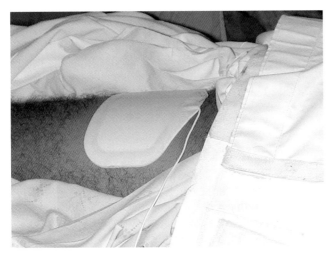

Figure 8-63 ■ Radiofrequency ablation grounding pad. A patch of skin on the patient's thigh is shaved and the grounding pad is affixed to the skin surface. If the lesion is in the lower extremity, the grounding pad should be placed on the opposite thigh.

beyond the tip of the biopsy needle. The Bonopty penetration cannula and drill stylet are well suited for this purpose (Fig. 8-64).

In addition to ensuring that the biopsy needle is adequate, the insulating cannula and electrode should be carefully inspected. The electrode should be sterile and straight with no bends or kinks. The electrode should be advanced through the insulating cannula to be utilized to ensure that only the tip of the electrode is exposed when the electrode is hubbed within the insulating cannula (Fig. 8-65). Exposure of too much of the electrode could lead to burns or excessive ablation of the tissues. If the electrode is too short or kinked and its tip does not protrude from the tip of the insulating cannula, inadequate heating will occur, leading to failure of adequate ablation.

Precise placement of the radiofrequency ablation electrode within the center of the osteoid osteoma is essential for successful treatment of the lesion. The Radionics radiofrequency electrode has a 1-cm-diameter zone of ablation. This equates to a 5-mm radius about the tip of the electrode.

Figure 8-64 ■ Insulating cannula through a Bonopty penetration cannula. The penetration cannula can be used to reach the lesion. The insulating cannula is then placed through the penetration cannula in a coaxial fashion. The insulating cannula should be long enough to protrude at least 1 cm beyond the tip of the needle used to reach the lesion to avoid unwanted heating of the metallic biopsy needle.

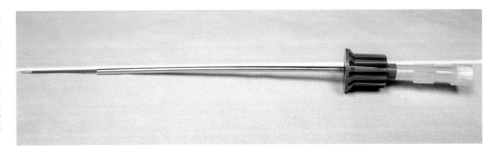

Figure 8-65 ■ Radiofrequency ablation insulating cannula and electrode. The length of the electrode is precisely matched to the insulation cannula (*A*). The electrode is placed through the insulating cannula in a coaxial fashion (*B*). The entire length of the electrode is then insulated apart from the distal noninsulated tip, which is exposed in the lesion.

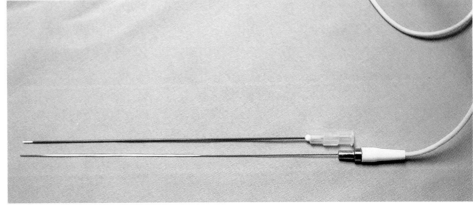

A

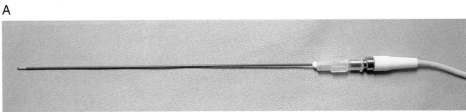

B

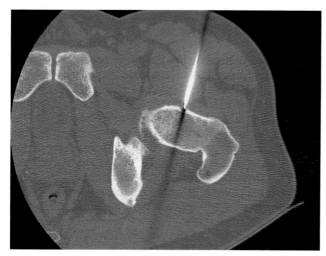

Figure 8-66 ■ Osteoid osteoma radiofrequency ablation. CT image depicting precise placement of the biopsy needle at the margin of a sub-periosteal osteoid osteoma involving the anterior cortex of the left femoral neck.

In order to place the electrode precisely, one must first place the biopsy needle precisely (Fig. 8-66). The Bonopty penetration cannula and stylet are advanced through the soft tissues toward the bone surface. When the bone is reached, the diamond-pointed stylet is exchanged for the drill stylet. The drill stylet is rotated clockwise until the drill is anchored in the bone. Imaging is then performed to verify the position and direction of the drill and penetration cannula. It is important to have the needle well aligned along the expected path before entering the bone. At this point, correction and minor adjustments of the position and angulation are easy; however, when the drill and cannula significantly enter the bone, changes in course of the biopsy system become more difficult. The drill is then rotated further in the clockwise direction, embedding the stylet and cannula further in the bone. When the drill has breached the cortex of the bone and

entered the softer medullary bone, the penetration cannula can be advanced by careful clockwise rotation to a point at which its tip is a few millimeters into the bone. The drill stylet is then removed and the penetration cannula can be used as a fixed pathway for placement of the radiofrequency electrode and insulating cannula. At this point a biopsy can be performed, although this is typically not necessary as the diagnosis is accurately made with history, clinical presentation, and imaging findings.

Precise placement of the insulating cannula (and subsequently the radiofrequency electrode) is necessary. The insulating cannula is advanced through the biopsy needle in a coaxial fashion until its tip is within the center of the lesion (Fig. 8-67). If this is not possible, the biopsy needle must be repositioned. If the lesion is more than 1 cm in maximum length, two ablations are necessary to ablate the entire lesion. Even a minute amount of residual nidal tissue typically results in recurrence.

When the insulating cannula is properly placed within the center of the osteoid osteoma, the biopsy needle is withdrawn several centimeters to avoid any contact between the metal biopsy needle and the exposed portion of the insulating cannula (Fig. 8-68). Contact between the biopsy needle and the exposed portion of the cannula can result in significant heating of the biopsy needle and result in soft tissue burns along the tract of the biopsy needle.

Once the insulating cannula is placed and the biopsy needle is withdrawn, the radiofrequency ablation electrode can be advanced through the insulating cannula (Fig. 8-69). When the electrode is fully advanced into the insulating cannula, only the distal tip should be exposed within the lesion. One final image of the position of the electrode and insulating cannula should be performed to ensure correct positioning. If the position is ideal, radiofrequency ablation of the lesion is performed at 90°C for 6 minutes.[14,15] It is often helpful to hold the biopsy needle in place to maintain stability and proper separation of the needle and ablation electrode and to ensure that no abnormal heating occurs along the metallic needle (Fig. 8-70). Subsequently, the biopsy needle, insulating cannula, and radiofrequency

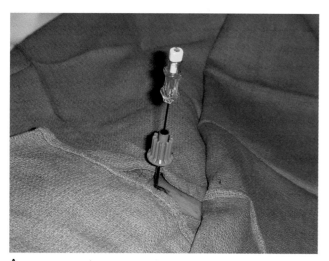

A

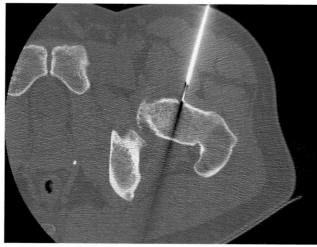

B

Figure 8-67 ■ Osteoid osteoma radiofrequency ablation. The insulating cannula is placed through the penetration cannula in a coaxial fashion (*A*). CT depicts precise placement of the insulating cannula within the center of the nidus of the osteoid osteoma (*B*).

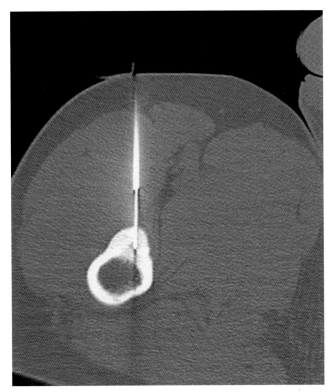

Figure 8-68 ■ Osteoid osteoma radiofrequency ablation. The penetration cannula is withdrawn several centimeters to avoid any contact with the distal noninsulated portion of the insulating cannula and electrode, which could result in unwanted heating of the penetration cannula.

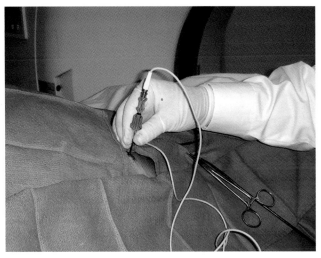

Figure 8-70 ■ Osteoid osteoma radiofrequency ablation. The nidus of the osteoid osteoma is ablated at 90°C for 6 minutes. It is often helpful to hold the penetration cannula to maintain stability of the cannula and ablation electrode and to ensure that no abnormal heating occurs along the metallic cannula.

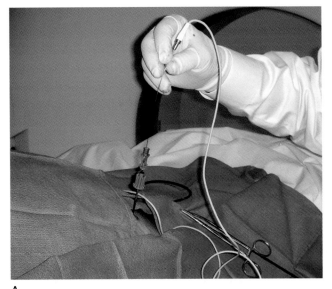

A

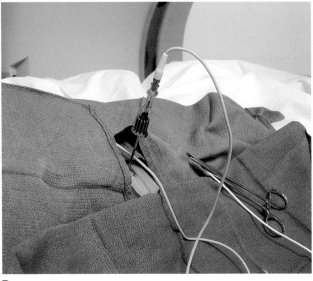

B

Figure 8-69 ■ Osteoid osteoma radiofrequency ablation. When the insulating cannula is placed and the biopsy needle is withdrawn, the radiofrequency ablation electrode can be advanced through the insulating cannula in a coaxial fashion (*A*). When the electrode is hubbed within the insulating cannula, the distal tip of the electrode is exposed within the lesion (*B*).

electrode are removed. A small amount (2-3 mL) of long-acting anesthetic can be instilled through the insulating cannula as it is withdrawn to alleviate some of the post-procedural pain. The skin is cleansed with hydrogen peroxide to remove the povidone-iodine, and an adhesive bandage is applied to the puncture site. The anesthetists should then be informed that the procedure is complete.

The patient is likely to have significant pain related to the procedure itself for approximately 24 hours. For this reason, patients are typically admitted for 23-hour observation for pain control.[18] If the patient reports no significant discomfort from the procedure and experiences no post-anesthesia difficulties, the patient can be discharged to home the same day.

POTENTIAL COMPLICATIONS[8]

In experienced hands, the complication rate with radiofrequency ablation is very low, depending on the size and location of the osteoid osteoma

- Bleeding
- Infection (cellulitis, septic arthritis, or osteomyelitis)
- Thermal injury
- Drug-related allergic reactions
- Inadvertent nerve injury
- Arterial or venous injury
- Vasovagal reaction

POST-PROCEDURE CARE/FOLLOW-UP[8]

Immediate

- The patient should be transferred to the anesthesia recovery unit for post-anesthesia care.

Post-Procedure

1. The patient should be admitted for 23-hour observation for pain control.
2. Diet and activity should be advanced as tolerated.
3. Pain medication should include:
   a. Ibuprofen 800 mg, one orally every 8 hours as required
   b. Percocet 325 mg, one or two orally every 4 to 6 hours as required
   c. Morphine sulfate 1 mg intravenously every 4 hours as required
   d. Antiemetic medications may be useful for anesthesia-related nausea

Discharge

1. The patient should be discharged into the care of a responsible person.
2. The patient is instructed not to drive or perform any other tasks that require clear thought and quick reactions for the remainder of the day.

3. A 2- to 3-day nonrenewable prescription for a narcotic pain reliever or a muscle relaxant, or both, may be given to the patient.
4. Patients are instructed to continue to take their prescription medication, although the pain medication may be tapered as indicated.
5. An adhesive bandage may be placed on the puncture site. The bandage should remain dry for at least 24 hours, at which point it can be removed.
6. A discharge sheet should be given to the patient outlining the following:
   a. The procedure performed
   b. Procedure-related symptoms that typically resolve in 7 to 10 days
      * Pain at the needle puncture site(s)
      * Mild stiffness with a feeling of fullness in the affected region
      * Deep pain in the region of the ablation
   c. Treatment for mild post-procedure symptoms
      * Rest the affected area for 3 to 4 days
      * Avoid movements that worsen the pain
      * Use cold compresses to the area that hurts
   d. Signs and symptoms of infection
      * Fever
      * Chills
      * Swelling or drainage from the puncture site(s)
      * New pain that is different from the usual pain
   e. Signs and symptoms of possible, more serious problems
      * Increasing pain
      * Motor dysfunction of the affected region or extremity
      * Bowel or bladder dysfunction
   f. Physician name and contact number if the patient has any concerns or if any problems were to arise as a result of the procedure
   g. Advice to schedule a follow-up appointment with the referring physician in 7 to 10 days

SAMPLE DICTATIONS

Fluoroscopically Guided Right Metacarpal Mass Biopsy

After the procedure was explained to the patient and informed consent was obtained, the patient was seated adjacent to the fluoroscopy table with his hand placed on the table in pronation. Preliminary imaging revealed a lytic destructive osseous lesion involving the right third metacarpal. The skin overlying the dorsal aspect of the hand was prepared and draped in the usual sterile fashion. Local anesthesia was obtained with 1% lidocaine with bicarbonate buffer. Under fluoroscopic guidance, a 14-gauge, 5-cm Ostycut needle was advanced into the lesion and a specimen was obtained. This was repeated three times for a total of four specimens. The specimens were delivered to members of the department of pathology. No complications were observed during or immediately after the procedure. The patient tolerated the procedure well and left the department in stable condition.

CT-Guided Left Iliac Bone Biopsy

After the procedure was explained to the patient and informed consent was obtained, the patient was placed on the CT table in the prone position. Intravenous versed and fentanyl were administered for sedation and pain relief. Electrocardiogram, pulse oximetry, and blood pressure were monitored during the examination. Preliminary scans demonstrate a mixed lytic and sclerotic lesion involving the left posterior ilium. The skin overlying this area was sterilely prepared and draped in the usual fashion. Local anesthesia was obtained with 1% lidocaine with bicarbonate buffer. Under CT fluoroscopic guidance, a Bonopty penetration cannula was advanced to the margin of the lesion. The extended drill stylet was advanced into the lesion and withdrawn. Bone fragments were obtained from the helices of the drill stylet and delivered to members of the department of pathology. This was repeated twice for a total of three passes through the lesion. No complications were observed during or immediately after the procedure. The patient tolerated the procedure well and left the department in stable condition.

Ultrasound-Guided Soft Tissue Mass Biopsy

After the procedure was explained to the patient and informed consent was obtained, the patient was placed on the table in the prone position. Preliminary imaging demonstrated a large soft tissue mass in the posterior thigh. The skin overlying this was sterilely prepared and draped in the usual fashion. Local anesthesia was obtained with 1% lidocaine with bicarbonate buffer. Under real-time gray-scale sonographic guidance, a 17-gauge, 6-cm coaxial needle was advanced to the margin of the lesion. An 18-gauge, 11-cm Temno biopsy needle was then advanced through the indwelling needle in a coaxial fashion. A core specimen was obtained and the biopsy needle was withdrawn. This was repeated three times for a total of four core biopsy specimens. The coaxial needle was then withdrawn. Specimens were delivered to members of the department of pathology. No complications were observed during or immediately after the procedure. The patient tolerated the procedure well and left the department in stable condition.

Osteoid Osteoma Radiofrequency Ablation

After the procedure was explained to the patient and the patient's parents, informed consent was obtained. The patient was placed on the table in the prone position. Members of the department of anesthesia administered general anesthesia. The skin overlying the left thigh was shaved and the grounding pad was affixed to the patient's skin. Preliminary imaging demonstrated an osteoid osteoma involving the left femoral neck. The skin overlying this area was sterilely prepared and draped in the usual fashion. Local anesthesia was obtained with 1% lidocaine with bicarbonate buffer. Under CT fluoroscopic guidance, a Bonopty penetration cannula was advanced to the margin of the osteoid osteoma. The drill stylet was then exchanged for the radiofrequency ablation insulating cannula, which was precisely placed in the center of the osteoid osteoma. The Bonopty penetration cannula was then withdrawn 2-3 cm. The radiofrequency ablation electrode was placed through the insulation cannula in a coaxial fashion. The osteoid osteoma was ablated at 90°C for 6 minutes. The penetration cannula, insulating cannula, and electrode were then withdrawn. No complications were observed during or immediately after the procedure. The patient tolerated the procedure well and reported complete relief of pain prior to discharge.

CASE REPORTS

CASE 1

Clinical Presentation

The patient was a 17-year-old female with left hip pain for nearly 2 years, which has gradually progressed. The pain was described as a dull ache that woke her up at night. The pain was constant with flares of worse pain. The pain was relieved by naproxen (Naprosyn); however, the pain always returned when the medication wore off. The pain did not correspond to activity, and there was no history of trauma.

Imaging and Therapy

Radiographs at an outside facility shortly after the pain began reportedly demonstrated no obvious abnormality. Six months later, a subtle periosteal reaction was seen along the proximal left femoral shaft. A subtle stress fracture was suspected clinically, and an MR study was obtained. MR depicted the periosteal reaction along the proximal femoral shaft to better advantage and demonstrated associated marked abnormal marrow signal throughout the proximal left femur (Fig. 8-71). A high-resolution CT scan of the left proximal femur (Fig. 8-72) was obtained and revealed periosteal reaction about the medial aspect of the left proximal femur with an 8-mm central lucency compatible with the nidus of an osteoid osteoma. Reformatted CT images (Fig. 8-73) depicted the lesion as elongated, measuring 1.2 cm in maximum craniocaudal dimension. The lesion was well away from surrounding vital structures and was amenable to percutaneous radiofrequency ablation. Because of the length of this lesion, two ablations would be necessary to cover the entire lesion completely and avert recurrence.

Under CT guidance, a Bonopty penetration cannula was advanced into the upper pole of the lucent nidus of the lesion and the radiofrequency ablation cannula and electrode were placed into the lesion in a coaxial fashion (Fig. 8-74A). The upper pole of the lesion was then ablated at 90°C for 6 minutes. The lower pole of the lesion was then targeted and the Bonopty penetration cannula was placed at the margin of the nidus. The radiofrequency ablation cannula and electrode were then placed into the lower pole of the lesion in a coaxial fashion (Fig. 8-74B), and the lower pole was ablated at 90°C for 6 minutes.

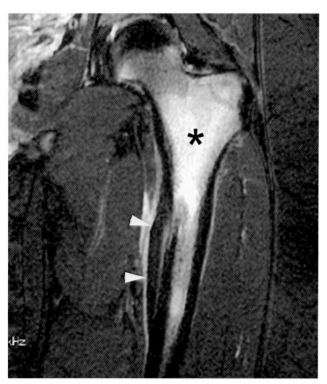

Figure 8-71 ■ Osteoid osteoma. Coronal T2-weighted image with fat saturation. MR depicted the periosteal reaction along the proximal femoral shaft *(arrowheads)*. This is associated with marked abnormal marrow signal *(asterisk)* throughout the proximal left femur although the nidus is not well appreciated, which is often the case with MR imaging with osteoid osteoma.

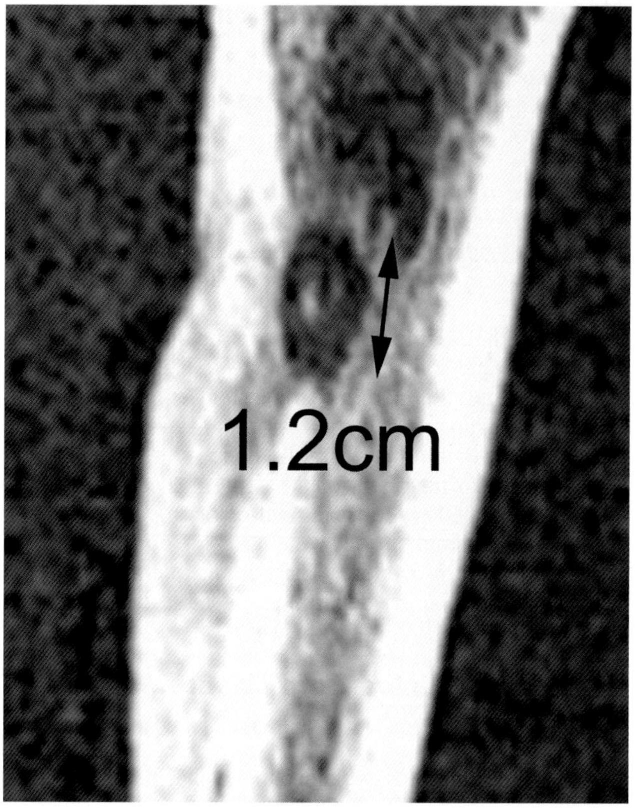

Results

As is often encountered, the patient had significant pain related to the procedure following recovery from general anesthesia. The patient was admitted for 23-hour observation for pain control. The pain improved, and the patient was discharged the following day. Over the next week the procedure-related pain improved. The previous pain associated with the osteoid osteoma resolved, compatible with successful treatment.

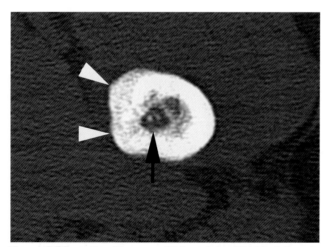

Figure 8-72 ■ Osteoid osteoma. High-resolution CT of the left proximal femur demonstrates periosteal reaction about the medial aspect of the left proximal femur *(arrowheads)* with an 8-mm central lucent nidus of an osteoid osteoma *(arrow)*.

Figure 8-73 ■ Osteoid osteoma. Reformatted CT image of the left femur shows the nidus of the osteoid osteoma to be elongated, measuring 1.2 cm in maximum craniocaudal dimension. This lesion will require two separate ablations to cover the entire lesion completely.

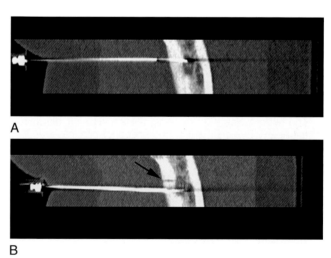

Figure 8-74 ■ Osteoid radiofrequency ablation. Reformatted CT image obtained during radiofrequency ablation of a large osteoid osteoma of the left proximal femur *(A)* depicts the insulating cannula and electrode precisely located within the superior pole of the lucent nidus. Reformatted image obtained later in the procedure *(B)* depicts the penetration cannula and drill stylet reaching the inferior pole of the lesion. The insulating cannula and electrode were then placed into the inferior pole of the lesion in a coaxial fashion. Note the previous tract used to reach the upper pole of this lesion *(arrow)*. Because of the length of this lesion, two separate ablations were necessary to cover the lesion completely.

CASE 2

Clinical Presentation

A 67-year-old man presented with a rapidly progressive lesion involving the left ring finger (Fig. 8-75). The digit was not painful but showed marked erythema and enlargement on physical examination. The patient had a remote history of cutaneous lymphoma but had been in remission for many years.

Imaging and Therapy

Radiographs were obtained showing a destructive lesion involving the left fourth proximal phalanx (Fig. 8-76)

corresponding to the abnormality on physical examination. The lesion was predominantly lytic with a suggestion of associated soft tissue extension of the lesion. An MR study was obtained and showed that the lesion had completely destroyed the overlying cortex with circumferential soft tissue extension of the lesion (Fig. 8-77A). The lesion encased the adjacent flexor tendons and extensor mechanism (Fig. 8-77B).

Fluoroscopic guidance was utilized for the percutaneous biopsy, as the lesion could be well

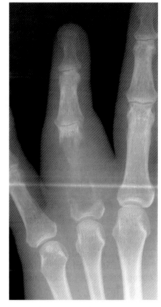

Figure 8-75 ■ Anaplastic lymphoma. Photograph reveals a rapidly progressive lesion involving the left ring finger. The digit was not painful but showed marked erythema and enlargement on physical examination.

Figure 8-76 ■ Anaplastic lymphoma. AP radiograph of the hand depicts a destructive lesion involving the left fourth proximal phalanx corresponding to the abnormality on physical examination. The lesion was predominantly lytic with a suggestion of associated soft tissue extension of the lesion.

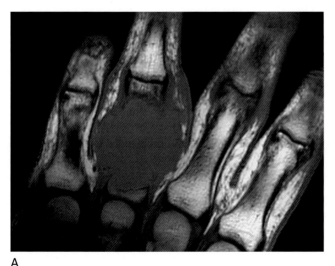

A

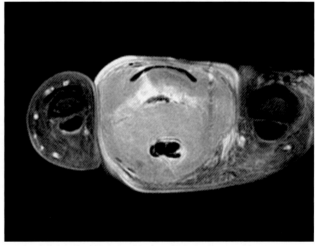

B

Figure 8-77 ■ Anaplastic lymphoma. T1-weighted coronal MR image (*A*) shows a large lesion arising from the fourth proximal phalanx with destruction of the overlying cortex and circumferential soft tissue extension. Axial post-contrast T1-weighted image (*B*) with fat saturation shows the lesion to encase the adjacent flexor tendons and extensor mechanism.

seen with fluoroscopy and could be easily reached (Fig. 8-78A). An 18-gauge SureCut needle was utilized for the biopsy using a single-pass technique (Fig. 8-78B). Three passes were performed, yielding adequate tissue for the diagnosis.

Pathology proved the lesion to be anaplastic lymphoma. The patient underwent radiation and chemotherapy with some improvement; however, eventually the digit was resected surgically.

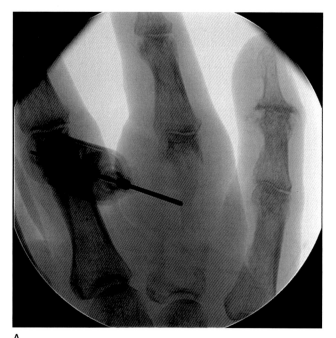

A

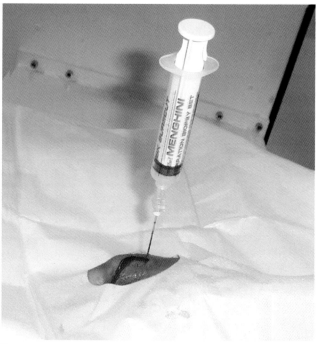

B

Figure 8-78 ■ Fluoroscopically guided biopsy of anaplastic lymphoma. In the fluoroscopic image (*A*) an 18-gauge SureCut needle has been inserted until its tip is within the lytic lesion involving the fourth digit. Photograph (*B*) depicts the SureCut needle embedded within the lesion. A single-pass technique was utilized to obtain three biopsy specimens, which yielded adequate tissue for the diagnosis.

CURRENT PROCEDURAL TERMINOLOGY (CPT) CODES[32]

CPT codes change often and sometimes are valid only for certain states or regions. It is best to consult with coding experts to make sure that coding for one's procedures is legitimate and complete. Below is a sample of codes that are being used for musculoskeletal biopsy and radiofrequency procedures at this writing.

Surgery

10021 Fine-needle aspiration; without imaging guidance

10022 with imaging guidance

(For radiologic supervision and interpretation, see 76942, 77002, 77012, 77021)

(For percutaneous needle biopsy other than fine-needle aspiration, see 20206 for muscle)

(For evaluation of fine-needle aspirate, see 88172, 88173)

Musculoskeletal System

20200 Biopsy, muscle; superficial

20205 deep

20206 Biopsy, muscle, percutaneous needle

(If imaging guidance is performed, see 76942, 77012, 77021)

(For fine-needle aspiration, use 10021 or 10022)

(For evaluation of fine-needle aspirate, see 88172-88173)

(For excision of muscle tumor, deep, see specific anatomic section)

20220 Biopsy, bone, trocar, or needle; superficial (e.g., ilium, sternum, spinous process, ribs)

20225 deep (e.g., vertebral body, femur)

(For bone marrow biopsy, use 38221)

(For radiologic supervision and interpretation, see 77002, 77012, 77021)

20982 Ablation, bone tumor(s) (e.g., osteoid osteoma, metastasis), radiofrequency, percutaneous, including computed tomographic guidance

(Do not report 20982 in conjunction with 77013)

23065 Biopsy, soft tissue of shoulder area; superficial

23066 deep

(For needle biopsy of soft tissue, use 20206)

24065 Biopsy, soft tissue of upper arm or elbow area; superficial

24066 deep (subfascial or intramuscular)

(For needle biopsy of soft tissue, use 20206)

25065 Biopsy, soft tissue of forearm and/or wrist; superficial

25066 deep (subfascial or intramuscular)

(For needle biopsy of soft tissue, use 20206)

26100 Arthrotomy with biopsy; carpometacarpal joint, each

26105 metacarpophalangeal joint, each

26110 interphalangeal joint, each

27040 Biopsy, soft tissue of pelvis and hip area; superficial

27041 deep, subfascial or intramuscular

(For needle biopsy of soft tissue, use 20206)

27323 Biopsy, soft tissue of thigh or knee area; superficial

27324 deep (subfascial or intramuscular)

(For needle biopsy of soft tissue, use 20206)

27613 Biopsy, soft tissue of leg or ankle area; superficial

27614 deep (subfascial or intramuscular)

(For needle biopsy of soft tissue, use 20206)

28050 Arthrotomy with biopsy; intertarsal or tarso-metatarsal joint

28052 metatarsophalangeal joint

28054 interphalangeal joint

Hemic and Lymphatic Systems

38220 Bone marrow; aspiration only

38221 biopsy, needle or trocar

(For bone marrow biopsy interpretation, use 88305)

Radiology

76942 Ultrasonic guidance for needle placement (e.g., biopsy, aspiration, injection, localization device), imaging supervision and interpretation

(Do not report 76942 in conjunction with 43232, 43237, 43242, 45341, 45342, or 76975)

77002 Fluoroscopic guidance for needle placement (e.g., biopsy, aspiration, injection, localization device)

(See appropriate surgical code for procedure and anatomic location)

(77002 includes all radiographic arthrography with the exception of supervision and interpretation for CT and MR arthrography)

(Do not report 77002 in addition to 70332, 73040, 73085, 73115, 73525, 73580, 73615)

77012 Computed tomography guidance for needle placement (e.g., biopsy, aspiration, injection, localization device), radiologic supervision and interpretation

77021 Magnetic resonance guidance for needle placement (e.g., for biopsy, needle aspiration, injection, or placement of localization device) radiologic supervision and interpretation

Pathology and Laboratory

88172 Cytopathology, evaluation of fine-needle aspirtate; immediate cytohistologic study to determine adequacy of specimen(s)

88173 interpretation and report

(For fine-needle aspirate, see 10021, 10022)

(Do not report 88172, 88173 in conjunction with 88333 and 88334 for the same specimen)

88305 **Level IV**-Surgical pathology, gross and microscopic examination

88333 cytologic examination (e.g., touch prep, squash prep), initial site

88334 cytologic examination (e.g., touch prep, squash prep), each additional site

Moderate (Conscious) Sedation

99143 Moderate sedation services (other than those services described by codes 00100-01999), provided by the same physician performing the diagnostic or therapeutic service that the sedation supports, requiring the presence of an independent trained observer to assist in the monitoring of the patient's level of consciousness and physiologic status; younger than 5 years or age, first 30 minutes intraservice time

99144 age 5 years or older, first 30 minutes intraservice time

99145 each additional 15 minutes intraservice time (List separately in addition to code for primary service)

(Use 99145 in conjunction with 99143, 99144)

99148 Moderate sedation services (other than those services described by codes 00100-01999), provided by a physician other than the health care professional performing the diagnostic or therapeutic service that the sedation supports; younger than 5 years or age, first 30 minutes intra-service time

99149 age 5 years or older, first 30 minutes intra-service time

99150 each additional 15 minutes intra-service time (List separately in addition to code for primary service)

(Use 99150 in conjunction with 99148, 99149)

References

1. Gupta S. Role of image-guided percutaneous needle biopsy in cancer staging. Semin Roentgenol 2006; 41:78–90.
2. Hau MA, Kim JI, Kattapuram S, et al. Accuracy of CT-guided biopsies in 359 patients with musculoskeletal lesions. Skeletal Radiol 2002; 31:349–353.
3. Hodge JC. Musculoskeletal Imaging: Diagnostic and Therapeutic Procedures. Montreal: Karger Landes Systems, 1997, pp 91–108, 189–201.
4. Murphy WA. Radiologically guided percutaneous musculoskeletal biopsy. Orthop Clin North Am 1983; 14:233–241.
5. Harish S, Hughes RJ, Saifuddin A, Flanagan AM. Image-guided percutaneous biopsy of intramedullary lytic bone lesions: Utility of aspirated blood clots. Eur Radiol 2006; 16:2120–2125.
6. Thanos L, Mylona S, Kalioras V, et al. Percutaneous CT-guided interventional procedures in musculoskeletal system (our experience). Eur J Radiol 2004; 50:273–277.
7. Jelinek JS, Murphey MD, Welker JA, et al. Diagnosis of primary bone tumors with image-guided percutaneous biopsy: Experience with 110 tumors. Radiology 2002; 223:731–737.
8. Fenton DS, Czervionke LF. Image-Guided Spine Intervention. Philadelphia: WB Saunders, 2003.
9. Fraser-Hill MA, Renfrow DL, Hilsenrath PE. Percutaneous needle biopsy of musculoskeletal lesions. Cost effectiveness. AJR Am J Roentgenol 1992; 158:813–818.
10. Martin HE, Ellis EB. Biopsy by needle puncture and aspiration. Ann Surg 1930; 92:169–181.
11. Ellis F. Needle biopsy on the clinical diagnosis of tumors. Br J Surg 1947; 34:240–261.
12. Anderson MW, Temple HT, Dussalt RG, Kaplan PA. Compartmental anatomy: Relevance to staging and biopsy of musculoskeletal tumors. AJR Am J Roentgenol 1999; 173:1663–1671.
13. Mankin HJ, Lange TA, Spanier SS. The hazards of biopsy in patients with malignant and primary bone and soft-tissue tumors. J Bone Joint Surg Am 1982; 64:1121–1127.
14. Rosenthal DI, Hornicek FJ, Wolfe MW, et al. Percutaneous radiofrequency coagulation of osteoid osteoma compared with operative treatment. J Bone Joint Surg Am 1998; 80:815–821.
15. Rosenthal DI, Hornicek FJ, Torriani M, et al. Osteoid osteoma: Percutaneous treatment with radiofrequency energy. Radiology 2003; 229:171–175.
16. Cantwell CP, Obyrne J, Eustace S. Current trends in treatment of osteoid osteoma with an emphasis on radiofrequency ablation. Eur Radiol 2004; 14:607–617.
17. Lindner NJ, Ozaki T, Roedl R, et al. Percutaneous radiofrequency ablation in osteoid osteoma. J Bone Joint Surg Br 2001; 83:391–396.
18. Woertler K, Vestring T, Boettner F, et al. Osteoid osteoma: CT-guided percutaneous radiofrequency ablation and follow-up in 47 patients. J Vasc Interv Radiol 2001; 12:717–722.
19. Ramnath RR, Rosenthal DI, Cates J, et al. Intracortical chondroma simulating osteoid osteoma treated by radiofrequency. Skel Radiol 2002; 31:597–602.
20. Goetz MP, Callstrom MR, Charboneau JW, et al. Percutaneous image-guided radiofrequency ablation of painful metastases involving bone: A multicenter study. J Clin Oncol 2004; 22:300–306.
21. Marchal F, Burnaud L, Bazin C, et al. Radiofrequency ablation in palliative supportive care: Early clinical experience. Oncol Rep 2006; 15:495–499.
22. Cardinal E, Chhem RK, Beauregard CG. Ultrasound-guided interventional procedures in the musculoskeletal system. Radiol Clin North Am 1998; 36:597–604.
23. Torriani M, Etchebehere M, Amstalden EMI. Sonographically guided core needle biopsy of bone and soft tissue tumors. J Ultrasound Med 2002; 21:275–281.
24. Dupuy DE, Rosenberg AE, Punyaratabandhu T, et al. Accuracy of CT-guided needle biopsy of musculoskeletal neoplasms. AJR Am J Roentgenol 1998; 171:759–762.
25. Genant JW, Vandevenne JE, Bergman AG, et al. Interventional musculoskeletal procedures performed by using MR imaging guidance with a vertically open MR unit: Assessment of techniques and applicability. Radiology 2002; 223:127–136.
26. Koenig CW, Duda SH, Truebenbach J, et al. MR-guided biopsy of musculoskeletal lesions in a low-field system. J Magn Reson Imaging 2001; 13:761–768.
27. Physicians' Desk Reference, 60th ed. Montvale, NJ: Medical Economics Company, 2006.
28. Torriani M, Rosenthal DI. Percutaneous radiofrequency treatment of osteoid osteoma. Pediatr Radiol 2002; 32:615–618.
29. Barei DP, Moreau G, Scarborough MT, Neel MD. Percutaneous radiofrequency ablation of osteoid osteoma. Clin Orthop Relat Res 2000; 373:115–124.
30. Pinto CH, Taminiau AHM, Vanderschueren GM, et al. Technical considerations in CT-guided radiofrequency thermal ablation of osteoid osteoma: Tricks of the trade. AJR Am J Roentgenol 2002; 179:1633–1642.
31. Venbrux AC, Montague BJ, Murphy KPJ, et al. Image-guided percutaneous radiofrequency ablation for osteoid osteomas. J Vasc Interv Radiol 2003; 14:375–380.
32. Derived from CPT 2007, CPT Intellectual Property Services. Chicago: American Medical Association, 2007.

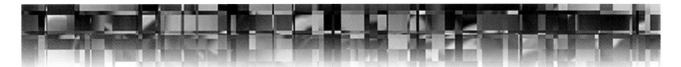

An Orthopedic Oncology Surgeon's Perspective

Percutaneous Image-Guided Biopsy and Radiofrequency Ablation

Mary I. O'Connor, MD

The role of biopsy is critical in the evaluation of many bone and soft tissue tumors. Some benign bone lesions with characteristic radiographic features do not require tissue for diagnosis (e.g., nonossifying fibroma). Lesions that are not completely benign in their radiographic appearance, however, typically require biopsy to establish the diagnosis. Biopsy may be performed with an open (surgical) procedure or by needle technique (fine-needle aspiration or core needle biopsy). Image-guided core needle biopsy is preferred for most lesions that require biopsy. With a needle of sufficient diameter, adequate tissue can often be obtained to establish the diagnosis with less morbidity and cost than an open biopsy procedure. With the proper guidelines, image-guided biopsy is highly safe and effective.

Placement of the needle for biopsy is critical to minimizing complications and obtaining diagnostic tissue. In our practice, the musculoskeletal radiologist and orthopedic oncologist review the imaging studies together and plan the location and orientation of the needle biopsy. Areas of potentially necrotic tumor are avoided. The surgeon discusses the potential operative approach for resection of the lesion and possible soft tissue reconstruction. Needle placement is oriented to minimize tissue contamination and permit resection of the needle biopsy tract with the specimen if subsequent excision is required. It is important to remember that the most direct approach to the lesion from a cross-sectional imaging standpoint may not be appropriate and may result in tissue contamination that negatively affects the surgical plan. Confirmation of neoplastic tissue on frozen section at the time of needle biopsy is ideal.

Needle biopsy is not appropriate for all lesions. With the limited amount of tissue obtained with a core needle biopsy, differentiation of a benign from a low-grade sarcomatous lesion can be quite difficult, particularly in cartilage lesions of bone and fatty soft tissue tumors. Such patients are not ideal needle biopsy candidates. Biopsy sample error can further compromise diagnostic accuracy of percutaneous needle biopsy in these lesions. If tissue diagnosis is clinically indicated, open biopsy of such cartilage or fatty neoplasms is typically performed. Finally, in some primary bone sarcomas (e.g., osteosarcoma), current national chemotherapy protocols require open biopsy for study enrollment to permit adequate pretreatment of neoplastic tissue for genetic study.

Finally, radiofrequency ablation of osteoid osteoma has greatly improved patients' care. I favor this therapy for all lesions amenable to this technique. In experienced hands, the risk of complications from radiofrequency ablation is very low. In lesions that are too close to vital structures for ablation to be performed, surgical excision of the nidus is effective but subjects the patient to the morbidity of an open surgical procedure.

In closing, collaboration and communication between the orthopedic oncologist and musculoskeletal radiologist are critical for achieving optimal clinical care for these patients. This teamwork has clearly advanced the care we provide our patients.

Index

Note: Page numbers followed by the letter f refer to figures.